HEALTH, MEDICINE, SOCIETY

PROCEEDINGS OF THE INTERNATIONAL CONFERENCE ON THE SOCIOLOGY OF MEDICINE

WARSAW (JABŁONNA), AUGUST 20–25, 1973

organized by the Polish Academy of Sciences, Institute of Philosophy and Sociology and co-sponsored by the Research Committee on the Sociology of Medicine, International Sociological Association

HEALTH, MEDICINE, SOCIETY

Editors:

MAGDALENA SOKOŁOWSKA
Polish Academy of Sciences

JACEK HOŁÓWKA
University of Warsaw

ANTONINA OSTROWSKA
Polish Academy of Sciences

D. REIDEL PUBLISHING COMPANY
DORDRECHT – HOLLAND / BOSTON – U.S.A.

PWN–POLISH SCIENTIFIC PUBLISHERS
WARSAW – POLAND

Library of Congress Cataloging in Publication Data

International Conference on the Sociology of Medicine, Jabłonna (Warsaw), 1973.
Health, medicine, society.

"Organized by the Polish Academy of Sciences, Institute of Philosophy and Sociology and co-sponsored by the Research Committee on the Sociology of Medicine, International Sociological Association."
Bibliography: p.
1. Social medicine – Congresses. I. Sokołowska, Magdalena. II. Hołówka, Jacek. III. Ostrowska, Antonina. IV. Polska Akademia Nauk. Instytut Filozofii i Socjologii. V. International Sociological Association. Research Committee on the Sociology of Medicine. VI. Title.
RA418.I53 1973 301.5 76-7916
ISBN-13: 978-94-010-1432-8 e-ISBN-13: 978-94-010-1430-4
DOI: 10.1007/978-94-010-1430-4

Distributors for the U.S.A., Canada and Mexico
D. REIDEL PUBLISHING COMPANY, INC.
Lincoln Building, 160 Old Derby Street, Hingham, Mass. 02043, U.S.A.

Distributors for all other countries
D. REIDEL PUBLISHING COMPANY
P.O. Box 17, Dordrecht, Holland

PREFACE

This volume contains a selection of papers presented at the International Conference on the Sociology of Medicine, held between August 20th and 25th, 1973 in Warsaw (Jabłonna).*

The Conference was organized by the Institute of Philosophy and Sociology of the Polish Academy of Sciences in collaboration with the Research Committee on the Sociology of Medicine of the International Sociological Association. The participants included medical sociologists from the United States, and from the countries of Western and Eastern Europe, including a delegation of general sociologists and physicians and also a group of young medical sociologists from Poland. Dr. Leo Kaprio, Director of the Regional Office for Europe of the World Health Organization, together with a member of his staff, was also present. The Conference was opened by the Deputy Minister of Health and Social Welfare of the Polish People's Republic, Dr. Ryszard Brzozowski. The first Chairman was Prof. Jan Szczepański, Vice-President of the Polish Academy of Sciences and Director of the Institute of Philosophy and Sociology. The first speech was delivered by Prof. Jivko Oshavkov from Bulgaria, then Vice-Chairman of the International Sociological Association.

The Conference had several objectives which, we believe, were successfully achieved. It was intended first to provide an occasion to bring participants of East and West together, and give them a chance to exchange information on the state of medical sociology in different countries. They found an opportunity to discuss their views in a relaxed and informal atomsphere. The second objective was to review with general sociologists and physicians the different theoretical sources from which the sociology of medicine has evolved. These discussions covered a wide area of problems concerning applied health care and their connection with social research, social planning and social engineering.

* A longer account of the Conference written by Maria Bartnik and Barbara Uramowska was published in *Medical Sociology Newsletter* edited by Research Committee on Medical Sociology of the International Sociological Association (October 1973, No. 3) – and in *Social Science and Medicine* **8** (1974) 469–472.

The third objective was to lay foundations for possible international collaboration in the future. Several projects for comparative or joint international studies were outlined and discussed during the Conference.

In order to achieve these goals the participants were asked to contribute a written paper. A number of additional papers were also received from scholars who were unable to be present. Altogether fifty-six papers were submitted to the Conference. They comprised research reports, theoretical analyses, teaching programs, policy studies, and, occasionally, historical investigations.

The Editors of this volume had a difficult task in selecting a limited number of these papers for publication. First of all, we had to forego publishing those short factual contributions which presented current developments and achievements in various scientific establishments in Poland. We also had to exclude a number of full-length papers in order to comply with the demands of the publisher concerning the size of this volume.* We decided, therefore, to present only those papers which can most adequately represent the five problem areas which we regard as most important and to which, in consequence, this book has been primarily devoted.

The first part of this volume concerns health and society. A consistent picture of the health status of a given society involves a number of complementary viewpoints. We tried to emphasize the complexity of this subject by including here epidemiological (Kostrzewski, Jablensky) and demographic (Klonowicz) studies, articles on attitudes of the society at large to problems of health and disease (Tahin *et al.*), a comprehensive analysis of health problems of immigrants to a new country (Haavio-Mannila) and a study of various aspects of medical behaviour of city inhabitants (Titkow).

* The materials which have not been included in this book are to appear in other publications. Two volumes in Polish we currently prepared. One will be published by PWN – Polish Scientific Publishers under the title *Socjologia a zdrowie* (*Sociology and Health*) and will embrace several papers presented in this volume together with reports on research programs in medical sociology conducted in this country and presented at the Conference as well as a bibliography of Polish literature on medical sociology published in years 1969–1974. The other volume *Polityka społeczna a zdrowie* (*Social Policy and Health*) to be published by Książka i Wiedza will comprise Conference papers devoted primarily to general sociological topics and questions of social policy.

The second part of this volume deals with the transformations which have taken place in the field of medical intervention. Its principal aim is to show that the basic repertoirs of medical techniques, skills, practices and norms changes with time under the influence of social events. This part includes papers that review the changing values and ideologies prevailing in medicine (Fox), the impact of scientific discoveries on medical practice (Wald), ramifications of epidemiological and ecological theories (Susser), and new ways of organizing medical care (Nagi, Herzlich).

The third part is devoted to sociological insights in the health sciences, and illustrates the most important ways in which the sociologist is involved with the problems of health and medicine. It includes both papers which discuss characteristics of the medical profession (Kelus and Sikorska, Illsley, Springer), and those which seek to find appropriate definitions of health (Pflanz, Elinson) and related concepts (Ostrowska, Mauksch).

The fourth part tackles the intricate problems associated with the functioning of the health system. It presents the difficulties connected with the proper delineation of the health system (Field), shows the dynamics of the health system in different social and historical circumstances (Bizoń, Freidson), discusses certain examples of the existing health systems (Gill, Badgley) or policies and strategies that they involve (Gallagher) and reviews the problems encountered by those who undertake to plan their functioning (Holst, Reader).

The fifth part has been devoted to teaching. It contains two trend analyses of the place that sociology has had in medical education in two countries with the longest tradition in this area – U.S.A. and G. Britain (Bloom, Jefferys), a paper on the development of the oldest institutions that teach sociology of medicine (Straus) and two articles discussing ideologies, methods and curricula of the sociology of medicine for undergraduate and graduate students of sociology in two European countries (Nuyens, Stacey).

We are very grateful to all who have contributed to the Conference held in Summer 1973 with their papers. We feel also an obligation to all those who took part in the innumerable discussions held in the course of the Conference. We hope that their views and knowledge are also indirectly reflected in this volume.

The Editors

TABLE OF CONTENTS

III. SOCIOLOGICAL INSIGHTS INTO THE HEALTH SCIENCES

IV. THE HEALTH SYSTEM

V. TEACHING

THE DEVELOPMENT OF THE SOCIOLOGY OF MEDICINE IN POLAND

MAGDALENA SOKOŁOWSKA

Institute of Philosophy and Sociology, Polish Academy of Sciences, Warsaw, Poland

As a distinct and separate enterprise within sociology the sociology of medicine has existed in Poland for about ten or twelve years, and this period will be covered in my report. As it is not possible to give here a complete account of all our endeavours and experiences. I shall limit myself to a survey of certain questions which seem to me particularly important. I must admit that the slightly inflated title of my report represents primarily the experience of a small group of medical sociologists from the Institute of Philosophy and Sociology of the Polish Academy of Sciences – and I may add that the Polish Academy of Sciences is a research institution not involved in university teaching. Had the sociological-medical orientation developed, for example, at the Department of Sociology of Warsaw University, our experiences would most certainly have been different. My report also includes some information on the activities of the Sociology of Medicine Section of the Polish Sociological Association. [1]

I must also stress that this report does not aim to be a concise presentation of the research conducted by either of these two groups. I wish rather to discuss the specific style of our work, to show how it is influenced by various factors and conditions, and to indicate the prospects for the sociology of medicine, its place within sociology and its relation to medicine.

I. THEORETICAL DETERMINANTS OF THE SOCIOLOGY OF MEDICINE

The nature of the sociology of medicine is primarily determined by sociology. Since there does not exist any developed exposition of the specific foundations of the Polish sociology of medicine, I shall therefore point to some issues to be found among the theoretical features of the present day sociology in Poland. I shall begin by referring to a paper by Jan Szczepański on the Polish school of sociology.[2]

Szczepański characterized Polish sociology in the following words: "the following theoretical assumptions which are coexistent, interrelating and overlapping in the social consciousness and in the works of sociologists and their interpretation of contemporary Polish society can be indicated as typical of Polish sociology: 1) ... a specific pragmatism ...vigilance against menace to national interests, concentration on the development of society as a whole; 2) ... the theories developed in the interwar period by sociologists like Florian Znaniecki, Stefan Czarnowski, Kazimierz Dobrowolski, Jan S. Bystroń, Józef Chałasiński and Ludwik Krzywicki... Znaniecki's theory of personality and his concepts of the sociology of education, Czarnowski's theory of culture, the methodological directives for linking history with sociology developed by Dobrowolski...; 3) At present in Polish sociology Marxist theories play an important role: the Marxist theory of sociology, the theory of the historical process, of the class struggle, of the role of the socialist state and of politics, etc. The influence of Marxism on academic sociology was very strong; it became weaker, however, in the Stalinist period when simplified concepts were presented as the only scientific ones. The postwar reception of Marxism was connected first of all with the traditions of Polish Marxism, represented in the interwar period by Ludwik Krzywicki, who ventured his own interpretation of historical materialism. The traditional approval of the historic method also favored this reception. The influence of Marxism on Polish sociology consisted in: a) selection of research issues and emphasis on the processes occurring in macrostructures and on the transformation of social classes and strata; b) philosophical assumptions admitting the thesis of the objective nature of the social process and its specific roles; c) the admission of the complexity of social phenomena with the consequent necessity of applying a combination of research methods and techniques; d) an intensification of the traditional practical attitude of sociology and a facing up to the task of pursuing works that serve the cause of economic development...; 4) The influence of the sociology developed in the U.S. and Western Europe... After 1956... new contacts with world sociology were established... and... the theoretical concepts of that sociology were brought to Poland... nearly all known middle-range theories approved by contemporary sociology would be mentioned as occurring in the works of Polish sociologists... supplying the authors with a selection of concepts and interpretation schemes... Theories developed in the Western countries emphasized these aspects of social processes that had been, so to speak, traditionally neglected by Marxist sociology and openly disregarded in the Stalinist period, namely the processes occurring in microstructures, psychosocial mechanisms."

The development of the sociology of medicine outside Poland has been the second most important factor influencing the development of the sociological-medical orientation in Poland. In the early sixties the American model of the sociology of medicine won the most widespread acceptance in the world. Theories, methods, conceptual frameworks, techniques and styles developed in the U.S.A. were adopted or imitated by sociologists in various countries. The works of Talcott Parsons and Robert Merton in the field of sociology of medicine were widely read; as were those of Eliot Freidson and several other prominent social scientists. In this context I should like to mention an American sociologist Bernard Stern, who died in 1956, the author of an interesting attempt to apply Marxist methodology to the sociology of medicine. In 1951 'the unchallenged father of medical sociology', as Robert Straus called him, published a chapter on the foundations of medical sociology,[3] which in his view (1) is a branch of sociology, (2) aims at solving social problems, (3) bridges micro- and macrosociology, (4) frequently uses historical and interdisciplinary approaches, (5) associates man's biological traits with his social surroundings, thereby finding room for strand within sociology, (6) counts among its main interests the effective distribution of medical services. It was the considered opinion of Bernard Stern that action is a proper part of the sociologist's role. He also stressed that the usefulness of medical sociology for medicine depends on its full integration with sociology.

Stern's published works are still awaiting recognition and there may not be many sociologists in several countries who know that there exists an alternative model of the sociology of medicine that could be at least partially applied. Of course our Polish model has to be determined by the reality in which we live, by the experiences resulting from the functioning of the basic institutions of our society.[4]

II. THE DEVELOPMENT OF THE SOCIOLOGICAL-MEDICAL ORIENTATION

Originally our orientation was more medical than sociological. The fact that the medical sociology unit was institutionally located outside medicine had little more than formal significance. The Institute of Philosophy and Sociology of the Polish Academy of Sciences comprised a number of loosely connected units dealing with specialized branches of sociology, each conducting their own researches and seeking their reference groups outside the Institute. Our reference group was initially medicine. Gradually, it became sociology, and it is to a description of the process whereby our orientation changed from being a medical to a sociological one, that this section is devoted. On the other hand the Medical Sociology Section of the Polish Sociological Association has always been oriented toward 'sociology in medicine'. These two approaches are coexistent, closely related and mutually helpful.

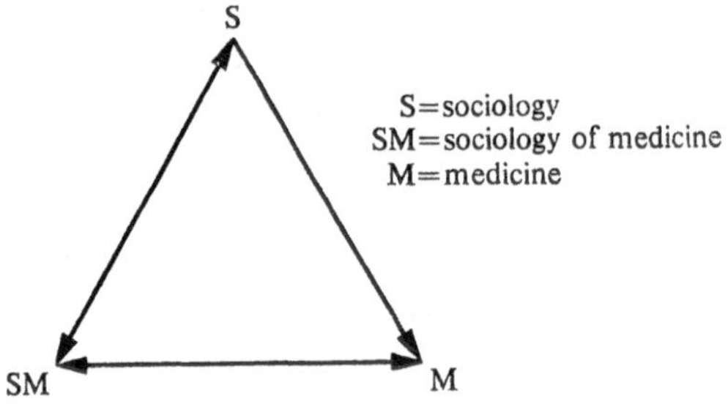

This diagram shows the basic types of interaction among the sociology of medicine, sociology and medicine. In the first phase of our work all relevant relations were limited to the connection between SM and M and our contacts with doctors consisted in supplying them with single variables isolated from their social or cultural context. Our main activities at that time consisted in teaching medical sociology in medical schools and research, whereas we were subcontractors of programs conducted by clinical departments of medical schools and research institutes attached to the Ministry of Health. [5] We were usually requested to complement their researches with a sociological survey [6] or to undertake a special study to solve a specific problem. We were once induced, for example, to find out why patients who had been completely rehabilitated clinically did not wish to return to work. This was the beginning of a lasting preoccupation on the part of our group with rehabilitation.[7] As can be seen from Notes 7 and 8, the titles of our publications, indicating our approach to rehabilitation have undergone several changes; reflecting the various stages of development of our sociological-medical orientation. We began by viewing rehabilitation in clinical terms. Next we adopted a different approach, treating rehabilitation as a social problem[8] or from a more theoretical, sociological point of view.

We also undertook research without any direct medical stimulus. However, we always choose to work on subjects that had direct application to medicine. We embarked, for instance, upon a laborious effort to describe socio-economic types of Polish urban families. The principal aim of that study was to supply epidemiologists with a multifaceted 'denominator' with which they could compare 'nominators' or, in plain words, populations under study. However our objectives changed during the four years spent on this project. When it was completed we found it to be above all a rich source of systematic knowledge on family life in Poland and a useful and promising tool for micro- and macrosociological, structural or cultural investigations.[9] And this rearrangement of objectives did not undermine the value of our family typology for the purposes of epidemiological investigations.

In 1968 the Institute of Philosophy and Sociology underwent a reorganization. Separate research units ceased to exist and fragmentary studies were discontinued. Three large teams were created, dealing with the Theory of Socialist Society, Class and Strata Structure Development and Social Change respectively. Soon complex macrosociological studies were initiated,[10] with the intention of building a platform on which two principal problems designated by the national research plan would be studied: (1) Evolution of the Structure of Socialist Society (with Elements of Demographic Analysis) in Poland and (2) Expected Changes in Consumption Patterns, Cultural Needs and the System of Values in Polish Society.

The Institute was appointed to act as a national coordinating agency and took direct responsibility for elaboration of a great number of issues. The former Sociology of Medicine Unit was incorporated into the team studying Class and Strata Structure Development. 'Health' was incorporated into both studies – as the correlate of structure, and as a social-cultural value.

The opening of this new period meant an activation of the 'S–SM' relation in the diagram shown above. 'S' was Polish society and we were expected to supply information about it in the field of health. In other words, we had to fit health into a macro-sociological study of social structure and life-styles. Thus our frame of reference shifted from medicine to society and we became 'medicine in sociology' rather than 'sociology in medicine'.

And immediately we were faced with the question of what we could offer the social researches. The answer was difficult both on (a) the medical and (b) the sociological aspect.

(a) As we know, medicine, universally, does not dispose of materials concerning the health of any general population, which would contain descriptions of individuals with regard to the features of their social situation, to say nothing of such data on a national scale. Official statistics, and scientific studies conducted on a country-wide basis in Poland, make use of average indices of clinically diagnosed cases of diseases. This problem could not even be solved by means of mass medical examinations of the whole population of Poland, with sociologists providing abundant information on the social traits of every individual studied and processing this material in the convention of sociological research. Quite apart from the organizational and financial problems involved in so prodigious an undertaking, the materials gathered would be of little use in studying the structure and life-styles of the whole society.[11]

(b) From the sociological point of view, introducing health into the picture was even more difficult. Admittedly, sociologists are committed to the study of society in all its aspects, and the sphere of health could certainly not be called indifferent to social development. Therefore it could hardly be neglected in any complex social planning. But on the other hand sociologists had never included the sphere of health in their structural studies in Poland and they were a little reluctant to do so. This fact we found to be an interesting point in itself. Why do sociologists consistently shrink from studying the field of health? This makes the position of medicine exceptional. It seems that the reluctance of sociologists to include the sphere of health in their studies stems from their feeling of unfamiliarity with the phenomena involved. The sociologist understands the issues involved in other areas of social life, because they are expressible in concepts, methods, and theories known to him. By doing so he does not pretend to exercise the specific knowledge of a given profession. He does not become a lawyer when he studies phenomena connected with the functioning of law, as in the course of such study he does not use the concepts and terms of legal theory. He uses his own notions which are alternative or complementary to the conceptual inventory of the field he is studying.

The sociological approach to law, education, industry, etc., helps to overcome specialist isolationism and gives a wider view of different spheres of social life and of the various connections between them. By offering alternative views of various spheres of social life sociology acquires significance in the formulation of social policies, and in a country widely employing centralized planning this is a prominent role.

But there is no such alternative approach towards medicine. Somehow it goes without saying that the sphere of health belongs exclusively to physicians while the sociologist may either rely uncritically on materials supplied by doctors or must altogether renounce the study of medical facts and phenomena. Sociologists usually opt for the second choice as they are unable to incorporate an 'alien body' into their research. Thus a vicious circle has arisen. Because the field of health 'is not the business' of students of society a sociological orientation within medicine has failed to develop. Consequently, for lack of any sociological approach, health is apprehended in terms of clinical disease which cannot as a rule be translated into behavioral definitions of illness and/or sickness. This only makes sociologists all the more reluctant to deal with health. The isolation eventually becomes so complete that one is tempted to think that medicine is ruled by special laws and must remain beyond the scope of both the study of society and general social policy.

Very often sociologists themselves are responsible for spreading the belief that health is something specific, remote and impossible to penetrate. Sociologists in Poland, as in most other countries, have no chance in the course of their university training, nor, as a rule, in their later career to become familiar with this field.[12] In a large proportion of sociological writings the concept of health is closely associated with such terms as 'pathological change', 'clinical norm' or 'state of an organism', i.e., with purely biological categories. Medicine is regarded in a narrow nineteenth-century manner exclusively within a naturalistic framework. Disease is explained by means of a mechanistic, closed system of reference formulated in the primitive universalist terms of a single cause-and-effect relationship, for instance the germ theory. Within such a conceptual pattern there is indeed no room for sociology. Apparently many sociologists fail to notice the fundamental changes occurring in medical science. Or perhaps they do notice them but remain fascinated by the biological and technological progress and fail to perceive other changes.

In the first place the causal model of disease has essentially changed. The single-cause, closed system is being replaced by an open, multicausal system that accounts – sometimes even too readily – for social factors. In some epidemiological studies these factors hypothetically considered as combined causes of diseases are already systematically treated as a social and cultural reality. There are also notable changes in the field of therapy. Alongside routine surgical and pharmacological therapy, more and more often attempts are being made to modify the social environment of medical institutions, for instance by creating 'therapeutic communities' in hospitals. The general trend is to throw open hitherto 'closed' institutions. Rigid rules are reformulated or abandoned, patients are allowed to receive visits more frequently than before, to keep their clothes and belongings during their stay in hospital, to leave the hospital from time to time, etc. Also more attention is being paid to the individual's natural habitat, especially if he or she is or was a patient or is considered to be a prospective one. The family, community and place of work have become the crucial places for prevention, treatment and rehabilitation. All these changes indicate that the process of 'de-professionalization' of medicine is continuing and the role of laymen in the system of health care becomes more important. While the physician still holds his unique position in the field of health in general and in the field of therapy in particular, the participation of nurses, social workers, psychologists, sociologists, and just people of good will, is increasingle felt to be necessary.

The most significant changes, however, are occurring at the theoretical level, in the concept of health, which is expressed more and more frequently in functional terms. For instance, the unique center for statistics relating systematically to the health of the general population, the U.S. National Center for Health Statistics, frequently uses the concepts of limited activity and bed disability as the only concepts defining ill-health. It is also significant that the Center attempts to reduce the group of causes of disease. In some surveys the causes are specified only with respect to acute cases, and within every group of diseases the number of possible causes is reduced to a minimum. It would appear that the question: 'who suffers from this or that?' is sometimes considered to be less important than the question 'what are the effects of this suffering?' It is also typical of the Center's mode of proceeding that the bulk of its data on health are obtained by means of home interviews.

Our proposals for studying the health of Polish society and its needs in this respect[13] postulate two different approaches to health: (1) behavioral, and (2) one involving clinical diagnoses, similar to the Health Examination Survey carried out by the National Center for Health Statistics. The behavioral study has already been completed.[14] We have also completed a project for a study of the second kind mentioned above. In 1974 the investigation of 'The Intellectual Performance of Polish Children (with Special Attention to Mild Mental Retardation)' will begin the field part of the study.[15]

We would like also to attempt a third approach in the future, to be based on the expected results of the arduous efforts currently being undertaken on sociomedical health indicators.[16]

I wish to make it clear that I am aware of the limitations of the functional approach to health inasmuch as it ignores etiology and the early, obscure stages of the disease process. We shall probably be looking in the future for still another sociological framework which will enable us to include in our researches social determinants of biological phenomena. However, I have ventured to discuss these questions here not in order to argue that functional terms are an ultimate tool, but to show that the essential realms of medicine seem to be no longer impenetrable to sociological exploration.

It is also possible that we shall find it desirable in the future to add a 'biological' slant to our research. If we in fact become interested in this area we shall be concerned to study not pathological but normal traits – the biological endowment of man. There are theorists of sociology who deprecate biological traits. However, on the border-line of the social sciences the biological investigation of man is developing, and this fact will perhaps, sooner or later, have some impact on sociological theory.

III. THE APPLICATION OF SOCIOLOGY TO MEDICINE

I should now like to discuss the 'S–M' relation of my diagram. This relation is referred to by different names: 'application', 'utilization', 'uses', 'problem solving', 'social engineering', 'sociotechnics'. None of these terms is unequivocal, but there can no doubt they all stand for practical applications of sociology. This multifaceted trend is developing dynamically in Poland. Its theoretical foundations were laid by Adam Podgórecki, who first used the term 'sociotechnics', [17] meaning a practical science, the general theory of effective social action. His is the first systematic attempt to work out such a technique of applying sociology and social research to various practical areas which would facilitate the scientific solution of practical problems. Podgórecki postulates an essential reorientation and modification of the patterns of thinking, of the methods and concepts used in contemporary sociology, whereby social engineering, in addition to the cognitive approach, would be accepted as an essential objective of this discipline.

Medicine was specifically the subject ot some of the articles published in several volumes of collected articles. [18] In one of these books I wrote some years ago that in my opinion there were three main ways of applying sociology to medicine: research, teaching and expert analysis. In the following years we tried to practise all three of these forms of collaboration with medicine. I would like to comment briefly on our experiences.

Neither research nor teaching – the two commonest and most important forms of applying sociology to medicine – are engineering or sociotechnical functions, in the sense these words may be used in other fields of social life. Sociotechnical activity can be performed in medicine mainly by doctors, (and by other health personnel), at least in Poland. If they are properly instructed in how to perform this role they will become real social engineers in their field. 'Application' means that the physician who was formerly familiar with the natural sciences only, today has his mental horizons expanded by psychology, sociology and the other social sciences and by the humanities. The sociotechnical component is closely combined with the professional one in an area such as medicine, where the main and uncontroversial goals are prevention, treatment and rehabilitation. In traditional medicine, occupied primarily with bedridden patients, the need for expanding the doctor's skills beyond the realm of traditional medical knowledge were not so obvious. Nowadays in the realms of human problems, mental health and social pathology, effective medical action is impossible without the methodology and conceptual framework of sociology and without the sociological imagination.

A. Research

To this day a sociologist in Poland seems to be of most use to medicine when he is working as part of a team doing basic research in etiology, the spread of disease, etc., or by undertaking specific studies suggesting or justifying some planned action like the reorganization of medical teaching, the opening of a new health institution, an improvement in the procedures for registering patients, etc. Participation in such endeavours offers a good opportunity for the sociologist to be helpful in practical situations by elaborating conceptual frameworks of research, specifying its goals, presenting original assumptions, suggesting hypotheses, choosing samples and techniques, assisting in the collection of data, deducing general conclusions and writing final reports. He may be very useful in providing an overall evaluation of some existing situation, which may either accelerate the trend towards change or stop it if change is unnecessary or undesirable.

The sociologist can be of great help in explaining the meanings of basic medical terms. The achievements of practical medicine and the individual disciplines composing it have left the general theory of medicine, concerned with general concepts and principles of action, far behind. The notions traditionally used in medicine – clinical observation, preventive procedures, treatment and rehabilitation – should all be redefined and critically analysed. A sociologist contributes by offering a fresh view of medicine from the perspective of society in general.

He may help the doctor to see his role in a new light, and convince him that the approach of the social sciences to health, illness and hospitals is also legitimate, and that both the sociological and medical approaches are theoretically interesting and practically useful.

The greatest value of the sociologist for medicine is the fact that he thinks unlike a doctor. The different nature of his approach is like a weak plant that should be carefully tended. If this plant takes root, what is today only a possibility may become a reality: medical prescriptions will contain recommendations based on the social sciences, as the prescriptions issued at present recommend therapy based on the natural sciences. But this chance depends on the sociologist's ability to make use of his special knowledge and his theoretical, methodological and conceptual equipment, in a word, on whether he is a good sociologist. But it also depends on the more or less favorable conditions provided by those who are 'hosts' in this field, i.e. the medical profession.

Harking back once again to my diagram, I should like to stress that a sociologist should be able to work effectively along all sides of the triangle 'SM–S–M'. In certain concrete cases this is downright essential. If one wants to find the reasons for high infant mortality, the high incidence of syphilis, high alcohol consumption or mild mental retardation among children, for instance – one has to know different subcultures and the different life-styles prevailing in various classes, social strata, groups or communities. One must know first of all where infants die, who contracts syphilis and where people drink excessively. Such phenomena must be studied against the total cultural and social background and never in isolation, as this makes preventive action ineffective. Medicine, also social medicine, throughout its history has used methods that did not involve analysis of social structures.[19]

The utilization of a social scientist in medicine only along the line 'SM'–'M', when he is unable to use his general sociological knowledge, is plainly short-sighted. Such tasks can be done by doctors and it is to be expected that in this sector social epidemiologists, social psychiatrists, family doctors, community doctors, etc. will replace sociologists in the near future. Routine statistics will probably include a great deal of data that in many countries are considered 'sociological' at the moment (the level of education for example). If the sociologist is to become useful and earn respect within the medical world, his wisdom cannot be merely of a common sense type, but it must also be clearly distinct from medical skill and knowledge.

B. Teaching

My remarks about teaching concern the training of sociologists.[20] In the European literature it is difficult to find works on teaching sociology of medicine to students of sociology. There is also a tremendous disproportion in the U.S. between the innumerable publications devoted to teaching the social or behavioral sciences to students of medicine, the endless conferences, discussions and disputes concerning this subject, and the relative silence about teaching students of sociology.[21] This situation is illogical and harmful, at least in Poland, where the social scientist is expected to understand all areas of social life and to teach health personnel in the social and cultural spheres.

The objectives of the Warsaw teaching program are connected with the general style of practising the sociology of medicine in Poland, given the present state of development in this field and with some ideas concerning the present conceptions of the role and aims of a sociologist of medicine. Besides the general knowledge common to all sociologists, he should have certain additional qualifications:

1. First of all, he should possess a specific knowledge of medicine. At present the vast majority of sociologists – like almost everyone else – possesses random scraps of information connected with medicine concerning, for example, the symptoms of certain diseases, organ transplants or mental illness. These matters are generally considered as extremely interesting (particularly if they involve specialized professional knowledge, technical advance in medicine and the like) but they are of little use in providing systematic knowledge of medicine. Knowledge of medicine should be formulated in accordance with the categories and traditions of sociology. The Warsaw program under discussion was called 'Medicine for the Sociologist'.

2. A sociologist of medicine should be problem-oriented, while acting in cooperation with other disciplines. As we know, any given problem will have an interdisciplinary nature and the phenomena under study within this framework require more than just a sociological approach.

The problems encountered by the sociologist in the field of medicine are no exception. The problem-oriented and interdisciplinary approaches can be useful, after all, not only in respect to medicine. At present university curricula in sociology generally do not sufficiently take this approach into account.

On the other hand, the necessity of expanding in Poland the classical sociotechnical role of the sociologist in medicine, the so-called policy-making role, at both local and national levels, is a somewhat controversial subject. This role, in the sense used by Polish sociotechnicians, and also by some Western sociologists of medicine, requires a more precise definition in relation both to medicine and to Polish realities.

3. In 1972/73 the main emphasis was put on the courses on macro-sociological formulation. In this connection, it was necessary to revise the content of the concept 'sociology in medicine' as defined by Robert Straus. This was because on the one hand we could not confine ourselves in our program to the 'sociology of medicine' (in the sense used by Straus) while, on the other hand, we wanted to avoid defining the field in terms of clinical concepts. Such a revision turned out to be quite feasible. As I said before, the concept of health of population, so far irrevocably linked for the sociologist with biology and the organism, is undergoing thoroughgoing changes; namely, it is being expressed with increasing frequency in behavioral terms. The development of the socio-medical health indicators will provide further possibilities. To put it briefly, the sociological approach to the study of medicine does not have to be limited to the investigation of 'the social behavior surrounding disease' (according to the well-known definition of Eliot Freidson) because 'disease', which is the essential realm of medicine, can also be expressed sociologically.

C. Expert analysis

Finally I should like to mention the latest function of a sociologist in Poland: that of an expert on different branches of social life. In this capacity his interests reach beyond the boundaries of individual sciences to cover the whole sphere of a given problem which is vital for society's interests. In 1971 a number of expert groups were created and entrusted with the task of analyzing various fields of social life and elaborating principles for an optimum policy on the part of the state in these fields. The first appraisal was completed by a committee working on the problem of education in Poland. Its final report was written under the guidance of a sociologist, who wrote at one point:[22] "The work of an expert appraising, for example, the value and social functioning of the school system is blocked by several obstacles which are seldom encountered by the social sciences in their everyday routine activities. These obstacles concern primarily the problem of finding criteria in order to evaluate the proposed changes. It is astonishing to see how various and how ill-thought out are the criteria of evaluation used by representatives of different educational systems, or by people who have become involved in their activities."

Recently the Presidium of the Polish Academy of Sciences set up an expert committee on the disability and rehabilitation in Poland which will produce its report in 1976.

* *
*

Ten years are a short time in the life of a scientific discipline. The body of knowledge accumulated, theoretical and empirical, must necessarily be modest. It should be borne in mind that, in contrast to other branches of sociology in Poland, it was necessary in this case to start from the foundation, to create an environment, a climate, an organizational framework. But by now the sociology of medicine is relatively well established within both sociology and medicine. It is attracting an increasing number of youthful talents. The establishment and functioning of the Medical Sociology Unit at the Institute of Philosophy and Sociology of the Polish Academy of Sciences and the Sociology of Medicine Section of the Polish Sociological Association have acted as catalysts in development of a definite need for this field in the country.

REFERENCES

[1] This Section was organized in 1965 and presently numbers 60 members, including both sociologists and physicians. Many of the sociologists are working in medical institutions: mostly in various departments of medical schools and research institutes. The Section meets once a month. It serves as a platform for contacts among

persons working in the broad area of medical sociology, providing them with the opportunity to exchange ideas and experiences related to their work. Through these contacts the author has become acquainted with a larger group of medical sociologists then the group mainly described here, and to some extent these wider experiences have been incorporated, in a generalized form, in the present paper.

[2] Jan Szczepański, 'Common Objectives of Sociology and the Polish National School', *Transactions of the Sixth World Congress of Sociology* **III** (1970).

[3] Bernhard J. Stern, 'Toward a Sociology of Medicine', in: *Historical Sociology*, New York 1959, pp. 410–419.

[4] "Should the sociologist wish to interpret these experiences into the language of theory, an assortment of the ideas within the theoretical tradition of historical materialism will not suffice nor will theoretical schemes set up in the technical civilization of Western societies. The characteristic feature of the changes experienced by this society is the fact that the ideas of Marxism were one of the forces transforming it, thus making its activities a sort of practical test of the ideas. Thus, in their investigations, the Polish Marxists have had to take into consideration the social action of what had been created only by Marx and what had not existed in the society described by him. On the other hand, we do not know enough yet about the real effects of a socialized economy or about how a socialized industry changes a society, therefore we cannot say what the features of Polish industrial society will be rising above the contemporary technique working in the framework of socialized and planned economy." Szczepański, *ibid.*

[5] With one exception where the sponsor was Commissioner of the City Health Department in Warsaw: 'A Survey of Patients' Opinions on the Functioning of the District Dental Clinics in Warsaw'. Janusz Bejnarowicz, unpublished report, Institute of Philosophy and Sociology, 1970 (in Polish).

[6] Within the broader scope of a series of studies on mental retardation, carried out by the Psychoneurological Institute: Irena Łabudzka, Magdalena Sokołowska, Maria Trawińska-Kwaśniewska, Ignacy Wald, 'The Knowledge and Attitudes of Warsaw Doctors towards Mental Retardation', unpublished report, Institute of Philosophy and Sociology, 1972 (in Polish).

[7] Within the broader study conducted by the Cardiological Institute, Warsaw Medical School: 'The Social Rehabilitation of Patients after the Myocardial Infarction', Janusz Bejnarowicz, Antonina Ostrowska, Magdalena Sokołowska, Final Report, 1969 (in English). Janusz Bejnarowicz, Antonina Ostrowska, Magdalena Sokołowska, 'Research on the Social Aspects of the Rehabilitation of Invalids', *Chirurgia Narządów Ruchu i Ortopedia Polska* 4 (1966) (in Polish). Janusz Bejnarowicz, Antonina Ostrowska, Magdalena Sokołowska, 'The Social Rehabilitation of Invalids', *Studia Socjologiczne* 2 (1967) (in Polish). Magdalena Sokołowska, 'Influencing the Social Process of Patient Rehabilitation', in: A. Podgórecki (ed.), *Sociotechnics*, Warsaw, 1970 (in Polish). Magdalena Sokołowska, 'A Sociological Interpretation of the Process of Rehabilitation', *Bulletin of the*

Research Institute of Invalid Cooperatives (1971) (in Polish). Antonina Ostrowska, 'The Use of the Concept of Socialization to the Study of Rehabilitation', in the present book.

[8] The approach to rehabilitation as a social problem is represented in the report of the expert committee preparing a report on disability and rehabilitation in Poland (see p. 15).

[9] Danuta Markowska, Peter Klemm, Janusz Bejnarowicz, 'The Types of Families in Polish Cities', Institute of Philosophy and Sociology, unpublished report, 1973.

[10] "Macrosociology may be defined as the study of large social groups, large-scale cultural systems, global societies, socio-economic formations in the Marxist sense and large-scale historical processes of social change – development or regression", Jan Szczepański, 'Some Remarks on Macrosociology', *Social Science Information* VII (1968).

[11] This question was extensively discussed in a paper by J. Bejnarowicz and M. Sokołowska, 'The Sociologist and the Concept of State of Health', in *Studia Socjologiczne* 3 (1973). Such examinations would be useful, indeed, in relation to e.g. cervical cancer, syphilis, TBC, mental retardation. It has become relatively simple to diagnose these diseases and to predict their occurrence within the population. Such examinations make it possible to identify those who are ill within the specified population and enhance more effective programs of prevention and other activities of health personnel. Such studies would also be recommended in relation to acute, severe diseases, injuries, etc. and in every instance where the clinical disease is synonymous with behavioral illness and sickness.

[12] Only in the academic year 1972–73 a course on medical sociology was introduced for undergraduate students of sociology at Warsaw University (see the last part of this paper).

[13] (a) Magdalena Sokołowska, Antonina Ostrowska, Janusz Bejnarowicz, 'The Health Needs of Polish Society', unpublished report, Institute of Philosophy and Sociology, 1972 (in Polish). (b) Magdalena Sokołowska, Antonina Ostrowska, 'Some Questions Related to the Study of the Health Needs of a Society', Unpublished Report, Institute of Philosophy and Sociology, 1973 (in Polish). These studies are based on two published works: 1. M. Sokołowska, S. Klonowicz, J. Bejnarowicz, 'The State of Health of the Polish Population – a Review of Medical and Demographic Publications', and 2. A. Ostrowska, 'The Health Needs of Polish Society. A Review of Sociological and Medical Publications' (both available in Polish in book form).

[14] As a Ph.D. Thesis by Anna Titkow, an extract from which is presented in this book.

[15] By the end of 1974 the data from the first part of the study, which was carried out in Warsaw, were in the final stage of processing: the cohort analysis of all children living in Warsaw that were born in 1963 (14,265). The study was carried out by a group of sociologists, psychologists and physicians (A. Firkowska-Man-

kiewicz, M. Sokołowska, A. Ostrowska, I. Wald, J. Kostrzewski, M. Czarkowski). The aim of the first stage was to define the intelligence levels of Warsaw children (by means of group intelligence tests) and to select a group for further investigation. Part of the project is financed by Fund PL-480, U.S. Government, Dept. of HEW, Social and Rehabilitation Service under the number 19-P-58334-F-01 – in cooperation with the Dept. of Epidemiology, Columbia Univ. School of Public Health (Prof. Z. Stein, Prof. M. Susser).

[16] See the paper by Jack Elinson in this book.

[17] In 1972 the Research Committee of Sociotechnics of International Sociologic Association was established.

[18] Magdalena Sokołowska, 'The Applications of Sociology to Medicine', in: A. Podgórecki (ed.), *Sociotechnics*: *The Practical Uses of Sociology*, Warsaw, 1968. Magdalena Sokołowska, 'Influencing the Social Process of Patient Rehabilitation', in: A. Podgórecki (ed.), *Sociotechnics*: *How to Act Effectively*, Warsaw, 1970. Magdalena Sokołowska, 'Two Modes of Health Policy', in: A. Podgórecki (ed.), *Sociotechnics*: *The Action Model*, 1972. Magdalena Sokołowska, 'Utilization of Sociological Research in the Area of Health' in: J. Kubin, A. Podgórecki (eds.), *Utilization of the Social Sciences*, 1973. Magdalena Sokołowska, 'Dysfunctions of Health Care Institutions' in: A. Podgórecki (ed.), *Sociotechnics*: *Functionality and Dysfunctionality of Institutions*, 1974. All in Polish.

[19] George Rosen, 'The Evolution of Social Medicine', in: H. E. Freeman, S. Levine and L. G. Reeder (eds.), *Handbook of Medical Sociology*, Englewood Cliffs, 1972.

[20] See Note 12. This is the so-called *monographic* course on this subject for students of the third year. There is also a seminar course leading to a master's degree in medical sociology. This is the beginning of the teaching of the sociology of medicine in Polish universities.

[21] See the paper by Ivo Nuyens in this book. Medical schools in Poland are not part of the universities. The curricula of training medical students in sociology have been in use for over ten years. Recently this training has developed considerably. Also training in psychology and sociology as part of nurses' training is developing dynamically, particularly in various postgraduate nursing schools, above all in the newly established Department of Nursing of the Lublin Medical School – the only one of its kind in continental Europe, leading to a Master's degree in nursing.

[22] Jan Szczepański, 'A Political Test of Social Science', in: *Utilization of the Social Sciences*.

I. HEALTH IN SOCIETY

HEALTH AND SOCIAL PLANNING

JAN KOSTRZEWSKI

State Institute of Hygiene, Warsaw, Poland

The title of my paper may seem to promise more than I will be able to offer the honourable participants of this conference. I am a physician without a sociological background. As the years go by I miss this kind of education more and more. I have devoted over thirty years of my professional work to epidemiology and to combatting communicable diseases in various conditions, in various countries and in various periods of peace and war. During the last twenty years I have been mainly involved in the organization of health care and the administration of the health service. The evolution of my work has undoubtedly been responsible for reinforcing my feeling that there is a growing need for cooperation between sociologists and the health service. The need for such cooperation originated primarily from failures in the implementation of certain disease control programmes and difficulties in the organization of prevention, treatment and rehabilitation. The organizer of health care works under the continuous pressure of the health needs of the population. Therefore the solution of individual problems does not bring him relief, as each problem solved is followed by a new one expecting solution. Despite the increasing number of health service employees: physicians, nurses and a whole range of other professions, despite the great number of newly built hospitals, sanatoria, institutions for chronic patients, out-patient clinics, health centres and centres for social and occupational rehabilitation, the scope of the population's health needs is not decreasing but changing and progressing. The health service is aware of this and this is the way how the situation is evaluated by the population demanding still broader range of health services representing higher and higher standards.

The health needs of a population and the problems arising from them depend on the social and economic development of the country in question, its geographical location, its natural and man-made conditions and, finally, on the degree of development of the health service and the resources made available by the government. I would venture the opinion that in all countries, regardless of their state of social and economic development, despite the differences in the organization and degree of advancement of their health services, the population claims that health care is inadequate. What is the reason for this and how far are those reproaches objective and justified? It is very difficult to answer these questions. A health service has two essential tasks to fulfil: one of them – to some extent technical – consists in diagonsis and treatment, application of proper preventive or curative measures and an appropriate rehabilitation system. The other – more difficult and complex – is the provision of adequate health care. The idea of health care comprises not only the provision of competent help but also the understanding of the mood and mental state of the patient, a display of consideration and showing him simple human attention. These two aspects of the work of a health service – professional and technical on one hand and protective and solicitous on the other – are in practice very often in conflict. It seems that, with the improvement of medical technique and the concentration by the health service on still more advanced equipment, methods of diagnosis and treatment, there is less time and place for the consideration due to the patient. The more excellent medicine becomes from the technical point of view, the colder and stiffer it is in its approach towards patients, and broadly speaking towards the whole population. I mention here the very important – in my opinion – problem of the assistance of sociologists and psychologists in medicine both at present and in the future. This is, of course, a group of problems very difficult to measure, and therefore may be considered, for the time being, as less important in comparison with the enormous number of health needs which can be objectively measured, but nevertheless these problems are of great significance from the point of view of the public – the recipient of health services.

Using the objective measures of public health one can divide countries into three groups: the highly developed with the longest life expectancy, lowest infant mortality rate where neither hunger nor widespread malnutrition exists, and where people are free from those diseases against which they can be successfully protected in view of the present progress of medical science. According to the definition accepted by the World Health Organization, citizens of those countries, apart from a satisfactory physical and mental condition, should also enjoy social well-being. However, in this respect there are alarming observations to be made and we are unable to discover any convergence between a good state of health (evaluated on the basis of criteria listed above) and social well-being. The Hippy phenomenon, drug addiction and suicide are spreading in those rich countries representing a high standard of living and the positive health indicators discussed above. Therefore we must be very careful in judging the state of health in various countries.

The second group of countries is composed of those where life expectancy is shortest, where infant mortality is highest, where people often suffer from hunger, where malnutrition can be widely observed and where infectious and preventible parasitic diseases are endemic.

Between these two groups of countries there are many various transitions. For example the longest mean life expectancy at birth amounted in Sweden (1967) to 76.5 years foı females and 71.9 for males, in India (1951–60) it was 40.6 and 41.9 and in Madagascar 38.3 and 37.5 respectively (Table 1). The average life expectancy in a given country depends, first of all, on the infant mortality rate. Usually the lower the infant

Table 1. Life Expectancy

Country	Year	Mean duration of life after birth (years)	
		Males	Females
India	1951–1960	41.9	40.6
Madagascar	1966	37.5	38.3
Egypt	1960	51.6	53.8
Peru	1960–1965	52.6	55.5
U.S.A.	1968	66.6	74.0
Sweden	1967	71.9	76.5

mortality rate the longer the average life expectancy. Differences between the infant mortality rate of individual countries are, however, much higher than differences between mean duration of life. In many African countries over 10% of children born alive die in their first year while in Sweden and other developed countries the infant mortality rate ranges from 1 to 2%. One should remember, however, that the average rate for the whole country does not reflect health and social differences within a given country (Table 2). Taking Republic of South Africa as an example,

Table 2. Birth and Mortality in 1969

Country	Population (thousands)	Live birth per 1000 population	General mortality per 1000 population	Infant mortality per 1000 population
Africa				
Egypt	32,500	36.8	14.4	119.0
Republic of South Africa				
Coloured population	13,300	38.2	14.2	134.6
White population	3,700	22.9	8.7	23.0
America				
Guatemala	5,000	43.0	17.0	91.3
U.S.A.	202,000	17.7	9.5	20.7
Europe				
Sweden	7,900	13.5	10.5	11.7
Yugoslavia	20,209	18.9	9.3	57.3

we find infant mortality rate among coloured people (134.6 per 1000 live births) almost six times higher than among the white population (23.0). This is a good illustration of the effect of social conditions on the state of health of inhabitants of the same country, living in the same geographical and climatic conditions.

Any attempt at a thorough analysis of demographic differences in relation to the average state of health in a population and vice versa should be supplemented by a sociological analysis. The demographic changes depend, first of all, on social and health changes in the country, and health and social living conditions are closely linked. This is an old truth which was already pointed out by the great philosophers and economists of the last century who created the background for the Marxist philosophy.

The analysis of diseases, injuries and causes of death is another kind of approach to the evaluation of the population's state of health for the needs of social planning. Investigations of this kind require the use of the whole arsenal of epidemiological methods. Epidemiology is in this respect a basic tool of those who administer and organize the health

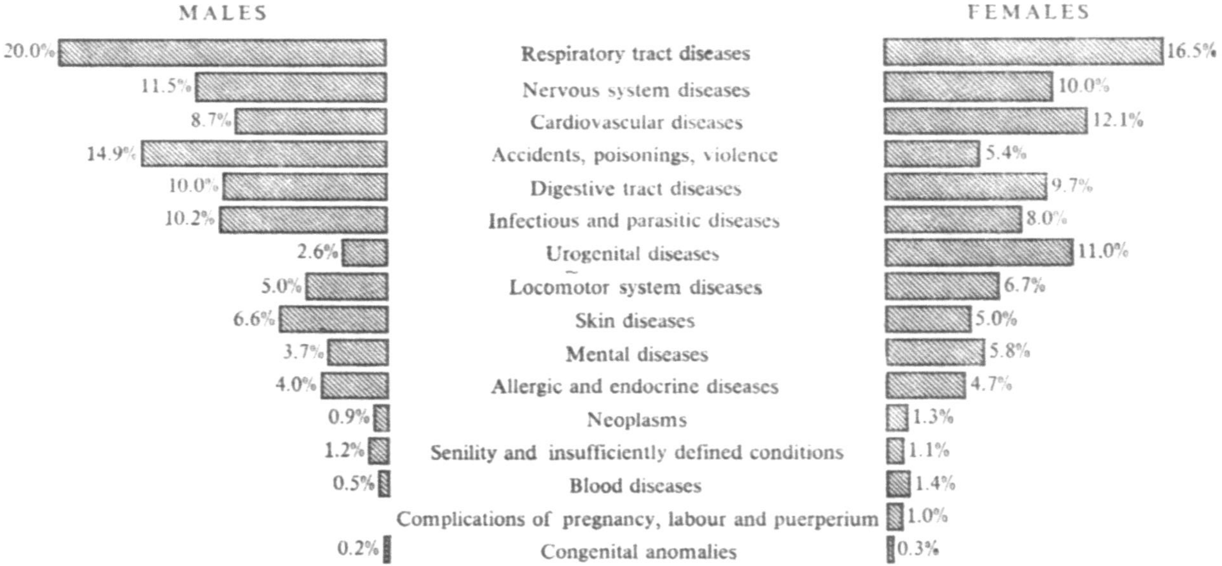

Fig. 1. Causes of visits in outpatient health service in Poland from July 1, 1967 to June 30, 1968 according to sex

service. I am talking, of course, about modern epidemiology, namely about the study of the distribution and determinants of disease frequency. Epidemiology is now understood to take within its scope all diseases, whether they are acute or chronic, physical or mental, communicable or non-communicable.

Epidemiology has three main aims:

1. To describe the distribution and size of disease problems in human populations;
2. To provide the data essential to the planning, implementation and evaluation of services for the prevention, control and treatment of disease and to the setting up of priorities among those services;
3. To identify aetiological factors in the pathogenesis of disease.

Having in mind the needs of social planning, the aims given in items 1 and 2 are of special significance. The implementation of these aims is not easy, however. Difficulties are faced at the very beginning when we start to select the criteria for making evaluations and establishing priorities. Moreover, the selection of criteria is connected with the selection of methods.

In the year 1967–68 an investigation was carried out in Poland based on a randomization (1) of all medical attendances in all types of health service institutions, including private practice. In this way information was obtained on diseases reported by physicians giving medical advice to inhabitants of Poland attending any sort of medical institution. This material was used for estimating the prevalence of various diseases in the population of Poland and in individual groups according to sex, age, place of residence, occupation and other characteristics.

The preliminary analysis indicated that respiratory diseases were the most frequent cause of medical attendance: 20% among males and 16.5% among females. Second on the list were, among males: accidents, poisonings, and violence (14.9%) and, among females, circulatory system diseases (12.2%). Third place was taken by nervous system diseases among males (11.5%) and urogenital system diseases among females (11.0%) (Fig. 1). In general, respiratory system diseases were first on the list both among males and females and next came nervous system diseases, circulatory system diseases and accidents, poisonings and violence (Fig. 2). This sequence provides a basis for establishing priorities in planning medical car e.

The question of priorities becomes complicated, however, when diseases of inpatients are analysed. Among the total number of patients treated in hospitals throughout Poland in 1967, diseases of the digestive

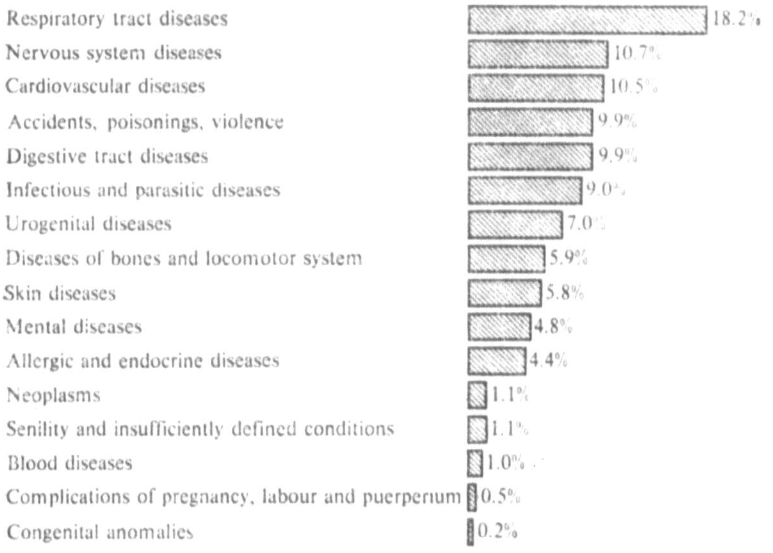

Fig. 2. Causes of visits in outpatient health service in Poland from July 1, 1967 to June 30, 1968

system predominated (16.6%), followed by accidents, poisonings and violence (12.2%), urogenital system diseases (10.2%) and respiratory system diseases (9.7%) (Fig. 3).

Further data were obtained when absenteeism at work as a result of illness, was considered. They are as follows: 1. accidents, poisonings and violence (18.8%), 2. respiratory system diseases (17.7%), 3. digestive system diseases (11.2%), 4. infectious and parasitic diseases (10.1%) (Fig. 4).

The fourth kind of analysis referred to causes of death, i.e. to the greatest losses suffered by the population as a result of illness. Almost one third of all deaths in Poland in 1967 were caused by circulatory system diseases (31.7%), followed by malignant neoplasms (17.5%), senility and ill-defined conditions (11.2%), and accidents, poisonings and violence (7.2%) (Fig. 5).

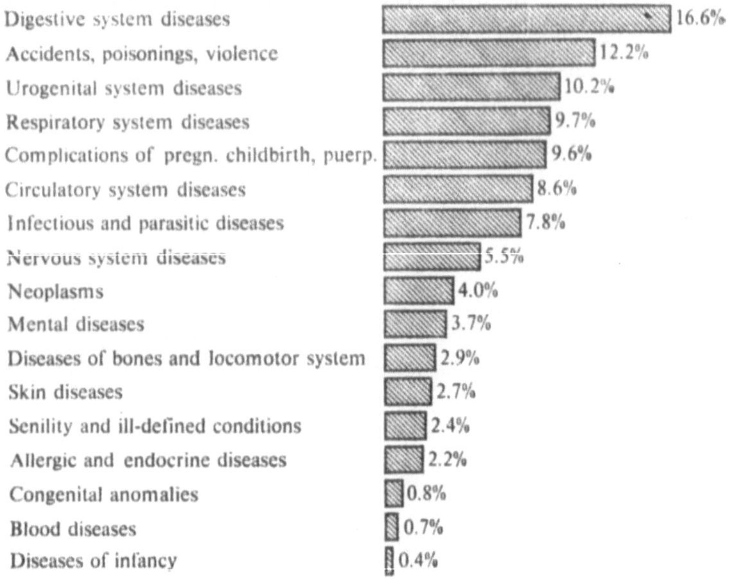

Fig. 3. Diagnoses in inpatiens in Poland in 1967

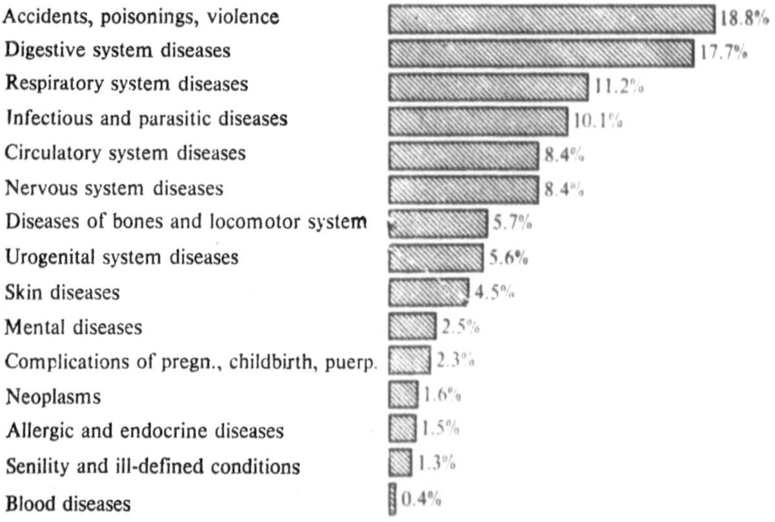

Fig. 4. Causes of sickness absenteeism in population aged 18–65 years in Poland in 1967

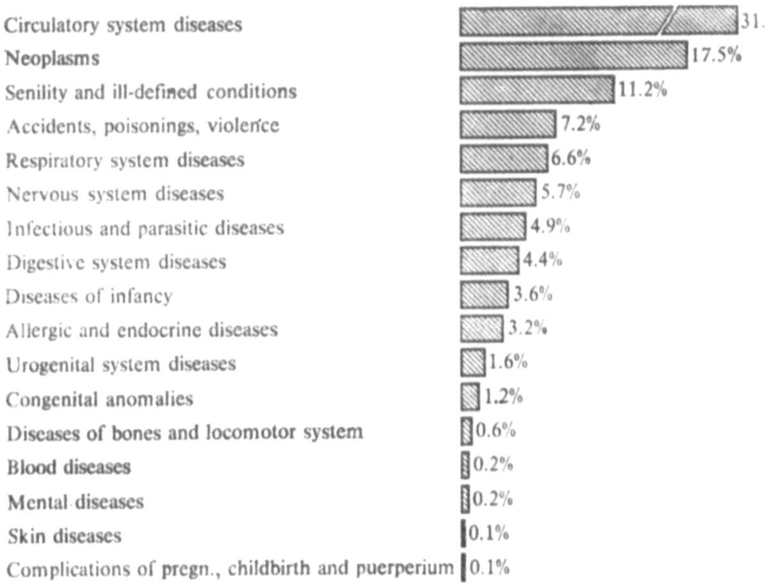

Fig. 5. Causes of death in Poland in 1967

Any final establishment of priorities in health and social planning should include all these analyses. In accordance with the results obtained from these analyses, the number of medical staff, its education and specialization, the number and distribution of hospitals, the number of hospital beds in various wards, the number of out-patient clinics and health centres and the financial provisions for preventive measures, treatment and rehabilitation in regard to individual categories of illness should be planned.

More detailed information about the frequency of individual diseases and the social significance of individual categories of disease can be found in the thorough epidemiological analysis reveal some hitherto undiscovered problems. In order to solve these problems, sociological analysis is also required. It is impossible to present here hundreds of tables and diagrams illustrating the prevalence of all the diseases among males and females estimated for the whole population of Poland, for various age groups and for inhabitants of urban and rural areas. I should like, therefore, to give only a few examples of diseases and traumas belonging to

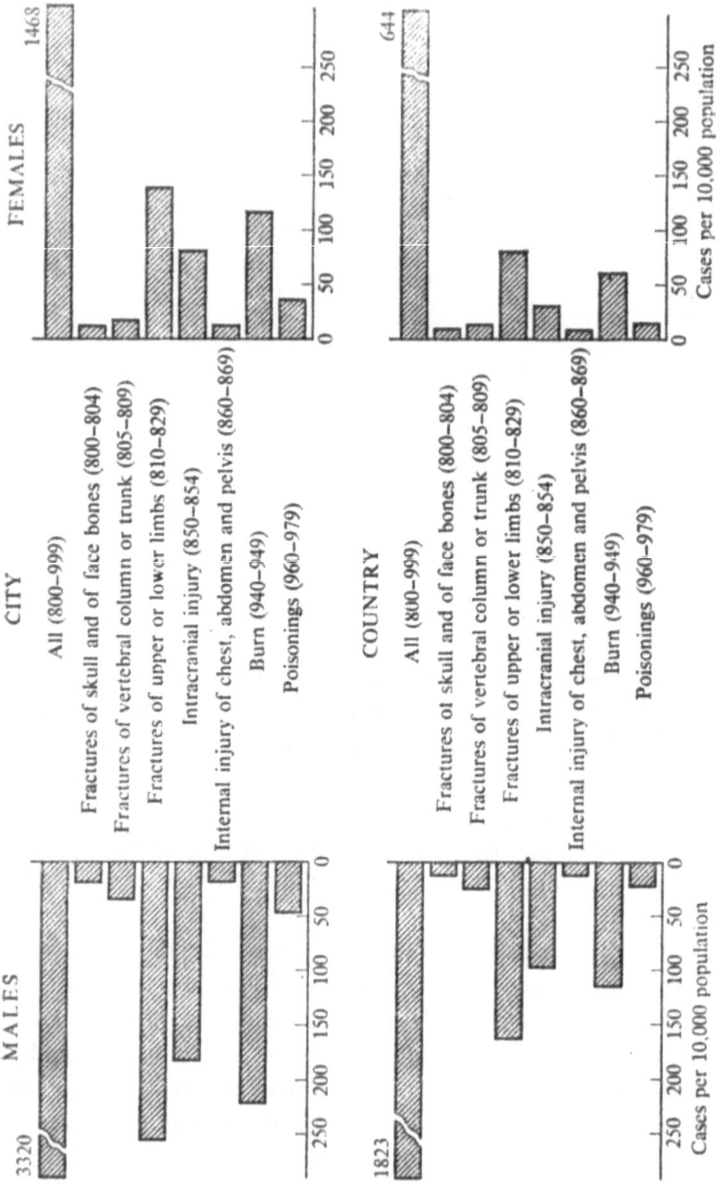

Fig. 6. Accidents, poisonings and violence in 1967–68 (N800–N999)

those categories which are of primary importance in view of their frequency and social significance.

Accidents, poisonings and violence come high on the lists of the above mentioned analyses (Figs. 1, 2, 3, 4, and 5); they occupy first place among causes of work disability, second place among causes of inpatient treatment, fourth among causes of death, although in the 1–30 age group they occupy first place among causes of death and fourth among causes of medical attendance. Probably they also come high among the causes of permanent disability. In planning health care and in the social planning, accidents, poisonings and violence must gain high priority. How do the results of epidemiological analysis shape up according to the 1967–68 study?

During one year 33 per cent of males living in urban areas sought medical advice because of accident, poisoning or violence, while in rural areas this figure was only 18 per cent; almost 15 per cent of females living in urban areas sought medical advice for the same reason, as against 6 per cent in rural areas (Fig. 6). The differences are great both between males and females and between inhabitants of urban and rural areas. If we divide all persons who met with accidents, poisonings or violence according to age we shall find further differences (Fig. 7). In males living in urban areas rates increase in the 1–25 age groups, then they gradually decrease, and only in the oldest over-60 groups can another increase be observed. Among boys aged 1–14 living in rural areas an evident increase in the beginning is followed by a slight increase. A dramatic rise is visible in the 14–25 age groups, which is in turn followed by a systematic decrease. In females, the differences between individual age groups are smaller. Slight increase can be observed in the 1–25 age groups but these rates, in the over-15 groups, are many times lower among females than among males.

An analysis of deaths shows a slightly different picture. Both in males and females, in rural and urban areas, mortality rates due to accidents, poisonings and violence are falling in the 1–15 age group. Then a slight increase of mortality is observed in females up to 20 years of age and it remains on the same level up to 60 years of age. Mortality due to accidents, poisonings and violence significantly increases above 60. Deaths among females living in urban areas occur a little more frequently than among those living in rural areas.

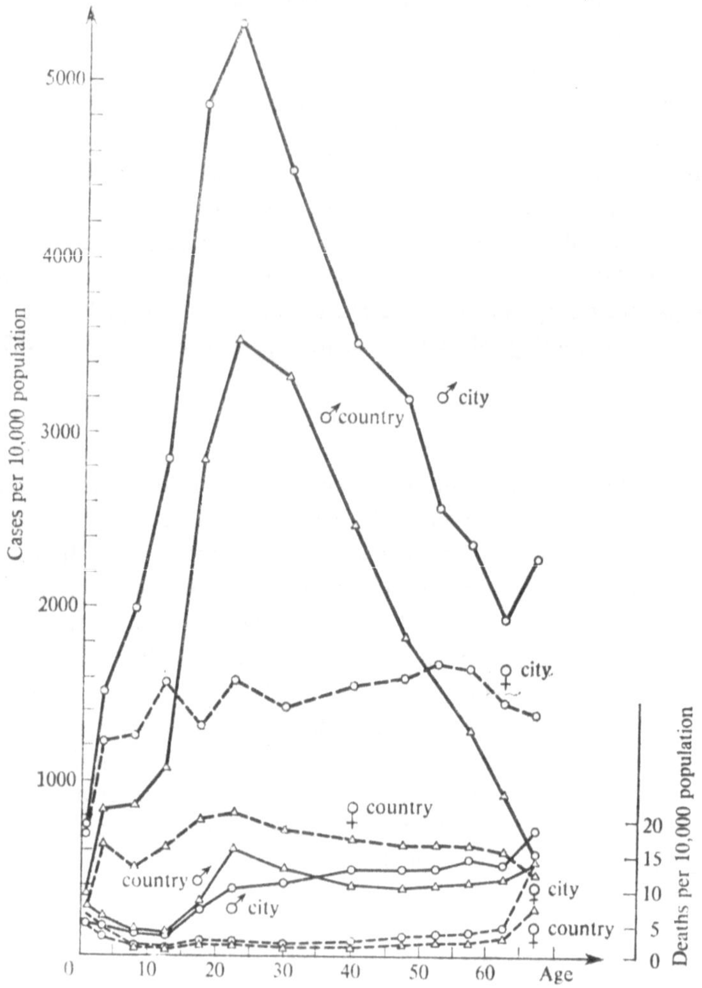

Fig. 7. Accidents, poisonings and violence in Poland in 1967–68 (N800–N999)

Among males living in urban areas a steady increase of mortality is observed from the age of 15 onwards up to a very advanced age. On the other hand, in rural areas a significant increase of deaths is found up to 25 years of age which, after a slight drop, remains on the same level up to 60 years of age and then increases again.

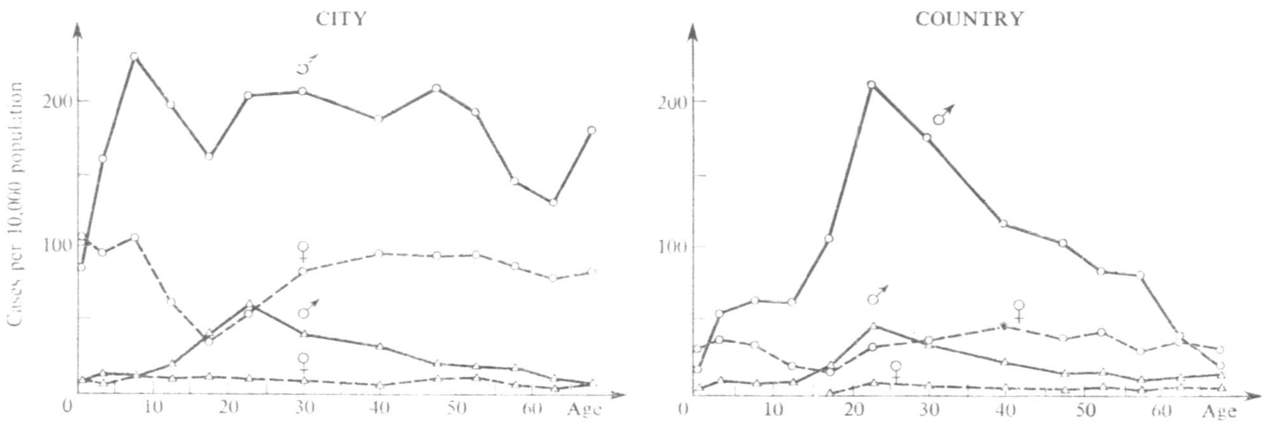

800–804 Fractures of skull and face bones

850–856 Intracranial injury (without fracture)

Fig. 8. Accidents and injuries in Poland 1967–68

In order to clarify the differences presented above, individual kinds of accidents, poisonings and violence, together with their causes, should be considered and supplemented by sociological analysis.

Fractures of the skull and facial bones and head injuries generally belong to the most serious injuries as regards social consequences. As to the frequency of medical consultations, these two categories counted as one are classified as fifth on the list (Fig. 8), but as regards fatalities, head injuries come out in first place among all injuries caused by accidents. This refers above all to males. With regard to medical consultations, fractures of skull or facial bones have a similar age distribution among males living in rural and urban areas (Fig. 8). Intracranial injuries without fractures have different distribution. In urban areas a considerable increase in the number of injuries is observed among boys aged from 5 to 15 years, but among males aged from 20 to 50 years the fre-

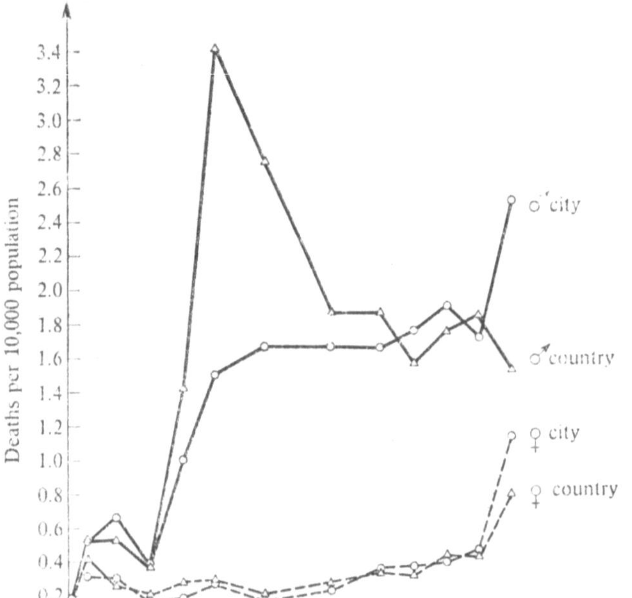

Fig. 9. Fractures of skull and face bones in Poland. Death in 1967–68 (N800–N804)

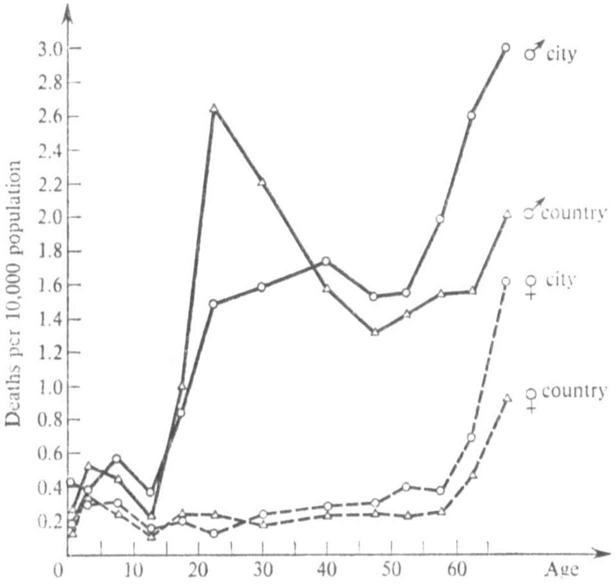

Fig. 10. Intracranial injury in Poland. Death in 1967–68 (N850–N856)

quency of these injuries does not show any considerable differences. In rural areas, in turn, there is no significant increase of head injuries in boys up to 15 years of age but a rapid increase is observed among males aged between 20 and 30. Differences in the incidence of death caused by head injuries among males living in rural and urban areas are even more significant (Figs. 9 and 10). The largest number of victims of accidents involving head injuries is observed among young men in the 20–35 age group living in rural areas. Among males living in urban areas, a rapid increase of mortality caused by head injuries is not found. Following a sharp growth from the ages of 10 to 25, the mortality rate remains almost the same up to 50 years of age to increase rapidly in older groups.

Sociological investigations are indispensable if these phenomena are to be explained. On the basis of epidemiological analysis only hypotheses can be formulated.

Differences in reporting head injuries in rural and urban areas can be explained to some extent, by the development of medical care in these areas. The larger number of medical consultations in cases of head injuries among boys living in urban areas results partly from the better organization of health care in urban than in rural schools. Similarly, the development of industrial health service contributes in some way to the increased number of medical consultations granted to industrial workers who are mainly inhabitants of urban areas. But differences in mortality rates cannot be explained by the development of the health service, since every severe case receives medical care regardless of the patient's place of residence and each death is presented in statistics. There are several reasons for a rapid increase of head injuries among young men living in rural areas. Just to mention a few: the rapid increase in the number of motor vehicles and especially the popularity of motor cycles used sometimes by young men under the influence of drink. Deaths of motor cyclists are reported almost daily by the press.

If we study the accident reports of newspapers we may often find notices about accidents involving aged people living in urban areas. These phenomena can affect the illustrations presented above. These are, however, only hypotheses which require further epidemiological studies, and are not strictly medical but rather sociological. They should indicate the causes of differences and recommend preventive measures.

I have paused over one example only, an example which stresses the necessity of the health service engaging in joint studies and activities together with sociologists. I should like this example to show the need for participation by sociologists in health service teams. There are hundreds of such examples which could be listed here, both in solving health problems and in organizing prevention, treatment and rehabilitation, as well as in environmental medicine. To succeed in environmental medicine it is necessary not only to involve government administration at all levels, industrial management and economists, but also to involve the whole population.

Therefore the future programme of health care will require an active contribution from the sociologists.

BIBLIOGRAPHY

J. Kostrzewski, Z. Branowitzer *et al.*, La Santé Publique, 1973, 16, 2, 165.

THE INFLUENCE OF THE LEGALIZATION OF ABORTION ON THE DEMOGRAPHIC REPRODUCTION IN POLAND 1956–72

STEFAN KLONOWICZ

Institute of Tuberculosis, Warsaw, Poland

The legalization of abortion in Poland, which took effect in 1956, made new, relatively reliable statistical data accessible to sociologists and demographers. I speak cautiously of 'relatively' reliable data because I am aware that even with the enactment of a free abortion law there still remain certain individual considerations which impel some women to seek the possibility of having an abortion performed outside the national health system. And in spite of the fact that doctors who privately perform abortions are obliged to report every case, if only for tax purposes, it seems perfectly justified to suspect that those 'individual considerations' occasionally prevail over the doctor's duty as a taxpayer, and some cases of abortion are never reported to the official statistical bureaux. Besides, there is no doubt that the official statistics do not include abortions undertaken by people unauthorized to practise medicine.

Hence, in order to adequately present the influence of abortion on demographic processes I shall complement the count of abortions made by the official statistics with an estimated number of interventions which have been presumably concealed. Such an assessment raises difficult problems, on which I shall elaborate later on. Here I may only remark that there is no evidence to support the view that the number of abortions not included in the official statistics surpassed in any single year after 1956 the level of one hundred thousand cases. It seems most probable that it always remained somewhere between fifty and sixty thousand cases annually [8].

Immediately after the enactment of the law sanctioning the termination of pregnancy for medical or social reasons the number of abortions performed rose dramatically. But as it now appears, the increase was only illusory. As J. Z. Holzer [9] correctly remarked it should rather be explained by "a transfer of a great number of cases that had been illegally performed before the abortion law was passed – frequently in unsanitary conditions – to the operating theatres of hospitals". Whereas the authors who believe that the fall in the birth rate was provoked by the enactment of the abortion law must be reminded that the falling trend which they have in mind had been observed at least four years earlier, in 1952.

According to all published statistical information, the number of abortions performed every year since 1960 only slightly surpassed 200,000 cases. It can be seen from the rates referring to abortion cases in the whole country that the number of terminated pregnancies was steadily decreasing. In 1960 it came to 223,800; in 1965 it was 223,700; in 1970 it was 214,000 and in 1971 it was 203,600. This means that in 1971 the number of arrested pregnancies was twenty thousand – or 16% – lower than it was in 1960 (see Table 1).

Table 1. Abortions and Other Arrests of Pregnancies Performed in Hospitals and Out-Patient Clinics (in thousands):

	Total	Abortions Performed in Hospitals			Abortions in Out-Patient Clinics
		For Medical Considerations	For Non-Medical Considerations	Other	
1960	223.8	4.0	146.4	74.4	
1965	223.7	3.1	121.6	65.1	33.8
1967	210.1	1.6	111.2	66.4	33.3
1970	214.0	1.8	107.4	65.7	39.2
1971	203.6	2.1	95.7	68.6	37.3

Sources: *Rocznik Statystyczny Ochrony Zdrowia 1945–1967*, GUS, Warszawa 1969, p. 410, and 'Ochrona Zdrowia 1971', *Statystyka Polski* **119** (1972) 83.

The data shown on Table 1 indicate that abortions performed for medical reasons played a marginal role in the overall pattern of terminated pregnancies. During the whole period covered by the official statistics they never constituted more than 2% of all cases. Approximately one half of all interventions (and before 1971 even more than half) were performed for non-medical reasons. Particularly interesting is the group classified under the heading 'other', since it includes cases of abortions initiated at home. This group represents therefore those women who were determined to terminate their pregnancies prematurely at all costs, and for this reason would be likely to seek abortion even when this kind of intervention is illegal.

I think, therefore, that among the cases attributable to the abortion law we can count only abortions performed in hospitals for non-medical considerations, abortions performed in out-patient clinics and some of the unregistered interventions. Even if we assume the highest possible estimate for this last figure – 100,000 cases annually – the total number of abortions performed under the sanction of the abortion law, including concealed interventions, amounts to approximately 200,000 cases annually.

For objectivity's sake I shall quote the opinion of M. Latuch [4], who says that in the period from 1956 to 1970 3,089,000 cases of abortion were registered, and that the number of unregistered interventions was even higher. However, he does not provide any evidence for this view.

In the literature on abortion, coefficients of the number of performed abortions per one hundred of live births are often used. In the opinion of opponents of the abortion law these coefficients manifestly indicate that legalized abortion has profoundly affected the rate of reproduction. It should be pointed out, however, that the use of such coefficients is gravely misleading since, in view of the spread of family planning and the universal availability of increasingly effective varieties of contraceptives, the number of live births is declining anyway. Nor do these coefficients take account of the number of still births and deaths in early infancy. Such births (although they influence the number of live births) are in no case connected either with the operation of the law on abortion or with any desire to limit the number of progeny. At the same time to leave those 'unsuccessful pregnancies' out of account distorts the empirical coefficient of miscarriages per number of deliveries. It would seem, therefore, that these coefficients should undergo certain adjustments.

Anyway, even if we use the traditional coefficients and calculate the number of miscarriages per 100 births, we shall still arrive at a conclusion which refutes the major arguments of the opponents of legalized abortion (Table 2).

The data cited show incontrovertibly that, after a certain rise in the years 1960–65, both coefficients (abortions in relation to the number of live births and in relation to the total number of pregnancies) showed

Table 2. Live Births, Still Births and Abortions in Poland

	1960	1965	1970	1971
Live births in thousands	669.5	546.4	546.0	562.3
Still births and deaths in early infancy in thousands	8.5	7.7	8.2	8.4
Abortions and other arrested pregnancies in thousands	223.8	223.7	214.0	203.6
Total of pregnancies in thousands	901.8	778.8	768.2	774.3
Abortions per one hundred livebirths	33.43	40.94	39.19	36.21
Abortions per one hundred pregnancies	24.81	28.77	27.86	26.29

Sources: *Rocznik Demograficzny 1971*, GUS, Warszawa 1971, p. 97, and *Rocznik Demograficzny 1972*, GUS, Warszawa 1972, p. 100, and computations of the author.

a definite drop in the years 1965–71. At the same time it should be noted that the number of pregnancies in 1971 showed a decrease of nearly 15% in relation to 1960. This is all the more significant in view of the fact that the number of women of childbearing age (15–49 years) increased markedly over the same period.

Hence it follows that the use of absolute figures is not enough and does not help in revealing certain essential features of the process taking place. I have in mind the already mentioned fact that the number of women of childbearing age has undergone major changes in the meantime. It should be noted that in the years 1960–71 (Table 1) the number of women in this age group in Poland increased by almost 1.5 million (an increase of over 20% in relation to 1960). For this reason it is best to use coefficients calculated in relation to the number of women of childbearing age (as a rule all data are calculated per 100 women in this age group).

Taking account of changes in the number of women of childbearing age, it has been found that the number of pregnancies per thousand was as follows: 126.9 in 1960, 101.2 in 1965, 90.1 in 1970 and 89.8 in 1971. The increasingly widespread use of contraception has brought about a decrease of almost 30% in the relative number of pregnancies. Such a major change can only testify to the utopian nature of the views of all those who support administrative measures against birth control. The contemporary model of the family has won such popularity that any medical change would appear to be impossible. Certainly there exist ways of influencing childbearing, but they have nothing in common with administrative prohibitions and injunctions; they require a complex assault on the totality of socio-economic conditions.

The use of relative coefficients permits the conclusion that the downward tendency is even somewhat more intensive than the absolute figures would suggest. The number of registered abortions and other miscarriages per thousand women of childbearing age was 31.4 in 1960, 30.8 in 1965, 25.8 in 1967, 25.1 in 1970 and 23.5 in 1971. The value of the coefficient fell by 25.2% over eleven years, and it appears that the rate of this process accelerated further in 1971, with a drop of almost 6.5% in comparison with 1970.

Let us recall in passing that the coefficient of fertility (the number of live births per thousand women of childbering age) in 1971 was almost 30% lower than in 1960. This is further evidence that the drop in the fertility rate took place in spite of a reduction in the number of abortions, which in itself suggests that the relationship between these two phenomena is not as simple as the advocates of legal prohibition of abortion sometimes seek to prove.

Nevertheless it is impossible to provide an answer to the fundamental question which I posed at the beginning without reference to other figures. In my view it is essential to compare the numbers of live and still births with the number of abortions performed in hospital conditions and the number of unregistered abortions. In order to obtain this last figure, it is essential to examine certain additional circumstances which are only indirectly connected with the subject under discussion.

In the conditions created by the law permitting abortion and given the genuinely easy access to its benefits, unregistered abortions can embrace only women for whom specific considerations – generally involving prestige – make this particularly important. The number of such women is limited to a certain extent by the comparatively high cost of obtaining an abortion from a doctor in private practice. It is therefore almost certain that their patients are predominantly recruited from among unmarried women. At the same time the percentage of single women (spinsters, widows, divorcees) in steadily decreasing as a result of the declining portion of women in the Polish population and amounts to less that a third of the total number of women of childbearing age.

I shall pass over the technical details involved in making further estimates and refer only to the family study conducted by Z. Smoliński [6] in 1972 under the auspices of the Polish Central Statistical Office. It transpired from this study that the incidence of miscarriages and abortions of all kinds among married women (only such were questioned) came to 37 per thousand annually. It can therefore be established that about 200,000 married women had abortions in 1970. As the total number of abortions in that year came to 214,000, single women must have accounted for about 14,000 cases.

If we go on to assume that the coefficient of abortions among single women is the same, or at the most one and a half times greater than that among married women, we may calculate that the former may account for 70,000–110,000 cases of abortion. After subtracting the 14,000 registered cases mentioned above, we should have to estimate the number of nonregistered abortions somewhere between 55,000 and 85,000 cases. In practical terms this figure should be somewhat lower, as women aged between 15 and 17 or over 45, or even over 40 – also age-groups in which childbirth is possible – would not in this case come into account.

On the basis of these estimates it may be assumed that the total number of abortions performed in Poland comes to 300,000 at the most, of which two thirds are accounted for in official statistics.

It would be wrong, however, to regard this as a uniform figure. As has already been mentioned, over 70,000 abortions performed on medical advice or other – i.e. initiated in the home – abortions do not testify a desire to terminate an unwanted pregnancy or that this termination was facilitated by the new law. Thus in examining the influence of legalized abortion on demographic processes we should operate with a figure of about 230,000. Assuming further that over the past eleven years this figure underwent the same fluctuations as the number of registered abortions, we may conclude that the corresponding figure for 1960 was 241,000.

In order to assess the significance of these figures, it is necessary to draw up a kind of 'balance-sheet of fertility'. We may take as our point of departure the quantity known as maximum fertility, i.e. the number of live births which would occur in a population where no recourse was taken to abortion or contraception. According to the abundant data to be found in the literature [1, 3, 6] on the subject, maximum fertility is estimated at somewhere between 200 and 220 per thousand. In other words, in hypothetical conditions, where no family planning methods or abortions are applied, there are 200–220 live births per 1000 women of childbearing age. This corresponds to a level of fertility of about 50 per thousand. It should be mentioned that even in contemporary conditions such fertility coefficients are to be found in some developing countries (Sudan, Niger, Rwanda, Dahomey, Pakistan, Swaziland, Afghanistan, Angola, Republic of Maldives, Yemen, Malagasy Republic), while in the distant past it may also have occurred in the countries beloging to European civilization.

Table 3. Balance of Potential Maximum Fertility in Poland in 1960 and 1970

	1960		1970	
	per thousand	per cent	per thousand	per cent
Maximum fertility	200.0	100.0	200.0	100.0
Total number of live births	93.0	46.5	64.0	32.0
Total number of abortions covered by the law	33.9	17.0	26.8	13.4
Total number of abortions not affected by the law	10.8	5.4	7.9	4.0
Birth control	62.3	31.1	101.3	50.6

Sources: *Rocznik Demograficzny 1971*, GUS, Warszawa 1971, p. 97, and *Ochrona Zdrowia 1971*, GUS, Warszawa 1972, p. 83.

In the Table 3 I have assumed that the level of maximum fertility will be somewhere in the region of 200 per thousand. I do not insist that this quantity be treated as absolute, for even if it should be revised upward to 220, the overall picture will undergo no change (apart from a rise in that proportion of 'unrealized fertility' which is determined by the use of various methods of preventing pregnancy). In order to simplify the argument which follows I have not taken account of the proportion of 'unrealized fertility' resulting from abstinence, a quantity which it would be impossible to estimate anyway. Nevertheless its omission – because of its insignificant size – should not influence the overall picture either.

As the data in Table 3 show, the proportion of live births in the overall balance of fertility declined over ten years from 46% to 32%, or by almost a third. There was also an insignificant decline in the proportion of abortions which were not affected by the abortion reform law. It is very significant that there was also a marked decline in the proportion of those abortions which were formally legalized: In 1960 it amounted to almost 17% maximum fertility, while by 1970 it was only 13.4%. Thus the structural index fell by about 20%.

It should be emphasized strongly that not only in 1970 were the coefficients of all arrested pregnancies and abortions taken together considerably lower than the coefficient of pregnancies averted by the use of contraception. The value of this last figure – according to my approximate calculations – was about 62 per thousand women of child-bearing age in 1960, whereas in 1970 it was 101. Thus in 1960 maximum fertility was reduced by almost a third and in 1970 by over half as a result of the use of contraception by women desirous of limiting the number of their children. At the same time arrested pregnancies and abortions of all kinds accounted for less than a quarter of maximum fertility in 1960, whereas in 1970 they accounted for somewhat more than a third.

This is incontrovertible evidence that the idea of consicious motherhood, spreading quite independently of the abortion law and being the result od socio-economic progress and the rise of the educational and cultural level of society as a whole, play an incomparably greater role in reducing the birth rate than the termination of unwanted pregnancies. The rise of this index against the background of a decline in the abortion coefficient shows moreover that in the near future – as a result of the steady improvement of the educational level of women – further favourable changes may be expected. There is every reason to suppose that the abortion coefficient and its share of the overall balance of maximum fertility will fall to negligible proportions. This assertion, based as it is on statistical estimates and studies, constitutes an additional argument in favour of legalizing abortion. It follows that as society

Table 4. Frequency of Abortions in the Major Cities and Voivodships of Poland (per thousand women of childbearing age)

	1960	1970	1971	Difference between 1960 and 1971 in %
National total	31.42	25.10	23.49	25.2
Warsaw	53.33	32.68	32.08	39.8
Cracow	38.65	28.65	23.19	40.2
Łódź	58.95	43.40	44.33	24.8
Poznań	38.50	28.94	30.56	20.6
Wrocław	47.49	26.15	27.36	42.8
Białystok voivodship	26.56	27.19	24.87	6.3
Bydgoszcz voivodship	20.91	21.28	20.15	3.7
Gdańsk voivodship	26.64	39.10	33.94	7.4
Katowice voivodship	38.35	28.73	27.16	29.2
Kielce voivodship	20.99	19.87	19.20	8.5
Koszalin voivodship	40.37	34.73	31.64	21.6
Cracow voivodship	16.65	14.43	12.97	22.1
Lublin voivodship	22.83	19.47	19.03	16.6
Łódź voivodship	31.27	20.54	19.05	39.1
Olsztyn voivodship	30.12	26.28	25.47	15.5
Opole voivodship	27.12	28.22	24.78	10.7
Poznań voivodship	18.06	14.01	14.41	20.2
Rzeszów voivodship	19.71	18.29	15.84	19.6
Szczecin voivodship	47.64	37.67	39.90	16.6
Warsaw voivodship	27.33	21.47	20.84	23.7
Wrocław voivodship	41.02	27.81	20.04	51.2
Zielona Góra voivodship	46.05	27.95	26.93	41.5

Sources: *Rocznik Statystyczny Ochrony Zdrowia 1945–67*, GUS, Warszawa 1969, p. 410–411, 'Ochrona Zdrowia', *Statystyka Polski* **119**, GUS, Warszawa 1972, p. 83, and computations of the author.

proceeds to more advanced phases of socio-economic and demographic development, which bring about a steady drop in the birth rate, the role of legalized abortion – even as a catalyst of this process – steadily declines.

I should like to mention here that these conclusions go a long way to supporting the results of the study carried out in 1972 by Z. Smoliński [7], who found that about 50% of married women regularly practise contraception.

Our assessment of the influence of abortion on the birth rate in the country as a whole would, however, be incomplete were we to omit the essential fact that there exist considerable regional differences in this respect, as may be seen from the data in Table 4.

Thus in comparing the figures for arrested pregnancies and abortions it should be noted first and foremost that there is not a single major town or voivodship in Poland in which their number has not fallen. The coefficients of arrested pregnancies and abortions (per 1000 women of childbearing age) in 1960 were highest in the cities of Łódź, Warsaw and Wrocław and in the voivodships of Szczecin, Zielona Góra and Wrocław; these coefficients were lowest, on the other hand, in the voivodships of Cracow, Poznań, Rzeszów, Bygdoszcz and Kielce.

By 1971 that order has changes relatively slightly. Łódź remained in first place, followed by the voivodships of Szczecin, Gdańsk and Koszalin and the cities of Warsaw and Poznań. The voivodships of Cracow, Poznań and Rzeszów continued to bring up the rear.

The period under discussion witnessed a decline not only in the value of the national coefficient, but also in the gap between the highest and lowest of the provincial coefficients (from 42.4 to 31.3, i.e. 26% less than the gap noted in 1960). It may therefore be supposed that a process of levelling out of regional differences is taking place. It is a slow process which is still far from completion (not only in the cities of Łódź, Warsaw and Poznań, but also in the voivodships of Gdańsk, Szczecin and Koszalin the coefficient in question is still over twice as high as in the voivodships of Cracow, Poznań and Rzeszów). Nevertheless the fading away of regional differences is an undeniable fact which should encourage further and more thoroughgoing research.

This process is probably favoured by the varying rates at which the value of the coefficient of arrested pregnancies and abortions is declining in individual voivodships. In the period under discussion it was highest in the cities of Cracow, Wrocław and Warsaw and in the voivodships of Wrocław, Łódź and Zielona Góra and lowest in the voivodships of Kielce, Gdańsk, Bydgoszcz and Białystok.

Particular attention should be paid to the way in which the coefficient of arrested pregnancies and abortions varies between the urban and rural populations. The data cited show that this coefficient is highest in large urban agglomerations. In 1960 over 42,000 abortions were performed in the five chief cities of Poland, or 19% of the national total. By 1970 this index had dropped to 16.6%, but in 1971 it had again risen to 17.4% of the total of nationally registered abortions. In 1970 the coefficient of arrested pregnancies and abortions in Poland's five principal cities was 66.5% higher than in the rest of the country, the figures being 39.04 and 23.44 per 1000 women of childbearing age respectively.

These data indicate that the abortion rate rises under the influence of the urbanization factor, although the level of education, a factor correlated with the spread of contraception, is undeniably higher in large urban agglomerations than in the rest of the country. This simple example demonstrates that the spread of arrested pregnancies and abortions and hence their relative influence on demographic processes as well, lies in very complex relationships with the operation of many factors which have still not been adequately studied. Nor in this connection should the very delicate matters associated with religion and morals be treated lightly. There cannot be the slightest doubt that the uncovering of all the complex determining factors and objective laws whereby the objective and subjective factors shaping the phenomenon in question interact, will be possible only in the event of comprehensive studies being undertaken with the participation of demographers, doctors, sociologists and psychologists.

Before concluding the present paper, I must confess that I have quite deliberately omitted one more very important problem. I have not said a word about the possible indirect influence which may be exerted on the birth rate by abortions which are sometimes considered a major cause of female infertility. It is may impression that it is not as yet possible to discuss this problem as no serious scholar has presented any convincing data which would either confirm or finally repudiate this long-standing hypothesis [2]. This of course constitutes a serious gap in our knowledge, but the statistical materials we have at our disposal are far from being ideal not only in this respect.

Nevertheless, the statistical information which it has been possible to obtain—and I should like to stress this point once more—only as a result of the legalization of abortion, make it possible to draw certain conclusions, which are, of course, tentative and in need of further verification.

CONCLUSIONS

1. The fall in the birth rate, which is determined by numerous objective and subjective factors, at a specific stage in the development of societies, constitutes a universally occurring demographic law.

2. Poland did not embark upon the road of demographic revolution until the eve of the Second World War, and hence belatedly in relation to many other countries within the ambit of European civilization. In the post-war period—after a few years of demographic boom partially caused by a compensatory upsurge of births—there occurred another, this time much steeper, drop in the birth rate, which was accompanied by an equally steep decline in the mortality rate. At present Poland's demographic characteristics place her in the category of countries with an average birth rate and a low mortality rate.

3. The post-war fall in the birth rate began in Poland before the legalization of abortion (in 1952), but underwent a marked acceleration in the period 1960–66.

4. Abortions are not a cause of the decline in the birth rate but constitute a means whereby women implement their objectively determined desire to limit the number of their children. At a specific stage of demographic development abortions may accelerate the process of transition to a lower birth rate, but they cannot initiate this process.

5. All attempts at prohibiting abortion through administrative fiat are doomed to failure, as such attempts do not change the character and intensity of the socio-economic and socio-psychological factors which determine demographic processes, including above all the decline in the birth rate.

6. The legalization of abortion has had no significant influence on demographic processes. What it has made possible, on the other hand, is reliable statistics, and, what is more important, it has reduced the number of abortions carried out in insanitary conditions by unqualified individuals.

7. In the period 1965–71 a significant reduction in the number of abortions occurred in Poland. The proportion of abortions carried out as a result of their legalization in the general balance of maximum fertility is declining steadily. In 1970 it came to a third of the number of averted pregnancies due to contraception.

8. Further research into this problem is essential in order to obtain objective information concerning the role of abortion as a possible factor causing infertility in women and also to discover the reasons for the regional variations in Poland's abortion rate.

BIBLIOGRAPHY

[1] V. Belova, L. Y. Darski, *Statistika mnenii v izuchenii rozhdaemosti*, Moscow 1972.
[2] B. Górnicki, M. Bulska, 'Medical Aspects of Birth Control' (in Polish), paper delivered at the conference sponsored by the Demographic Committee of the Polish Academy of Sciences, Warszawa (Jadwisin), March 15–18, 1972 (typescript).
[3] L. Henry, 'Etude statistique de l'abaisement des naissance', Population 3 (1951).
[4] M. Łatuch, Elements of Population Control Policy in Poland (in Polish), paper delivered at the conference sponsored by the Demographic Committee of the Polish Academy of Sciences, Warszawa (Jadwisin), March 15–18, 1972 (typescript).
[5] Y. A. Sadokvasova, Rol aborta w osushchestvlenii soznatelnogo maternistva, in: *Izucheniye vozproizvodtsva naseleniya* (ed. A. J. Wolkow), Moscow 1968, pp. 221–212.
[6] Z. Smoliński, *The Size of Families: the Present Situation and Future Prospects – Family Poll*, GUS, Warszawa 1973.
[7] Z. Smoliński, *op. cit.*
[8] Z. Smoliński, in a conversation with the author.
[9] Z. Smoliński and J. Z. Holzer, *Problems of Population Reproduction in Poland* (in Polish), GUS, Warszawa 1968, p. 61.

HEALTH AND DISABILITY IN A TOTAL POPULATION

A. JABLENSKY

Department of Psychiatry, Medical School, Sofia, Bulgaria

J. OSHAVKOV

Institute of Sociology, Bulgarian Academy of Sciences, Sofia, Bulgaria

In the framework of a large-scale sociological survey in Bulgaria the health status and the prevalence of disability in the population were assessed in relation to certain major demographic, social and environmental variables.

The study was based on a random sample of the total population of the country over 16 years of age. The sample included 18,994 persons and its representativeness was checked against census data and other statistics. Confidence intervals were determined and the sample was evaluated as highly representative.

Each subject in the sample together with a number of key informants were extensively interviewed by a social worker using a questionnaire designed to cover important areas of personal history and social functioning.

To assess the health status of each subject in the study, a total of 1,274 physicians participated in the project. Most of them were general practitioners who were required to examine personally those subjects in the sample who were residents in the area of their practice. Each subject was given a physical examination and a number of laboratory tests (routine blood count, blood pressure, electrocardiogram, chest X-ray and respiratory function tests). Health information was also obtained from medical records. On the basis of these data, the physicians were asked to record any specific disability and also give an overall rating of the subject's state of health or degree of disability using a scale consisting of the following major categories:

1. Good general health: subject has had no serious illnesses, or has had only trivial or infrequent health problems which have not resulted in any complications, or in physical or mental impairment.

2. Satisfactory state of health: subject has had illnesses which have resulted in mild impairment of a particular function but his social functioning has not been affected and he is not in need of continuous medical supervision or social assistance.

3. Unsatisfactory state of health: subject has a chronic illness or defect, seriously limited work capacity or social functioning and requires long-term medical care, rehabilitation and social assistance.

4. Poor state of health: subject has a long-term serious illness or defect, has lost his capacity to work, may be bed-ridden. Social functioning is severely impaired; needs continuous medical, nursing and social care at home or in an institution.

Complete sets of data were obtained on about 90% of the subjects in the sample. The analysis of the data made it possible to estimate the overall prevalence of disability and the different categories of health status in the population. It aslo indicated several groups of variables which appeared to be strongly associated with health and disability.

OVERALL PREVALENCE OF DISABILITY

The overall rates for the four levels of health and disability as defined above were: 0.8% were assessed to be in a poor state of health and another 4.6% in an unsatisfactory state of health. A satisfactory state of health was found in 17.9% of cases and good general health in 76.7%.

Extrapolating from the sample to the general population over 16 years of age, it may be estimated that about 5% are severely disabled and are in need of longterm treatment, rehabilitation, nursing care and social assistance.

Equally important is the finding that over three quarters of the population over 16 years of age have never had any serious health problems.

HEALTH AND DISABILITY BY AGE AND SEX

The prevalence of disability rises almost linearly with age, and approximately one-half of the subjects whose state of health was assessed as poor were in the over-69 age group. 76.8% of those rated as being in good general health were aged between 18 and 48.

The sex differences in the rates of disability were highly significant ($p<.001$, χ^2 test) in all age groups: females had more illnesses and disability than males. This difference was even more marked in advanced age. This finding should be interpreted in association with the demographic statistics which indicate an excess mortality rate among men in older age groups. Thus, women seem to have a higher survival expectancy than men, in spite of the higher prevalence of ill-health and disability among women. On the other hand, those men who survive into corresponding old age groups tend to be generally healthier than women in the same age groups.

Some sex differences in the prevalence of specific disorders were also highly significant ($p<.001$). More women than men were suffering from cardiovascular disorders, arterial hypertension, psychiatric disorders, arthritis and other musculo-skeletal diseases. Men had a higher prevalence of peptic ulcer and tuberculosis.

TYPE OF ILLNESS AND DEGREE OF DISABILITY

Cardiovascular disease was most strongly associated with overall disability: of all subjects in whom a cardiovascular disorder was present, 21.7% were in the 'unsatisfactory' or 'poor' general health categories. Disability was also highly associated with psychiatric disorder of a chronic kind: 15.9% of those in whom a psychiatric diagnosis had been made were in the two disability categories, and most of them were suffering from chronic psychotic or organic cerebral disorders.

Apart from these two groups of conditions which were strikingly associated with serious disability, the majority of the subjects assessed as disabled had clusters of various conditions which were difficult to separate diagnostically.

HEALTH AND DISABILITY BY URBAN VS. RURAL RESIDENCE

The general health state of urban residents was slightly better than that of the rural population (Table 1). However, this difference could be largely attributed to the excess of old age pensioners in rural areas (40.6% of all rural residents, compared to 33.7% of the urban residents).

Table 1. Health and Disability in Urban and Rural Populations
Urban Residents ($N=7{,}162$)

Health status	Good	Satisfactory	Unsatis-factory or poor	Total
Working	72.9	50.0	19.9	66.3
Not working or pensioners	27.1	50.0	80.1	33.7
Total (%)	100.0	100.0	100.0	100.0

Rural residents ($N=10{,}226$)

Health status	Good	Satisfactory	Unsatis-factory or poor	Total
Working	67.7	40.1	12.8	59.4
Not working or pensioners	32.3	59.9	87.2	40.6
Total (%)	100.0	100.0	100.0	100.0

There were no differences in the health status of urban and rural residents who were actively employed. Old age pensioners in rural areas tended to suffer more disability than urban pensioners. This might be a result of selective migration: healthier old people are more likely to move to the town, along with the younger members of their families.

The rural population had a higher prevalence of cardiovascular disorders, while peptic ulcer was more frequent among urban residents. These differences were age-related but did not disappear entirely after standardization for age. The prevalence of psychiatric disorders did not show urban-rural differences.

HEALTH, DISABILITY AND OCCUPATION

Neither length of occupational record nor the major sphere of occupation were associated with any significant differences in the health status and prevalence of disability, other than the differences that could be attributed to age and sex. The prevalence of disability was of the same order of magnitude among those employed in industry, services and agriculture.

Table 2. Health and Disability Related to Level of Occupational Skills (N=18,456)

Occupational categories	1	2	3	4	5	6	7	Total
Health status:								
Good	68.2	81.0	76.2	83.4	78.0	81.9	84.1	76.9
Satisfactory	23.7	15.1	18.7	13.3	17.2	14.3	12.8	17.8
Unsatisfactory or poor	8.1	3.9	5.1	3.3	4.8	3.8	3.1	5.3
Total (%)	100.0	100.0	100.0	100.0	100.0	100.0	100.0	100.0

Occupational categories:
1 – low-skilled agricultural workers,
2 – skilled agricultural workers (e.g. technicians, mechanics, etc.),
3 – low-skilled industrial workers,
4 – skilled industrial workers,
5 – low-skilled sales and services workers,
6 – skilled services workers, supervising jobs, managers,
7 – professionals, engineers, etc.

Within each sector of occupation, however, there were significant differences clearly related to the level of skill. Table 2 shows the tendency of individuals with an unsatisfactory or poor state of health to accumulate in low-skilled occupational categories. This relationship cannot be explained simply as the effect of a drop in occupational level as result of illness because a considerable proportion of the sample were pensioners who had already completed their occupational record. The association between low-skilled occupation and a higher rate of disability was particularly marked in this group, and this would support the suggestion that a number of factors whose nature is yet to be investigated are associated with low-skilled work in a way that increases the risk of disease and disability.

The low-skilled occupational groups had higher rates for cardiovascular and psychiatric disorders, as well as for a number of other conditions. The only disorder which was found to be strikingly associated with higher occupational skills was peptic ulcer.

HEALTH, DISABILITY AND EDUCATION

Health state and disability were strongly associated with educational level: lower grades of completed education were significantly related to poorer health and more disability. The critical point in this respect seemed to be completed primary school (4 years). The disability risk in later life was increased mainly for those who had failed to complete primary school. They were almost exclusively in the older age groups but their contemporaries who had obtained better education were found to have significantly less disease and disability.

HEALTH AND DISABILITY IN RELATION TO INCOME AND HOUSING CONDITIONS

The relationship between state of health, rates of disability and personal income was of the same type as that between health and occupational skills or education. Since income, level of occupational skills and level of education are intercorrelated, this finding would be anticipated.

Less expected was the very weak association between poor health and housing conditions. None of the several measures used to assess the quality of housing was significantly correlated with rates of disability. For example, the coefficient of association (Goodman and Kruskal's gamma) between unsatisfactory and poor health and overcrowding was .13. This may be the effect of housing policies which give rehousing priority to the chronically ill and disabled.

HEALTH AND DISABILITY IN RELATION TO HOUSEHOLD SIZE AND MARITAL STATUS

There was a strong association ($p<.001$) between state of health and household size (Table 3). People living alone or in two-member households tended to have more illnesses and disability. It was interesting to note that the optimum size of household with regard to health status was between 3 and 5. Households containing more than 5 persons showed no association with the state of health of their members.

Table 3. Health and Disability Related to Size of Household (N=17,542)

Health status:	Good	Satisfactory	Unsatis-factory or poor	Total
State of household:				
Living alone	2.4	5.5	7.9	3.3
2 members	12.7	22.0	28.0	15.2
3–5 members	67.1	55.8	46.5	63.9
More than 5	17.8	16.7	17.6	17.6
Total (%)	100.0	100.0	100.0	100.0

Marital status was significantly associated with health and disability only in the over 28 age groups (Table 4). In the older age groups poor health and disability were more prevalent among the widowed and divorced. Single men were as healthy (or slightly healthier) than married men of the same age group but single women had poorer health than married women.

Table 4. Health and Disability Related to Marital Status over 28 Age Group

Marital status:	Married	Widowed	Divorced	Single	Total (%)
Health status:					
Good:					
Men	94.4	2.2	0.6	2.8	100.0
Women	89.6	6.7	1.4	2.3	100.0
Unsatisfactory or poor					
Men	82.6	14.3	1.3	1.8	100.0
Women	61.4	32.9	2.1	3.6	100.0

Among those of pensionable age the relationship between marital status and health was strongest, and widowhood seemed to be associated with a particularly increased risk of illness and disability. However, there was a marked difference between the two sexes in this respect. 15.5% of the men, and 31.1% of the women of pensionable age were widowed.

Widowers constituted 16.3% of all men whose health was unsatisfactory or poor, while widowed women constituted 40.2% of all women in the unsatisfactory and poor health categories. At least in part, this difference may be due to the higher mortality rate among men in advanced age groups.

CONCLUSIONS

The results of this cross-sectional survey of health and disability are important in two main respects.

First, the size and representativeness of the sample studied make it possible to estimate the prevalence of different degrees of disability in the total population. Different degrees of disability are present in a sizable proportion of the population, although only a small number are disabled to a degree which makes them entirely dependent on continuous medical care and social assistance. Equally important is the fact that the vast majority, i.e. about three quarters of the adult population, have never had serious health problems.

Secondly, the distribution of disability conforms to a pattern in which social factors play a major role. Most of the associations found are in agreement with hypotheses and findings reported in other studies, but further work will be necessary to determine cause-and-effect relationships and, possibly, identify the social mechanisms whose monitoring and control in the framework of health services and policies would result in a reduction of the prevalence of disability and an increase of positive health.

IMMIGRATION AND MENTAL HEALTH

ELINA HAAVIO-MANNILA

Institute of Sociology, University of Helsinki, Finland

KERSTIN STENIUS

Institute of Sociology, University of Helsinki, Finland

CONTENTS Page

Emigration from Finland to more economically developed Sweden in the late 1960's reached large proportions. Since then the wave of migration has somewhat subsided. About 300,000 Finnish-born persons are currently living in Sweden. Many of them are industrial workers with a poor knowledge of the Swedish language.

Earlier studies, such as Ødegaard (1932) on Norwegian emigrants and migrants and Malzberg (1969) on immigrants to New York indicated that migrants crossing national borders have a higher incidence of mental illness than people who remain in their home country. Further, Salokangas (1973) found in Finland that persons who were forced to migrate against their wishes (i.e. Karelian refugees) had a high rate of mental illness. However, as a general conclusion from a review of the literature on immigration, migration, and mental illness (with special emphasis on schizophrenia), Victor D. Sanua (1970, 336–337) writes: "... some migrations are related to greater risks in mental health and some migrations are related to favorable mental health".

This paper will explore the mental health problems of Finnish immigrants in Sweden, through examination of unpublished empirical data from three different studies: (1) the physical and mental health of Finnish immigrants as compared with their Swedish 'twins' in comparable positions, (2) the emergence and background of neurotic symptoms in the families of Finnish immigrants in a middle-sized industrial town as compared with similar Swedish families, and (3) a study on immigrant mental patients in the psychiatric clinic of the same town. On the basis of these data, we shall try to obtain some kind of picture of the factors related to mental health in this particular immigrant situation.

1. THE HEALTH SITUATION OF FINNISH IMMIGRANTS IN SWEDEN

The data on the general health status of Finnish immigrants in Sweden relate to the year 1968 when the mass migration from Finland to Sweden as an economic phenomenon was just beginning. The results thus represent the health situation of migrants in 'low migration' years [1]. Their health status is compared with that of their Swedish 'twins', that is, persons similar as to sex, age, and occupational position.

According to all indicators used, the Finnish immigrants had poorer health than the Swedes (see Table 1). Of course this can be attributed to the fact that people in Finland in general have a lower level of health than the Swedes. Because there was no control group involved in the survey of the Finnish health situation, we must rely on information about general health differences between these neighboring countries.

Table 1. Health Situation and Consumption of Health Care Services among Finnish Immigrants and Native Swedes, Matched according to Sex, Age and Occupational Group 1968. Percentages for Different Illnesses and Averages Number of Days in Care

	Finnish immi-grants (95)	Swedes (95)
Obstacles to movement (patients unable to walk at a reasonable speed or negotiate stairs without difficulty)	14	6
Tiredness (patient has felt particularly tired during daytime over period of two weeks preceding the interview in June 1968)	20	14
Psychological problems (has suffered of problems with sleep or depressions during the last year)	17	10
Ache (ache in some of the following areas (a) shoulders, (b) back, (c) hands, arms, legs, knees)	17	6
Dental problems (acute dental problems, i.e. has no teeth or badly functioning loose teeth or own teeth in bad condition)	14	5
Circulation problems (at least three of the following problems: blood pressure, dizziness, swollen feet, varicose veins, heart weakness, pains in chest, dyspnea)	14	7
Average number of days spent in hospital in 1967 according to hospital data	5.0	0.6
No days spent in hospital in 1967 according to hospital data	91	96
No days registered as ill in 1967	45	58
Average number of days registered as ill during 1967	23	7

Source: Sten Johansson, *Finska invandrare i Sverige*, Institute for Social Research, Stockholm 1973, p. 3.

Thus, according to the preliminary results from "The Scandinavian Survey on Welfare and Need Satisfaction", both material conditions and the health situation are better in Sweden than in Finland (Research Group for Comparative Sociology 1972). We can therefore theorize that from the beginning Finnish immigrants may have been in worse health than the Swedes, but because migration is selective, we cannot be too certain about that. Further we may speculate that the high material standard in Sweden and the problems connected with adjustment to the new environment would have had counterbalancing effects on the physical and mental health of the Finnish immigrants. On the basis of this 1968 material, we can only say that individually the Finnish immigrants were more prone to illness and made greater use of health care services than Swedes in comparable positions.

2. IMMIGRATION, MARRIAGE, AND NEUROSIS

2.1. Frame of Reference for the Analysis

Migration means of profound change in life: the material resources of an individual or a family may improve, but former ties with kin, fellow workers, and friends are usually disrupted. The group under study here – Finnish immigrants to Sweden – usually took their families with them. This at least allowed them to maintain close human ties with one important primary social group. But the migrant situation makes the pressure of this group especially pronounced. The immigrant family unit has to function satisfactorily without support from other close groups such as relatives, neighbors, fellow workers, and friends. If the family as a group cannot fulfil its tasks, there are no other groups to compensate for its defects.

The importance of family and the marital group as regards the mental and physical health of an individual has in many connections been pointed out. Clark E. Vincent (1970, p. 255) remarks in his article 'Mental Health and the Family' that it is "difficult to conceive of any degree of marital stress which does not have some repercussions with reference to the physical and emotional states of the two people involved". He introduces the concept *marital health* and discusses marital dynamics as a factor in the etiology of illness. The relationship between quality of marriage and health is of course a two-way one: illness also has some impact upon the marital relationship. It is often difficult to say which comes first: marital problems or ill health. They usually support each other: marital problems make people ill and illness worsens marital relations.

However, family is not the only social factor that affects the immigrant in the new country. Material resources, type of work, and human relations outside the family have an impact on the life of an individual and his mental health. As a frame of reference in discussing the social factors related to mental health, we shall use the trichotomy introduced by Erik Allardt. Allardt sees the satisfaction of certain basic human needs as corresponding to three general values that are assumed to be central to welfare. These are ***having***, ***loving***, and ***being***. "***Having*** refers to the resources an individual has and can command in order to satisfy his physical and safety needs. Lists of components of the level of living can be viewed as operationalizations of having. ...*Loving* as a value pertains to many kindred terms such as companionship, affection, belongingness, and solidarity. The realization of this value comes about as a person reciprocally relates to individuals and groups that *he cares for* and in which he *is cared for*. He is socially anchored, and with some justification the satisfaction of needs related to loving may be regarded as the opposite to anomie. ... *Being* as a value is related to many other concepts such as personal growth, satisfaction of growth needs, self-individuation, and self-actualization at the other. Since alienation refers to a state in which an individual is a thing or a commodity, we can proceed to look for something which is its opposite. ...We assume that insubstitutability is an attribute of self-actualization and the opposite of alienation. A person who is easily substitutable is in a sense treated as a thing, a machine or as something which more or less mechanically can be replaced. ...(Being) has to do with man's ability to master his own fate, ... to participate in decisions on matters concerning his own personal life." (Allardt–Uusitalo 1972, p. 6–7, Allardt 1973, p. 11–12).

We try here to relate some characteristics of the total social situation – as defined by these basic values – of the Finnish immigrant families in Sweden to the mental health status of the husbands and wives in these families. In the *having* dimension, we examine the influence of social status, income, and dwelling density. In the *loving* dimension, special consideration is given to the marital relationship. We interviewed both spouses in all the families studied. In this way, we can correlate the characteristics and feelings of both husband and wife with the emergence of ill health in either of them. But loving needs can be satisfied also in other connections than in the family. People can feel solidarity and companionship with their friends, fellow workers, and kin. Or they may even fall in love with nonfamily persons. We shall investigate how these other social relationships, in addition to the marital relationship, affect the mental health of the immigrants. In the *being* dimension, we study the impact of work satisfaction, the importance given to work relations, and career success, as well as feelings of nonsubstitutability and a lack of opportunity to decide about one's own life. Some of our measures of having, loving, and being have been adopted from the Scandinavian Survey of Welfare and Need-Satisfaction directed by Erik Allardt at the University of Helsinki.

The material was collected in 1972 in Västerås, an industrial town in central Sweden with 118,000 inhabitants. The population consists of married couples with children of school-age, except for families in the highest social strata. Both spouses were interviewed by two interviewers simultaneously in different rooms using the same questionnaire. Thirty-six Finnish immigrant families and twenty-eight Swedish families were interviewed. The response rate for the Finnish families was 93%, for the Swedish 57%. Most of the immigrant families had migrated recently: 70% had lived in the town for less than six years; 16% could speak no Swedish. The basic education of the Finnish families was somewhat lower than that of the Swedish families: only 14% of the Finns had more than primary education, whereas of 29% the Swedes had. In both groups, 75% of husbands and 57% of wives had some kind of vocational education. In both groups, the same proportion of wives – 70% – were employed outside the home. The social status of the Swedish families was a little higher than that of the Finnish: this was particularly true for many Finnish wives, who belonged to the lowest social stratum because they were working as cleaning women. Most husbands in both groups were industrial workers. The family income of the Finns was somewhat higher than that of the Swedes, even though the Finnish husbands had lower incomes than their Swedish fellows. This was because of the higher income of the wives and more social security benefits such as children's allowances. The average number of children in Finnish families was 2.9, whereas in the Swedish families it was 2.2.

As an indicator of mental health, we use the emergence of neurotic symptoms (see Table 2). Immigrant husbands had such symptoms somewhat more often (47%) than Swedish husbands (32%). Wives

Table 2. Appearance of Neurotic Symptoms among Swedish and Finnish Husbands and Wives in Västerås in 1972

	Husbands		Wives	
	Swedish	Finnish	Swedish	Finnish
	%		%	
Somatic symptoms:				
Frequent spells of complete exhaustion or fatigue	18	18	21	43
Suffers often from pressure or pain in the head	11	16	18	30
Is often bothered by thumping of his/her heart	10	8	7	16
Heart often runs like mad	11	5	7	5
Shakes or trembles often	7	5	4	5
Psychic symptoms:				
Is constantly keyed up and jittery	11	18	18	16
Thinking gets completely mixed up when he/she has to do things quickly	7	5	29	16
Wears him/herself out worrying about his/her health	4	5	4	16
Feels usually unhappy or depressed	7	8	11	16
Frightening thoughts keep coming back to his/her mind	4	–	14	5
Summary:				
Both psychic and somatic symptoms	14	18	25	32
Only somatic symptoms	11	24	21	27
Only psychic symptoms	7	5	18	5
Neither	68	53	36	35
	100	100	100	99
Mean number of symptoms	0.89	1.03	1.32	1.83
Number of respondents	28	36	28	36

Source: Data compiled by Elina Haavio-Mannila in 1972. The reseaich was financed by the Finnish Ministiy of Labour.

in both groups had more symptoms than husbands, 65% of them having had at least one. The main difference between the Finnish immigrants and the Swedes was that the immigrant group suffered more from somatic symptoms: headache, palpitations, and fatigue. The Swedish wives often had only psychological symptoms, such as getting mixed up when they had to do things quickly, or having frightening thoughts. The mean number of neurotic symptoms is higher for the immigrant than the Swedish wives, even though an equal number of women in both groups suffer from them. This means that if the immigrant wives have neurotic symptoms, they have many of them.

2.2. Material Resources and Neurosis

The relationship between material resources of the family and number of neurotic symptoms reported by individual members proved to be weak (Table 3). Low social status and disadvantageous economic position were associated with neurosis. But there were exceptions to this general rule. In the Swedish families, for example, the wife's high in-

Table 3. Correlations Between Some Having, Loving, and Being Variables and Neuroses in the Groups of Swedish and Finnish Immigrant Husbands and Wives in Västerås

	Husband's neurosis		Wife's neurosis	
	Swedes	Finns	Swedes	Finns
Having				
Husband's income	−.09	−.18	−.06	−.10
Wife's income	.15	−.07	.11	−.19
Family income	.20	.10	.15	−.08
Low dwelling density	.35	−.05	−.15	−.19
Husband's social stratum, high	−.27	−.09	.27	−.06
Wife's employment	−.05	.02	.10	.02
Wife's social stratum if she is employed	−.40	−.21	−.22	−.27
Loving:				
marriage and family relations				
Husband considers his marriage happy	.14	−.33	−.24	−.31
Wife considers her marriage happy	−.13	−.17	−.11	−.07
Husband considers sexual life happy	−.18	−.39	−.03	−.30
Wife considers sexual life happy	−.13	−.26	−.15	.25
Husband considers family relations important	.10	.11	.25	−.16
Wife considers family relations important	−.39	−.02	−.19	−.02
relations with friends				
Husband has different types of friends	−.18	−.01	.14	−.11
Wife has different types of friends	−.12	.25	−.29	.05
Husband has intensive relations with fellow workers	−.31	−.16	.18	−.20

	Husband's neurosis		Wife's neurosis	
	Swedes	Finns	Swedes	Finns
Wife has intensive relations with fellow workers	−.32	.16	−.06	.04
Husband has extramarital love relations	−.07	−.16	.16	−.10
Wife has extramarital love relations	−.15	.46	.20	.39
Husband is satisfied with friendships	−.30	−.00	.07	−.22
Wife is satisfied with friendships	.21	.13	−.39	−.12
Husband has good possibilities to get contact with people	−.42	−.16	.14	−.02
Wife has good possibilities to get contact with people	.12	.01	−.21	−.23
Husband feels no pressure toward conformity	−.14	−.33	−.21	−.17
Wife feels no pressure toward conformity	0	.03	−.37	−.05
Being				
Husband is satisfied with work	−.04	−.27	−.16	−.06
Wife is satisfied with work	.10	−.01	−.13	−.36
Husband considers work relations important	−.25	.13	−.12	.06
Wife considers work relations important	−.22	.14	.17	−.19
Husband considers success in career and high income important	−.32	.02	.15	−.16
Wife considers success in career and high income important	.47	.12	.07	.21
Husband feels himself insubstitutable	−.04	−.14	.07	−.28
Wife feels herself insubstitutable	−.13	−.30	−.21	.00
Husband has good opportunities to decide about own life	−.26	−.20	.43	−.39
Wife has good opportunities to decide about own life	0	−.30	−.27	−.42

Source: Data compiled by Elina Haavio-Mannila in 1972.

come and the resulting high total family income were associated with neurosis. Changing sex roles, because of the wife's employment, clearly contributed to a continuing strain in the family. The Swedish wife's employment was found to be strongly correlated with unhappiness in marriage. However, this was not the case among the immigrant families, since in Finland the working wife is much more common than in Sweden. This cultural pattern may partly explain why the wife's employment and high income in the Finnish immigrant families were not associated with marital disorder and neurosis.

In the Swedish families the husband's neuroses were common even when dwelling density was low, although the dwelling standard is supposed to measure a family's economic position. A high material standard thus seems not to have been a guarantee of good mental health, particularly in the Swedish families.

High social stratum and lack of neurosis go together in most of our research groups, but even here we find one exception. Wives of high status Swedish husbands had more neuroses than those of low stratum husbands. We shall return to this finding later.

The families studied here were homogeneous as regards material resources, that is, income, dwelling density and social stratum. This may explain why the correlation between indicators of material standard and neurotic symptoms remained low. On the other hand, one may also conclude that in our families in Västerås the basic material needs were so well satisfied that there was no 'real' poverty or economic misery that might make people ill. Other variables than those connected with living standards, the *having* values, must be studied to find out what social factors are related to mental health problems.

2.3. Human Relations and Neurosis

Unhappiness in marriage and in sexual life generally seem to go together with neurosis. In our study, the correlations of these conditions were particularly high in the Finnish immigrant families. The only exception was the Finnish wives, who were reported as being neurotic yet also indicated a happy sexual life. Another quite interesting divergence from the general pattern that a good family life is combined with lack of neurosis became apparent when we looked at the importance given to the family by the individual respondents. The family-centered husbands were often neurotic, and in the Swedish group they even had neurotic wives. Consideration of family, marriage, and children as being important in life is apparently not congruent with the traditional sex role expectations which demand that men concentrate on their careers and work. But for a Swedish woman, on the contrary, it was considered 'good' for mental health to be family-centered. Sex role expectations were not as clear in the immigrant families; there was no correlation between the wife's family orientation and any neurosis of either of the spouses; furthermore, a low negative correlation existed between a husband's family orientation and his wife's neurosis.

Close and multifarious relations with friends and fellow workers seemed to be associated with good mental health. This relationship was more pronounced among the Swedes than among the Finnish immigrants. The great importance of marital dynamics on the mental health of the spouses can be seen in the Finnish group. If the wife had many friends, intensive relations with fellow workers, was satisfied with friendships, and particularly if during her marriage she had been or was still in love with somebody else than her husband, the husband had many neurotic symptoms. A wife's close relationships outside the marriage seemed to give rise to mental health problems for the husband.

The Finnish immigrant husbands were in some ways less well adjusted than their wives to Swedish society. The wives for example mastered the Swedish language better and had more friends of the opposite sex. The husbands often became jealous about the satisfactory human relationships of their wives outside the family even when these were not love relationships. The neurotic husbands often felt compelled to repress their opinions, an indication of high pressure toward conformity.

Another example of the influence of marital dynamics on the mental health was the relationship between the wife's neurosis and the husband's friendship relations in the Swedish families. The more friends the husband had, the closer were his ties to his fellow workers, the more satisfied he was with his friendships, the better opportunities he felt he had to make contacts with people with whom he could have a real feeling of companionship, and the more extramarital love relationships he had, the more neurotic symptoms his wife exhibited. The pattern of the Swedish wives was very similar to that of the Finnish husbands. If one spouse had close personal ties with other people, the other spouse was neurotic. For the Finnish husbands, we suggested as an explanation jealousy of the wife's successful integration with the community. For the Swedish wives the explanation may be connected with the finding mentioned above: that upper status husbands had neurotic wives. Among the Swedes, a husband's high social status was associated with a wide circle of friends and close work relations which seemed to leave the wife outside so that she might feel deserted and become neurotic. In the same way as the Finnish neurotic husbands, the Swedish wives felt great pressure toward conformity if they were suffering from neurotic symptoms. We have here interpreted neurosis as a consequence of the other spouse's close ties with outsiders. The connection is, however, a two-way one. Spouses of neurotic persons may have sought outside human relationships because they were tired of the complaints of their marital partners.

Swedish husbands with neurotic symptoms were socially isolated. They were also dissatisfied with their friendships and felt that they had poor opportunities to make contacts with people. In the fourth group, the Finnish immigrant wives, correlations between loving variables and neurotic symptoms were low. The husbands of neurotic wives seemed isolated. The wives themselves often had extramarital love relationships and maintained good relationships with friends and fellow workers. However, they said they had not good opportunities to make rewarding contacts with other people.

2.4. Alienation and Neurosis

Alienation seemed to be more connected with the emergence of neurotic symptoms among the Finnish immigrants than among their Swedish 'twins'. Satisfaction with work and feelings of having control of decision-making in matters concerning one's personal life correlated negatively with neurosis, especially in the immigrant group. Among the Finns, the spouses of neurotic persons of both sexes felt that they were easily replaceable and that nearly everybody could do their jobs without special schooling, examinations or personal qualities.

The neurotic Swedish wives also feel that they are easily replaceable. But they also had husbands who felt able to master their own fate. This is related to our earlier finding that the husbands of neurotic Swedish wives had a high social status and close human relationships outside the family. They seemed married to self-sufficient men.

The neurotic Swedish husbands did not regard success in one's career and high income important in life, although their wives clearly did. This discrepancy in values between husband and wife resembled the value conflict described by Cleveland and Longaker (1967) in a study about neurotic patients in a small Canadian community. They found that many neurotic patients had parents who to a differing degree paid attention to the so-called 'striving' and 'being' values that were prevalent in the community. Such value conflict in the family seemed disastrous both to the spouses and the children.

The Swedish non-achievement oriented husbands with achievement-oriented wives didn't believe in 'masculine' success value, although they considered 'feminine' family relations as important. Probably the achievement-oriented wives exerted pressure on these husbands to try to reach goals they had not aspired to nor which were even possible for them. The result seems to be that the husbands became neurotic.

2.5. Characteristics of Neurotic Spouses in the Immigrant and Non-immigrant Families

We may summarize the typical characteristics of the neurotic persons in the four groups studied in the following way:

1. *Swedish husbands.* Even though the husband himself had a fairly low social status and income, the material conditions of the family were quite good thanks to the wife's high income. The husband lacked close human relationships outside the family. His wife regarded career success and high income important, but she did not value as important warm family relations. The husband didn't appreciate economic or social achievement, but was more family-oriented. The neurosis in this group was thus related to *isolation from human relations outside the family and a value conflict between the spouses.*

2. *Swedish wives.* Neurosis in this group was related to the husband's high status and the family's having fairly good material conditions. The husband had many close relations outside the family and was not alienated. The wife herself was dissatisfied with her friendships but felt strong pressure toward conformity. *Relative social isolation and marriage with a socially active and self-sufficient husband* characterized the background of neurosis in Swedish wives in Västerås.

3. *Finnish immigrant husbands.* The husband himself usually had a fairly low income, but otherwise the material conditions had little to do with the emergence of neurotic symptoms. *Marital and sexual unhappiness and the wife's having close human relationships outside the*

family characterizes the Finnish husbands who exhibited many neurotic symptoms. Their wives felt themselves alienated perhaps as an expression of strain in the family. That this situation arose only in the immigrant families may be due to the Finnish wives good knowledge of Swedish and integration with the community compared with that of their husbands.

4. *Finnish wives.* More than any other group, *low material standard* here was related to neurotic symptoms. The husbands of the Finnish neurotic wives were unhappy in marriage and sexual life. The wives themselves had extramarital love relationships and were satisfied with their sexual life. Alienation was characteristic of both spouses. *Dissatisfaction with the marriage on the part of the husband, her own extramarital relationships and the alienation of both spouses* characterize the background of neurosis in immigrant wives.

When we compared the Swedish and the Finnish families in Västerås we found that unhappiness in marriage was more closely associated with mental health problems in the Finnish families. In the beginning we hypothesized that the role of the family was especially important in the immigrant situation in which the relations with the outside community were weak. We have shown that this is the case, especially when the wife succeeds in making friends and even in falling in love with people outside the family.

Of the three value dimensions – having, loving, and being – having was least, and loving was most closely connected with mental health in the Swedish city studied. In general, however, low status, isolation, and alienation are associated with the emergence of neurotic symptoms.

3. FINNISH IMMIGRANTS AS MENTAL PATIENTS IN SWEDEN

3.1. Introduction

The problematic life situation of an immigrant is reflected in disturbances in his health. As was shown, Finnish immigrants in Sweden have had more physical and mental illnesses than non-migrant Swedes in comparable positions. This may have been the result of poor health in their country of origin, or alternatively to or in combination with adjustment problems in the new environment. The family seems to have a more important function in preserving the mental health of its members among the immigrants than among the non-migrants who are more dependent on relations with their fellow workers and friends.

We shall next investigate the situation of the Finnish mental health patient in Sweden on the basis of material collected by a Hungarian visiting psychiatrist at the Västerås Central Hospital. He interviewed all the 170 immigrant patients visiting the hospital during January–August 1971. Of them, 87 were of Finnish origin. We will try to find out which social factors are associated with different types of mental problems among these Finnish immigrants. We have no control group of Swedish patients. The material on other immigrants groups, which is available, arrived too late to be included in this report.

Even though Finnish immigrants, as we have seen, have a poorer mental health status than native Swedes in comparable positions, as a total group they visit mental health institutions to a lesser degree than the Swedes. Only 0.5% of all the Finns in Västmanland province in central Sweden ($N = 19{,}000$) contacted the psychiatric clinic in Västerås during 1971, as compared with 2% of the whole population ($N = 275{,}000$). This is related to the advantageous age structure of the immigrant population from the point of view of mental health: the majority of them are in early middle age. There is no significant differences in the frequency of seeking medical care for illnesses in general between immigrants and comparable Swedes (Haavio-Mannila 1973). The large difference in seeking mental health care shown above may, however, in addition to the difference in age structure be caused by reluctance on the part of immigrants to seek psychiatric care because of linguistic and cultural obstacles. The patients studied here may thus represent the most severely ill group of immigrants.

Mental illness may be defined as a deviation from 'normal' cultural, social, psychological, or biological standards. Of course, in different cultures and societies the same behavior may be looked on and labelled in different ways. The resources of an individual or a group in solving its problems, and the reactions of other people have to be taken into consideration when the kind and degree of psychological problems and the reliance on different sources of help are examined. Aware of the cultural relativity of psychological problems we only can report here the diagnoses and symptoms given in the material. Those persons are defined as psychiatric patients who visited the psychiatric clinic of the Central Hospital in Västerås. Of the 87 Finnish immigrant patients, 10% were diagnosed as psychotic, for 6% the diagnosis was uncertain, and 84% had only neurotic symptoms of some kind. Two-fifths of the patients were given hospital care, mainly in Västerås. Ten percent were sent to a mental hospital outside the town. Most of them were first treated at the psychiatric ward of the Västerås clinic. A majority of the immigrant patients studied here were thus persons with neurotic symptoms who in almost 60% of cases were treated only at the outpatient clinic of the general hospital.

3.2. Patients with Pre- and Post-migration Problems

The characteristics of the mental patients who had psychological problems in Finland before immigration, and those who fell ill in Sweden will be examined first. In this way, we may find out the specific social conditions that made the originally healthy persons fall ill after the migration experience. We may also examine how mentally disturbed persons got along as immigrants in Sweden, as compared to nondisturbed ones: what were their resources (having); human relations (loving); and what the possibilities were for self-actualization (being). After that we shall examine three groups of patients: those who suffered from stress-neurosis, family conflicts, and feelings of persecution. These three symptoms may be differently related to the three value dimensions of having, loving, and being. Finally, a typology of immigrant patients is presented as a result of a factor analysis.

One-third of the Finnish immigrants visiting the psychiatric clinic in Västerås during the first part of 1971 had some mental health problems already in Finland. 22% had received psychiatric care in Finland. In the following pages we shall describe differences and similarities in the social and demographical background of the two patient groups – the pre-emigration and post-immigration patients. We will look at how they function in the existing social situation. And most important we shall examine the type and severity of the psychological problems of these two patient groups, the first one having, the second one not having had mental health problems before emigration from Finland.

In the pre-emigration problem group there were more (64%) men than in the post-immigration group (48%). The previously ill group had arrived to Sweden considerably later, 40% after 1967, than the originally healthy group (17%). On the average, the members of the first group were much older at the time arrival in Sweden than these of the second group, and consequently also at the time of the investigation, as can be seen from Table 4.

Table 4. Demographic Characteristics of Patients Having/not Having Psychological Problems Before Migration (Data for One Patient are Lacking)*

		Psychological before migration		All
		yes (28)	no (58)	(87)*
		%	%	%
Year of migration	-1950	–	11	7
	1950–54	18	11	13
	1955–59	14	13	14
	1960–64	14	22	19
	1965–69	36	41	39
	1970–	18	2	7
		100	100	99
Age at arrival	0–9	–	11	7
	10–19	11	19	15
	20–29	54	60	58
	30–39	29	11	17
	40–49	7	–	2
		101	101	99
	average	26	19	22
Age in 1971	20–29	32	43	40
	30–39	36	41	40
	40–	32	16	21
		100	100	101
	average	35	32	33
Age at time of first psychological problem in Sweden	15–19	–	5	4
	20–29	41	50	47
	30–39	37	33	34
	40–	23	12	16
		101	100	101
	average	31	27	29
No. of years spent in Sweden before emergence of first psychological problems		5.0	7.9	7.0

The immigrants with previous mental health problems had to seek help fairly soon after coming to Sweden: 49% sought help during the three first years as against 26% of those who had no such history. Those first falling ill in Sweden did so between one and five years after immigration or after thirteeen to seventeen years' stay (Figure 1)

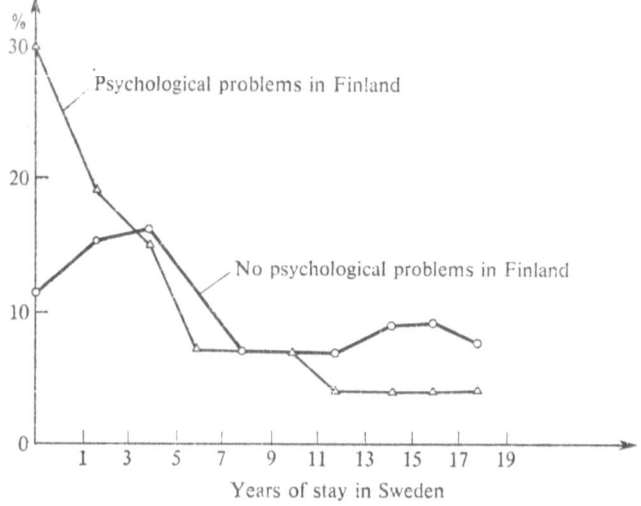

Figure 1. Years spent in Sweden before first mental health problem

The large immigration wave in the late sixties brought to the psychiatric clinic many patients of relatively advanced age who had had previous mental health problems in their home country. Those who fell ill first in Sweden immigrated earlier, and at an earlier age.

A higher proportion, 82%, of those immigrants who had psychological problems in Finland had been employed in their former home country than of the post-immigration patients (46%). If we look at the occupations of those employed, we find that 48% of pre-emigration and 41% of post-immigration patients had been working in 'better' occupations (i.e. technicians, skilled or service workers). Members of both patient groups had a similar educational background, with only about 15% having had more than a primary education.

Poor mental health on arrival in Sweden had as a consequence a decline in social position: 21% of those with pre-immigration problems ended in a job worse than the one they had held in Finland, on the other hand, only 5% of those with post-immigration problems settled into a worse job in Sweden than they had had in Finland (Table 5). However, one must notice that 33% of those becoming ill first in Sweden had no occupation in Finland because they had migrated at an early age. Almost all (93%) of those with problems in Finland had some kinds of job or occupation there (including that of housewife).

Table 5. Occupational Position in Sweden Compared with That in Finland in Relation to the Presence or Absence of Psychological Problems before Migration

Comparison of occupational position in Sweden and in Finland	Psychological problems before immigration yes (28) %	no (58) %	All (87) %
Better occupation in Sweden	7	9	8
No change	36	26	29
Change to similar level occupation	29	27	28
Worse occupation in Sweden	21	5	11
Retired in Sweden	–	6	4
First occupation in Sweden	7	27	20
	100	100	100

Table 6. Occupation in Sweden in Relation to the Presence or Absence of Psychological Problems before Migration

Occupation in Sweden	Psychological problems before migration yes (28) %	no (58) %	All (87) %
Technical or professional	3	4	4
Skilled worker	25	17	20
Service worker	4	12	9
Unskilled worker	64	43	50
Housewife	4	17	13
Retired	–	6	4
	100	99	100

Table 6 shows the current occupations of the patients at the time of survey. There were many immigrant workers, both unskilled and skilled, among those who had mental health problems in Finland. Those who were without such problems, however, often were housewives, or old age pensioners, or in service occupations.

Looking at another aspect, there was only a small difference in knowledge of the Swedish language between those who had first had psychological problems in Finland and those who had not (see Table 7). Contacts with Swedes were, however, clearly less common in the pre-migration problem group. Psychological problems preceding migration seemed to reduce the capacity to integrate into Swedish society.

Table 7. Knowledge of Swedish and Contacts with Swedes in Relation to the Presence or Absence of Psychological Problems before Migration

	Psychological problems before migration		All
	yes (28) %	no (58) %	(87) %
Knowledge of Swedish:			
good	43	50	48
poor	36	22	27
none	21	28	25
	100	100	100
Contacts with Swedes:			
good	18	28	25
poor	25	30	28
none	57	42	47
	100	100	100

Finnish immigrants with a previous history of psychological problems were also isolated in other respects: 39% were not married, as compared to 28% of the ones who had no such history. In both groups, 75% had children. The possibilities to love and to be loved were therefore less for those immigrants who had been ill in their home country: they had fewer contacts with people in the new country, and were less often able to found a family of their own.

Starting with a fairly advantageous occupational background in Finland, the immigrant who already had mental problems thus found himself in a lower social position, with fewer human contacts than the healthy immigrant. But what were these mental health problems? Was he able to communicate them, or was he totally alienated?

The problems of those falling ill for the first time after immigrating to Sweden were more severe than were the problems of those arrivals who had histories of previous problems (see Table 8).

Table 8. Type of Psychosis in Relation to the Presence or Absence of Psychological Problems before Migration

	Psychological problems before migration		All
	yes (28)	no (58)	(87)
	%	%	%
No psychosis	93	81	85
Paranoia	4	12	9
Schizophrenia	–	7	5
Manic depression	4	–	1
	101	100	100

The younger the immigrant was when he arrived in the new country, the more time it took before he become mentally ill (the correlation between age at the time of immigration and the time elapsing before the emergence of the first psychological problem in Sweden is −.36). But those who were young when they arrived fell victim to the most serious types of mental health problems (Table 9). This may be due to the great vulnerability of children and young people to the process of migration. Another explanation would be that migration is selective so that only those persons who were relatively healthy mentally dared to emigrate at an advanced age. People who have migrated as children or young persons have remained in Sweden despite their mental health problems.

Table 9. Proportion of Psychotic Patients According to Age at Arrival to Sweden

	Age at time of migration					All	Average age, years
	0–14	15–19	20–24	25–29	30–		
	(8)	(11)	(28)	(21)	(16)	(87)	
	%	%	%	%	%	%	
Psychosis	38	9	14	–	6	10	17
Uncertain	12	–	11	5	–	6	20
Neurosis	50	91	75	94	94	84	22
	100	100	100		100	100	21

Type of neurosis was somewhat different in the group that had problems in Finland than in the mentally healthy group of immigrants (Table 10). Finnish immigrants with previous illness were more often diagnosed as suffering from neurasthenia, alcoholism, angoris, or phobia, whereas those who became ill first in Sweden are classified as neurotic, hysteric, or hypochondriac.

Table 10. Type of Neurosis in Relation to the Presence or Absence of Psychological Problems before Migration

Type of neurosis	Psychological problems before migration		All
	yes (28)	no (58)	(87)
	%	%	%
Neurasthenia	25	12	17
Alcoholism	21	16	17
'Angoris'	7	2	3
Phobia	4	–	1
Neurosis	21	24	23
Hysteria	–	10	7
Hypochondria	4	12	9
Other (drug addiction, delinquency, adjustment problems, etc.)	11	12	12
Psychosis	7	12	11
	100	100	100

In this study a special question about adjustment problems in Sweden was presented to the patients. 67% of the total admitted to having some kind of adjustment problems; they were reported by 79% of those having had psychological problems in Finland, and by 63% of the others. Problems at work and in the use of alcohol can be looked on as examples of adjustment problems characteristic to those having pre-migration mental health problems (see Table 11).

Those Finnish immigrants falling ill in Sweden were troubled in their relationships with family and friends, or they suffered from loneliness. Feelings of persecution were more common among those who had no history of previous problems. The Finn immigrant situation seemed to give rise particularly to mental health problems in the *loving* area. The same result was achieved when the patients were categorized according to their *main* problem (Table 12).

Table 11. Problems Expressed by the Patients in Relation to the Presence or Absence of Psychological Problems before Migration

Problem	Psychological problems before migration yes (28) %	no (58) %	All (87) %
Alcohol problems	29	24	26
Financial and work problems	29	26	27
Somatic symptoms	54	53	53
Conflict with the law	—	3	2
Problems in human relations	32	46	42
Feelings of persecution	7	26	20
Diffuse problems only	57	59	58

Table 12. Main Problems in Relation to the Presence or Absence of Psychological Problems before Migration

	Psychological problems before migration yes (28) %	no (58) %	All (87) %
Distress, depression	21	26	24
Somatic symptoms	29	24	26
Financial and work problems	18	5	9
Disturbed relations with family or friends	21	28	26
Conflict with the law	—	4	2
Some combination of the above	11	14	13
	100	101	100

Problems of work and of a financial nature (having) were characteristic of the pre-migration patients, whereas difficulties in human relations (loving) were most common among those only falling ill after migration. This is connected with our earlier finding that those who arrived with mental health problems relatively often experienced downward social mobility. Mental problems related to the satisfaction of their material needs tended to appear among pre-migration patients. Neurasthenia or stress neurosis, a symptom related to a difficult work situation and low status, was twice as common among pre-migration patients as in the post-immigration patients (Table 10). Post-migration patients had relatively good material conditions, close family ties and good relationships with the social environment (see also Table 13 below). Either way, their mental health problems were related to the satisfaction of their *loving* needs. We shall soon try to interprete this result.

Table 13. Low Status, Isolation and Alienation in Relation to the Presence or Absence of Psychological Problems before Migration

	Scale value	Psychological problems before migration		All
		yes (28) %	no (58) %	(87) %
Low status (financial reasons for migration, only primary education, decline in social status after migration or totally unqualified job in Sweden, bad dwelling, poor or no knowledge of the Swedish language)	1–2	18	17	18
	3	36	28	30
	4	32	50	44
	5	14	5	8
		100	100	100
Average		3.42	3.35	3.36
Isolation (not married, or family problems, or feelings of persecution, mechanical job or work problems, limited or non-existent contacts with Swedes, adjustment problems)	0–1	15	31	26
	2	39	31	33
	3	32	28	29
	4	14	10	12
		100	100	100
Average		2.34	2.08	2.15
Alienation (vague problems only, admits no adjustment problems even though possesing some of the following: new occupation or mechanical job, bad dwelling, limited or non-existent contacts with Swedes, limited or non-existent knowledge of the Swedish language)	0	22	26	24
	1	64	53	58
	2	14	21	18
		100	100	100
Average		0.92	0.95	0.94

To combine the variables measuring the basic dimensions used in this paper we constructed three additive scales. They were called '*Low status*' (lack of *having*), '*Isolation*' (lack of *loving*), and '*Alienation*' (lack of *being*) scales. The *Isolation* and *Alienation* scales were partly composed of the same items, and they are thus technically negatively correlated. That is why we have mainly used marital status and contacts with Swedes as indicators of isolation, and the expression of only diffuse problems as an indicator of alienation. In any event we can see from Table 13 that the pre-migration problem patients have lower status and that they are more isolated than the post-migration patients. On the *Alienation* scale the means are almost the same in the two groups. This accords with our earlier results: nor did we find in Table 11 above any difference in the percentages of patients expressing only vague problems.

The severe illnesses of some of the patients who fell ill in Sweden resulted in some very long stays in the hospital (Table 14). As a whole, patients who had had problems prior to migration received more psychiatric treatment: a long history of mental health difficulties often made the need of psychiatric care most pronounced.

Table 14. Psychiatric Care Received in Relation in the Presence or Absence of Psychological Problems before Migration

	Psychological problems before migration		All
	yes (28)	no (58)	(87)
	%	%	%
Days in hospital care:			
None	54	58	57
Less than 2 weks	11	14	13
2 weeks – less than 2 months	28	14	18
2 months or more	7	14	12
	100	100	100
Visits to the outpatient department, average	12.1	9.3	10.2
	%	%	%
Amount of care received:			
Small (1 visit to outpatient dep. per year or at most twice in hospital for less than 2 months)	22	37	32
Medium (2–6 visits to outpatient dep. per year or more than twice in hospital)	56	46	49
Large (more than that)	22	17	19
	100	100	100

Migrants with pre-migration psychological problems seem to settle into materially disadvantageous and socially isolated positions in the new country. Their problems often were related to bad economic situations, and the main diagnosis given to them was neurasthenia (stress-neurosis) and alcoholism. Poor mental health before arrival in the new country seems to cause problems in the *having* area of life. These problems were, of course, difficult but could not be considered hopeless. Need of mental care was considerable, but these patients could probably be helped to a certain degree by practical health and welfare measures. Few of them were really psychotic. Migration undoubtedly was selective in that deeply disturbed persons did not emigrate at an advanced age.

The problems of immigrants falling ill after migration were in some cases really serious, and those who had migrated at a very early age especially were often psychotic. It is difficult on the basis of this patient material alone to say how important the factor of age at the time of migration was in the development of mental illness. We have no data on the proportion of young immigrants who have remained healthy. However, we can state that many of the psychotic immigrants were forced to move with their parents while still children. The new demands and environmental stress may have influenced the young person's identity in an important way.

Patients who became ill for the first time in Sweden had problems concentrated in the *loving* area. They suffered mainly from family and friendship problems and often had paranoiac symptoms. Their material needs were reasonably well satisfied, they often had their own family, and they had good contacts with the Swedes. We may interprete their problems just in the loving area by referring to the theory of Abraham Maslow (1943) which was the starting point of Allardt's trichotomy of *having*, *loving*, and *being*. Unsatisfied material needs seem to concentrate or focus the expression of psychological problems upon the *having* area, as was the case in the pre-migration problem group. But if the material needs were better satisfied, problems can be expressed on the second level of the value or need hierarchy. That is on the *loving* level, even when from the outside it looks as if the need for human relationships could be met satisfactorily.

Diffuse problems, an indication of alienation, are equally common in both the groups studied here. We have not yet in this part of the paper been able to clarify the role of the third basic variable, *being*, for the mental health syndrome of immigrants. It is notable, however, that more than half of the patients cannot pin down their problems to any specific area even though it is likely that they have many concrete ones to solve.

3.3. Stress, Family Conflicts and Feelings of Persecution as Mental Health Problems of Immigrants

In this section we shall try to illustrate somewhat more concretely three types of mental health problems afflicting Finnish immigrants in Sweden. We assume that those problems are related to two of our concepts, *having* and *loving*. We have seen that neurasthenia or stress-neurosis was a common symptom among the immigrants who had mental health problems in their country of origin and who in Sweden suffered from financial and work problems, that is, problems related to the *having* dimension. Relationship problems, and feelings of persecution, arose usually after migration. These problems represent difficulties in getting along with other people, that is – problems in the *loving* dimension.

3.3.1. Stress-neurosis patients. Patients diagnosed as suffering from *neurasthenia* had symptoms related to stress: exhaustion, difficulties with sleep, concentration problems and irritability. The situation of the immigrant could easily evoke these symptoms: the vast amount of new, foreign experiences and demands, the great pressure to succeed, all combined with slight opportunities of receiving family or peer group support.

Out of our sample fourteen patients were considered to have these problems. One of two (or 50%) had already had psychological problems in Finland, while of the others only 29% had exhibited such symptoms. We may thus presume that the abilities of these patients to handle the difficulties of the immigrant situation were not too good.

Patients with stress-neurosis symptoms (SNP) were a little older and had come to Sweden some years earlier than the others. At the time of immigration, 61% of them were over 24 years of age, as compared with 38% of the non-SNPs. In Sweden however the psychological problems of this group were present after seven years, as in the case of the others.

The material resources of the stress-neurosis patients were somewhat more limited than those of the other patients. Starting often as unskilled workers in Finland (43% as against 26%), and not knowing the Swedish language well (36% as against 51% spoke it well), they ended up in mechanical jobs more often than the non stress-neurosis workers. As many as 64% of the SNPs as compared with 46% of the non-SNPs had mechanical jobs, whereas only 7% SNPs as against 33% non-SNPs had non-mechanical jobs. The SNPs also often experienced problems with their work of financial situation: 43% reported dissatisfaction with their work, inability to cope with it, complained it was hard, or mentioned financial trouble, as compared with 23% of the non-SNPs. On the scale measuring low-status situation, SNPs achieved an average score of 3.57 compared with 3.36 in the other group.

The strenuous situation of neurasthenia patients can also be seen in their family conditions. Most of them were married. They had larger families than the non-neurasthenia immigrants: 43% had at least three children compared with 25% of the patients without this diagnosis. They were also quite isolated from contacts with Swedes: only 14% had good contacts as compared with 27% in the other group. Even though stress-neurosis patients had their family life from which they could find company and human proximity, their human relations are in other ways restricted. The SNP group had failed to integrate with Swedish society, even though they had been living in it longer than the non-SNP group. However, problems related to human contacts are few in this group: only 14% reported such problems as against 47% in the other group.

Thus far we have found out that although stress-neurosis patients were not well off in the *having* dimension, they did not suffer openly from human relations problems despite being isolated from the Swedish community. Our scale of alienation measures difficulties in communicating one's problems. In this respect neurasthenia patients are more alienated (average 1.14) than the other patients (average 0.90). Mechanical work, which was studied in connection with the *having* dimension, can also be looked upon as an indicator of an *alienated* situation. Stress-neurosis patients thus suffered both from an alienating working environment and from difficulties in expressing their mental health problems.

Low status, isolation from the larger society, lack of relationship problems, and alienation were all characteristic of stress-neurosis patients. Mechanical, unsatisfying work plus a large family to support and take care of seemed to give rise to stress that led the immigrant to seek help from a psychiatric clinic. His need of care was, however, not very great. He was seldom taken into hospital for any length of time and the extent of other kinds of treatment did not differ from that of the other patients. This SNP group was not psychotic and thus its situation was not disastrous. Better working conditions and family allowances might lessen its problems.

3.3.2. Married immigrants with relationship problems. Human relations caused problems for about 40% of the patients, especially unmarried women and divorced patients of both sexes. Husbands married to non-Finnish women had rather more relationship problems than those who had a Finnish wife. For wives, on the other hand, it made no difference whether the husband was Finnish or not. Table 15 gives the percentages of patients having relationship problems according to marital status and nationality of the spouse. The amount of material is small so the differences are not considered statistically significant.

Table 15. Emergence of Family or Other Human Relation Problems or Loneliness According to Marital Status and Sex

Marital status	Men %	Women %
Single	36 (14)	50 (4)
Divorced or widowed	100 (3)	57 (7)
Married to a Finn	33 (21)	39 (18)
Married to a non-Finn	44 (9)	37 (11)
	40 (47)	42 (40)

Relationship problems afflicting married patients are so different that it is advisable to examine them separately. Because of the small number of non-married patients, we shall leave them outside our analysis and study only the problems of the married patients. This is in keeping with the discussion at the beginning of this paper in which we looked at the mental health problems of married persons in Västerås. We wished to find out under which circumstances the married immigrant patients had mental health symptoms which were connected with family conflicts. This can in some way reflect the functioning of the immigrant family.

45% of the married patients with relationship problems (MPRP) were diagnosed as neurotics (15% of the other married patients) or alcoholics (24% vs. 12%). Every fourth MPRP (24%) has feelings of persecution compared with only 5% of the other married patients. Here are some examples of their problems:

- Anxiety, restlessness, difficulties with sleep, marriage conflict.
- Moodiness, ill-tempered, aggressive toward wife.
- Moodiness, suspicious, performed coitus with wife 15 times a day, hit her.
- Irritable, deprived, anxious, does not like to be with husband.
- Wife frigid, wants to divorce, depressed, difficulties with sleep, brooding.
- Jealousy on part of wife, restlessness, anxiety, fatigue.
- Wife mentally ill, suspicious, depressed, tired, cannot cope with his job.
- Suicide attempts with pills, wife cannot have children, depressed, not satisfied with work.
- Restless, depressed, suicide attempts with pills, tired, cannot stand husband's friends.
- Husband consumes large quantities of alcohol and is violent in the home, depression arising therefrom, palpitations.

Aggressiveness, fights, jealousy, sexual problems, and inability to have children seem to be the main marital diffiiculties among our immigrant patients. Alcohol problems were very often connected with them.

Married patients with family problems were significantly younger than the other married patients, for example, 45% with problems vs. 17% were under 30 years of age. 51% of the MPRPs (vs. 28% of the other MPs) came to Sweden after 1965. The MPRPs had seldom had mental health problems in Finland (24% vs. 36%). Family problems seemed to appear relatively soon after immigration: the average time lapse before seeking help from a psychiatric institution was 5.4 years for the MPRP, and 8.5 years for the other married patients.

There were no differences in the material resources of married patients with family problems and those without them. The MPRPs had mechanical jobs as often as the other married patients. Neither did they have more work problems. Their lack of knowledge of Swedish is greater due to their recent immigration; only 32% knew Swedish well as compared with 46% of the other married patients. This fact was related to their few contacts with the Swedes: 68% had no contacts at all. In the group without family problems, 'only' 42% were totally segregated from the Swedish community. Even though the occupational position of the patients with family problems is not worse than that of the others, they were isolated from Swedish society because of their recent arrival and poor linguistic skills. Their problems clearly were concentrated in the *loving* dimension. They had neither close relations at home nor in the social environment. But they fortunately had few problems in the *being* dimension. Their jobs were not alienating and they were able to communicate their problems in the interview situation.

It seems as if this group would consist of *recently immigrated, young spouses with few contacts outside the family*. We may assume that some of their problems were projected from the outside world on the family. It is also probable that a new and not yet stabilized family life was easily wounded when the pressure on the family members was great.

3.3.3. Feelings of persecution. Feelings of persecution can easily arise in the immigrant situation. In an environment where what is going on is hidden from one, such a reaction is quite understandable. One may be handicapped by not knowing the language and thereby being barred from any verbal activity. Or one may possess considerable technical knowledge of a language and still not manage to catch the different 'levels' of a message or the subtle shades.

Not to understand what is happening around one, what is being said, makes one powerless. Things happen which concern one, but one is unable to take any action or one cannot understand why they happen. This is like being manipulated. 'The others' have a language that one does not share. Theey shut one out, they decide what will happen to one, they may be enemies. For refugees from economic hardship this reaction is quite 'rational'. This kind of immigrant *is really* shut out and manipulated.

These kinds of difficulties were expressed by seventeen persons in our material, that is by 20% of all patients. Paranoiac problems affected most of these persons' activities; as many as 53% of patients experiencing feelings of persecution were considered psychotic, while the corresponding proportion among the other patients is 6%. Paranoiac symptoms are connected with immigration at an early stage: the correlation between age at the time of immigration and appearance of feelings of persecution is −.15. Conflicts between self-evaluation and the negative reaction of society towards the immigrant before the basic identity is formed may have created a thorough insecurity. Fifty percent of the paranoiac patients are at present under 30 years old (while 36% of the others are in this age group). These patients arrived in Sweden approximately during the same years as the others. They were forced to seek help in the psychiatric clinic at an earlier stage following immigration than the others (6.0 vs. 7.2 years). Only 12% of them compared with 30% of the others had psychological problems in Finland. *Feelings of persecution seemed to emerge as a consequence of immigration, especially when it took place at an early age.*

There is no clear difference in the material resources between patients with and without paranoiac symptoms. Both had similar social status and similarly they seldom had work problems. In some respects, persons with ideas of persecution had even more resources than non-paranoiac patients: they mastered the Swedish language better and less often had mechanical jobs (Table 16).

Many of the patients with symptoms of paranoia had never been married (48% as against 14% of the non-paranoiac patients). This is not totally explained away by their relative youthfulness. Even though they knew Swedish fairly well, they were in little actual 'good' contact with the Swedes. Isolation from both family life and contacts with the larger human environment to a greater degree than would be attributable to linguistic reasons were characteristic of persons with persecution ideas. Their problems were concentrated around their human relationships: as many as 82% reported relationship problems as compared with 31% of the non-paranoiac patients.

Patients with feelings of persecution were able to express their problems. Our scale of alienation shows almost no difference between them and the non-paranoiac patients. As was noted earlier, their work situation wasn't especially alienating. We may conclude that *immigrants with ideas of persecution did not differ from the others in the satisfaction of having and being needs. Their difficulties were associated with loving, with their human relationships.* Having migrated at an early age, they were not able to create satisfactory ties with their social environment.

Table 16. Knowledge of Swedish, Contacts with Swedes, and Type of Work Among Patients with and without Feelings of Persecution

		Feelings of persecution yes (17) %	Feelings of persecution no (70) %	All (87) %
Knowledge of Swedish:	good	59	46	49
	poor	29	26	26
	none	12	28	25
		100	100	100
Contacts with Swedes:	good	18	27	25
	poor	41	25	28
	none	41	48	47
		100	100	100
Mechanical work:	yes	41	50	48
	uncertain	18	24	23
	no	41	26	29
		100	100	100

Even though they managed quite well in the Swedish language, they felt threatened and persecuted. Many of them became psychotic and had to undergo hospital care for longer periods. The correlation between the appearance of feelings of persecution and the length of time spent in hospital is +.43, and the extent of treatment of all kinds comes to +.30.

3.4. Dimensions of Mental Health Problems among Finnish Immigrant Patients

Having thus far only treated a few characteristic immigrant mental health syndromes, the picture of the whole patient group may have remained obscure. That is why the dimensions of psychological problems among immigrants will also be explored with the help of a factor analysis. Social background, mental health and health care variables are included in the same analysis. The correlation and the rotated factor matrices for 19 variables are presented in the appendices. Rotation with five factors gave the best results.

The first factor is related to *low integration* with the Swedish community and a high frequency of expressed *adjustment problems*:

Factor loading	Variable
–.86	Good contacts with Swedes
–.85	Good knowledge of the Swedish language
–.62	Long time in Sweden before appearance of first psychological problem
.38	Adjustment problems

Lack of contacts with native residents and poor knowledge of the language of the new country seem to make immigrants ill soon after arrival and to create problems in adjustment. The causal chain may also be in the other direction. Persons falling ill soon after migration do not make contacts and learn Swedish as easily as those who remain healthy for a longer time.

The second dimension can be called the *psychosis*-factor:

–.69	Feelings of persecution
–.67	Psychosis
–.49	Ample treatment
–.37	Long time in hospital
.33	Marital status: married

The only social background variable on this factor is marital status. Psychotic and paranoiac patients who need plenty of treatment are seldom married. Isolation from close human relationships in the family may be both a cause and a consequence of severe mental illness, which in the immigrant patient population is often expressed by paranoiac symptoms.

The third dimension is composed of *alcohol problems* and several social background variables:

.52	Marital status; married
.49	Sex: female
−.46	Alcohol problems
.42	Good housing conditions
.36	Long time in Sweden before appearance of first psychological problem
.31	Old age
−.31	Adjustment problems

The unmarried young male patient who has his first psychological problem soon after immigration, is living in a poor dwelling and acknowledges that his adjustment problems are probably a 'prototype' of the Finnish 'problem' immigrant. He is visible and people frequently talk about him as a typical example of an unwanted immigrant. One-fourth of the patients studied had alcohol problems (see Table 11); this patient group is numerically quite large.

Alcoholism emerges also in the fourth factor, which is a combination of different *symptoms* studied:

.51	Somatic symptoms
.48	Neurasthenia
−.36	Relationship problems
−.36	Alcohol problems
.36	Financial or work problems

Somatic symptoms and stress-neurosis are combined with work problems, as was pointed out earlier. These problems in the *having* area [2] are negatively correlated with relationship and alcohol problems, which represent difficulties in the *loving* area. *The fourth factor illustrates how the having and loving problems are almost mutually exclusive.*

The fifth factor combines *old age and psychological problems before migration with lack of severe human relations problems*:

.49	Old age
.46	Mental health problems in Finland
−.38	Relational problems
−.34	Psychosis
−.31	Feelings of persecution

This dimension was discussed in detail in Chapter 3.2 (patients with pre- and post-migration problems). The results of the factor analysis clearly indicate that young immigrants falling ill in Sweden suffer mainly from relationship, *loving* problems.

Other immigrant studies show that three of the psychological problem dimensions revealed by factor analysis, feelings of persecution, psychosomatic symptoms and alcoholism, are typical of people arriving in new environments. The *paranoiac* reaction is understandable for the isolated, powerless immigrant who is excluded from communication with the natives of the country. For immigrant laborer life in the new country often means even psychological changes. Since the functioning of his body is important for his life, it is natural that he keenly observes its reactions. Psychological and physical functions are closely interrelated. The natural and accepted way to be ill is to feel bodily pain, i.e. *somatic symptoms*. *Alcohol* problems reflect the most usual means resorted to in our culture to escape from distress and insoluble difficulties.

4. CONCLUSION

The mental health status of Finnish immigrants in Sweden is worse than that of Swedes in comparable positions. It is not possible to say that this is caused by adjustment problems simply because the general health situation in their country of origin is poorer than in Sweden.

In addition to a nation-wide survey we have here used material collected by personal interviews of married individuals in Västerås, Sweden, among Finnish immigrants and Swedes. We also had access to interview material collected at the psychiatric clinic of the central hospital in the same city. On the basis of these fairly limited data some preliminary results can be summarized:

Neurotic persons suffer more from marital problems in the immigrant than in the Swedish families. Value conflicts between the spouses, related to sex roles and achievement orientation, and lack of close contacts with people outside the family, correlated strongly with neurosis in the Swedish families. The immigrant marriage seems to be under particular pressure in a foreign environment. If one of the spouses, in our families usually the wife, becomes too closely integrated into the extra-familial community, marital and psychological problems seem to arise, especially for the husband.

In the prosperous Swedish society material conditions do not correlate strongly with the emergence of mental health problems. In the case of immigrants who have already had psychological problems in the home country, mental illness is related to financial problems and material conditions of relative poverty. But on the level of relatively high material need satisfaction, personal relations begin to account for most mental health problems. We studied stress-neurosis patients as an example of a group with problems related to *having*, i.e. to material need satisfaction. The other two groups studied, those with family conflicts and feelings of persecution, had no particular difficulties in their material conditions. By using factor analysis we were able to find clear dimensions in the patients population. Feelings of persecution, somatic symptoms, and alcoholism were related to different social background variables. Because of lack of some basic variables, the factor analysis remained somewhat incomplete.

More than half of the patients visiting the psychiatric clinic were unable to link their problems to any definite trouble or symptom; we classified them as having only diffuse problems. They may be called alienated, lacking means of communicating their difficulties. In the family study we also found that neurotic persons often felt themselves alienated, without the opportunity of deciding about their own life. All our three basic concepts, *having*, *loving*, and *being* are thus in some way related to mental illness.

In this preliminary report we have only been able to show some connections between mental health problems and certain other social phenomena in two limited groups. Keijo Kata at the Research Group for Comparative Sociology at the University of Helsinki has representative data on neurosis for four Scandinavian societies (Research Group for

Appendix 1. Correlation Matrix. Finnish Immigrant Mental Patients in Västerås Central Hospital, Jan. – Aug. 1971

Correlations are significant at .05 level if $r=20$

	18	17	24	22	33	26	47	46	3	2	32	16	35	28	36	1	20	37	10
18 Contacts with Swedes	–																		
17 Knowledge of Swedish	**75**	–																	
24 Time spent in Sweden before emergence of first psychological problem	**46**	**52**	–																
22 Adjustment problems	**–35**	**–29**	**–31**	–															
33 Feelings of persecution	–02	14	–08	08	–														
26 Psychosis	–03	02	–04	14	**57**	–													
47 Amount of treatment	**24**	**30**	12	11	**30**	**24**	–												
46 Hospital treatment	–14	02	–08	01	**20**	**28**	13	–											
3 Marital status: married	–13	**–23**	10	**–23**	**–26**	**–28**	–14	**–25**	–										
2 Sex: female	15	08	**21**	–11	01	05	07	07	15	–									
32 Alcohol problems	–01	03	**–22**	12	–02	–12	02	03	**–24**	**–38**	–								
16 Good housing conditions	–01	01	18	–10	03	11	–07	–10	**–26**	01	–02	–							
35 Somatic symptoms	–04	–10	–01	03	–12	**–22**	–09	–05	**29**	13	**–25**	06	–						
28 Neurasthenia	–12	–08	01	–03	–06	**–29**	–17	–17	07	–03	–18	–02	**29**	–					
36 Financial and work problems	–13	–01	–02	18	03	–00	–18	–02	04	13	–11	03	15	16	–				
1 Old age	14	**21**	**34**	–16	–14	**–22**	08	01	**28**	18	04	18	11	03	–03	–			
20 Psychological problems in Finland	–14	–01	**–23**	15	**–22**	–18	06	–01	–15	–07	05	–02	00	16	03	**20**	–		
37 Relationship problems	–01	02	**–20**	–03	**41**	**20**	18	16	–10	02	–01	–00	**–38**	**–24**	–03	–18	–14	–	
10 Education	06	01	–11	–01	–13	19	00	–17	10	01	–12	–08	**20**	10	–13	18	07	–08	–

Comparative Sociology 1972). The best feature of the material presented here is that we are able to study marital dynamics because we have interviewed both spouses and have also had access to unique hospital data.

Appendix 2. Varimax-rotated Factor Matrix for Five Factors. Finnish Immigrant Mental Patients in Västerås Central Hospital, Jan.–Aug. 1971

	I	II	III	IV	V	H
18 Contacts with Swedes	−86	−02	−03	−05	−05	.75
17 Knowledge of Swedish	−85	−18	−08	−07	08	.78
24 Time spent in Sweden before emergence of first psychological problem	−62	03	36	03	03	.51
22 Adjustment problems	38	−24	−31	18	10	.33
33 Feelings of persecution	−01	−69	−02	−04	−31	.57
26 Psychosis	05	−67	0	−06	−34	.57
47 Amount of treatment	−23	−49	−03	05	26	.36
46 Hospital treatment	11	−37	08	−30	09	.26
3 Marital status: married	11	33	52	08	12	.42
2 Sex: female	−14	−08	49	14	−10	.30
32 Alcohol problems	03	04	−46	−36	17	.38
16 Good housing conditions	−03	−03	42	−04	08	.19
35 Somatic symptoms	05	06	26	51	27	.40
28 Neurasthenia	04	12	−02	48	15	.27
36 Financial and work problems	07	−04	01	36	−06	.14
1 Old age	−22	05	31	−10	49	.40
20 Psychological problems in Finland	13	0	−18	03	46	.26
37 Relationship problems	08	−27	02	−36	−38	.36
10 Education	−01	12	04	12	20	.07
Eigenvalues	2.18	1.67	1.39	1.06	1.09	7.40

BIBLIOGRAPHY

Erik Allardt, 'Relation of Welfare Values to Culture and Economy', *Research Reports, Institute of Sociology, University of Helsinki* **188** (1973).

Erik Allardt and Hannu Uusitalo, 'Dimensions of Welfare in a Comparative Study of the Scandinavian Societies', *Research Reports, Institute of Sociology, University of Helsinki* **173** (1972).

E. J. Cleveland and W. D. Longaker, 'Neurotic Patterns in the Family', in: Gerald Handel (ed.), *The Psychosocial Interior of the Family*, Aldine, Chicago 1967.

Elina Haavio-Mannila, 'Migration and Competence to Handle Health, Economic and Work Problems in the Family', *Research Report of the Institute of Sociology, University of Helsinki* **207** (1973). This report is based on data collected simultaneously and using the same questionnaire and sample as the data analyzed in the present paper. It includes comparative material from Helsinki, too, which was gathered for the International Research Studies on the Family, directed by Marvin B. Sussman, sponsored by the International Sociological Association, and financed by the National Institute of Child Health and Human Development, U.S.A.

Sten Johansson, 'Finska invandrare i Sverige', Institutet för social forskning, preliminary report in stencil, Stockholm 1973.

B. Malzberg, 'Are Immigrants Pathologically Disturbed?' in: S. C. Plog and R. B. Edgerton (eds.), *Changing Perspectives in Mental Illness*, New York 1969.

Abraham Maslow, 'A Theory of Human Motivation', *Psychological Review* **50** (1943) 370–396.

Research Group for Comparative Sociology, *The Scandinavian Survey on Welfare and Need-Satisfaction*, Questionnaire with Marginal Distributions for Denmark, Finland, Norway and Sweden, University of Helsinki, March–May 1972.

Raimo Salokangas, 'Mielisairaus yhteiskunnallisena ilmiönä' (Mental Illness as a Social Phenomen), *Turun Yliopiston Sosiologian laitos, Monisteita* **57** (1973).

Victor D. Sanua, 'Immigration, Migration and Mental Illness: A Review of the Literature with Special Emphasis on Schizophrenia', in: Eugene B. Brody (ed.), *Behavior in New Environments, Adaptation of Migrant Populations*, Sage Publications, Beverly Hills, California 1970.

Clark E. Vincent, 'Mental Health and the Family', in: Paul H. Glasser and Lois N. Glasser (eds.), *Families in Crisis*, Harper and Row, New York 1970.

C. Ødegaard, 'Immigration and Insanity: A Study of Mental Disease among Norwegian-born Population in Minnesota', *Acta Psychiatrica et Neurologica Scandinavica*, Supplementum **4** (1932) 1–206.

REFERENCES

[1] The data were collected for a nation-wide 'low income survey' directed by Sten Johansson in Uppsala. The Finnish Ministry of Labour paid for the expenses of the secondary analysis.

[2] Type of work and occupational status were left out of this factor analysis for technical reasons. They will be included in future.

PROFESSIONAL AND LAY ATTITUDES TOWARD MENTAL ILLNESS AND MENTAL PATIENTS

T. TAHIN, GY. KÓCZÁN, J. PÖRCZI,
K. OZSVÁTH, I. KISS, B. KÉZDI

Institute of Marxism-Leninism, Medical School of Pécs, Hungary

According to unanimous estimates and statistical data the number of mental disorders is on the increase in our country. Year by year more and more people consult doctors about mental problems. Special medical offices, out-patient clinics and hospitals are overcrowded and specialists are overburdened. The development of mental health services cannot keep pace with the increasing demands. On the contrary, it has significantly fallen behind other branches of the Health Service. Health education has only paid attention to the prevention of somatic diseases. Mental health has remained *terra incognita* in the framework of health education. Medical training is one sidedly somatic oriented. Future doctors are not adequately prepared to deal with mental disturbances associated with social problems.

Practical experiences show the man on the street is not only averse toward mental patients but also towards those people and institutions dealing with them professionally. Fear, hatred and rejection, are frequently encountered reactions toward mental patients. They can be met with within the medical profession, too. Everyday speech offers a large assortment of pejorative expressions concerning mental disorder. Crazy, mad, insane, nut case etc. words used with intent to stigmatize, show that the everyday thinking – though it considers mental and behavioral disturbances to be illnesses – sharply differentiates them from somatic illnesses. The mentally ill represent a particular class of patients who are subjected to isolation and segregation. The labeling of somebody as a mental patient – whether or not complete recovery or significant improvement takes place – may deprive him of his previous social status. Besides these practical problems and the recently initiated official efforts to change the situation, there are some general considerations, too, which motivate the research into the beliefs and attitudes concerning mental patients and mental disorders. This kind of knowledge may contribute to a conceptual understanding of patients' behavior and that of the social behaviour connected with illness in various social and cultural groups (Mechanic 1969). In the field of mental health especially, beliefs and attitudes may influence the course of the illness, the success of treatment and social readjustment. They may have a significant effect on the epidemiology of mental illness. They may determine the success of educational efforts regarding mental health (King 1962, Maclean 1969).[1]

In this paper, we shall present the methods and some of the results of an investigation carried out in four social groups. The target population were medical practitioners, city dwellers, relatives of mental patients and village residents.

METHOD

The survey was conducted in four samples. The first was obtained from the register of medical practitioners working in the town of Pécs. The number of randomly selected doctors was 135. Residents of the Third District of Pécs made up the second sample. It consisted of 400 names taken randomly from the electoral lists. The third sample included 100 relatives of mental patients undergoing treatment in Pécs. The fourth sample was made up of residents of the village of Bóly. This sample consisted of 175 people selected at random.

The questionnaire used in the survey, was constructed by the Likert method (Likert 1932, Likert *et al.* 1934). The final questionnaire was worked out after analysing the results of two pilot studies. Attitude items used in the pilot studies originated partly from the scales worked out by Cohen and Struening and by Maclean respectively (Cohen and Struening 1962, Maclean 1969). We decided to adopt these items on the basis of a preceding opinion poll. The other part of the attitude statements was also composed with regard to the results of this poll. Statements concerning the causes of mental illness were phrased and selected similarly.

The final questionnaire included 37 attitude statements, one question offering a choice of 15 possible opinions on the causes of mental illness, and 12 questions concerning the demographic, soical and other variables of the samples. The attitude statements, on the basis of certain logical considerations, were grouped as follows: potential danger from mental patients (5 items); handling of mental patients (8 items); social rejection and degradation (8 items); social acceptability of former mental patients (5 items); possibility of rehabilitation (6 items); prognosis (5 items). We have used the term 'attitude' according to Sprott's definition (Maclean 1969). We accepted as expressing attitudes those items which were more emotionally charged than the 'opinions'. Throughout the study, we have used the terms 'mental illness' and 'mental patient' consistently, defined as: "Mental illness is a state which sooner or later results in the patient entering a mental hospital: a mental patient is one who gets into such a state." This definition originated from the one used by Cohen and Struening (Shaw and Wright 1967). We decided to adopt this because it emphasizes practical criteria. In our experience these criteria work as a unifying and collaboratory means of defining a state or behavior as mental illness and to label somebody as mental patient in everyday thinking.

The survey – with the exception of the professional sample – was conducted in the form of personal interviews. The names of the subjects were kept strictly confidential. The entire study began in November 1969 and was completed in the spring of 1970.

RESULTS

We received altogether 736 completed questionnaires. Their distribution according to the samples was as follows: medical practitioners returned 106 of the 135 questionnaires sent by mail; Third District dwellers of Pécs 379; relatives of mental patients undergoing treatment 100; residents of the village of Bóly 151. The subjects interviewed were classified into three age groups: 18–30, 31–55, and over 56. The distribution among our four samples was as follows: medical doctors 33, 63, and 4% respectively; dwellers of Pécs 18, 61 and 21%; relatives 16, 52 and 32%; residents of Bóly 22, 52 and 26%. The male-female ratio was: medical practitioners 67 : 33; dwellers of Pécs 52 : 48; relatives 34 : 66; residents of Bóly 53 : 47.

The subjects were divided by education into the following four categories: 7 grades completed, 8–11 grades completed, secondary school certificate, college or university, and the following breakdowns were achieved: residents of Pécs 20, 39, 27, 14%; relatives 44, 32, 15, 9%; residents of Bóly 37, 46, 13, 4%. The composition of the samples according to social strata was studied using four categories: I. Managers and those with higher education; II. Administrators and other non-manual workers; IIIa. Industrial manual workers; IIIb. Agricultural manual workers – and yielded the following results: residents of Pécs, 14, 44, 41, 1% respectively; relatives 9, 32, 59, 0%; residents of Bóly 5, 26, 37, 32%.[2]

The reliability index for the questionnaire was calculated on the basis of the Spearman–Brown formula: r_{xx} odd/even = 0.86/0.89. The responses given to every item of the samples significantly differed from one another with the exception of Nos. 7, 9, 18, 23, 24.[3] In regard to the responses received to item groups mainly under the heading of the 'social acceptability of former mental patients' we could find a significant degree of identity. However, significant differences could be demonstrated among the four samples in the responses to every item using the Kolmogorov–Smirnov formula (Siegel 1965). The positive nature of the attitudes – considering the responses to every item – decreased in the order of professionals, residents of Pécs, relatives and residents of Bóly.[4]

The primary sources of information about mental illness in regard to non-professionals were: in the sample of Pécs: personal experiences (45%), hearsay (21%), reading (19%), mass media (6%), other (9%), in the sample of village residents: personal experiences (43%), hearsay (28%), reading (11%), mass media (6%), other (7%); in the sample of relatives: personal experiences (79%), hearsay (7%), reading (7%), mass media (1%), other (6%).

Opinions concerning the etiology of mental illness were investigated with a list consisting of fourteen etiological factors and an open possibility of response. We asked the respondents to mark the five most important causes which, in their opinion, lead to mental illness. The five most frequently chosen factors were: physicians – heredity (92%), excessive alcohol consumption (83%), changes in the function of the organism in puberty and old age (67%), head injury (60%), severe mental shock (53%) in the sample from Pécs – severe mental shock (84%), excessive alcohol consumption (78%), head injury (70%), heredity (69%), excessive mental work (35%); in the sample of relatives – severe mental shock (80%), excessive alcohol consumption (68%), heredity (63%), head injury (45%), excessive mental work (45%); in the village sample – excessive alcohol consumption (78%), severe mental shock (75%), heredity (70%), head injury (68%), excessive mental work (42%). It is interesting to note that as long as the population attributes an important role to heredity, mental shock, extreme alcohol consumption and head injury, the factors representing the interpersonal etiology of mental illness (e.g. stresses and strains at home and at work, lack of parental love and care in childhood) were chosen very infrequently.

RESPONSES TO ATTITUDE STATEMENTS IN THE FOUR ITEM GROUPS

In the following pages we describe the responses received in the item groups: the potential danger from mental patients, the social acceptability of former mental patients, the possibility of rehabilitation, prognosis. The distribution of responses will be analysed in every item group according to professionals and laymen (samples of Pécs and Bóly together $N=530$), non-professional subgroups with higher or lower education (non-professionals $N=630$, subgroup with higher education $N=206$, subgroup with education $N=424$), professionals and non-professional subgroup with higher education.[5]

On this basis we wish to answer three questions:

a. Are there any differences in the attitudes toward mental illness and patients between physicians and laymen (excluding relatives of patients)?[6]

b. Are there any differences in attitudes between subgroups representing different levels of education?

c. Are there any differences in attitudes between physicians and the subgroup with higher education?

The Potential Danger of the Mentally Ill

Items No. 6, 8, 19, 23, and 27 compose the various aspects of the potential danger of the mentally ill. Table I shows the distribution of the responses.

The table shows that the laymen consistently chose the positive alternative considerably less frequently as regards every item expect No. 23, where the difference in the responses is not significant. The biggest difference between the physicians and laymen responses can be seen in item No. 27. This is understandable since the hospital and the mental ward are the doctors' place of work. On the other hand, the popular conception of the hospital in general and the mental ward in particular is one of fear and anxiety because of the negative stereotypes attached to them. The responses given to item No. 23 show that the stereotype of the dangerous nature of former mental patients thrives both in the minds of professionals and laymen. The contagion of mental illness, expressed in item No. 8 was found to be strongly refuted by doctors but received a relatively high rate of endorsement from laymen. The unpredictability of mental patients received a high rate of endorsement from laymen: (71 %). This is similar to the results obtained by Nunnally, where the biggest difference between normal and mentally disturbed persons was found in the scale of predictability-unpredictability (Nunnally 1969). Differences in the responses given by the subgroups possessing higher and lower education were significant except for items No. 23 and 19. Higher education is accompanied by a more positive attitude regarding every item. It is interesting to note that the subgroup with lower education holds the view that mental patients are always dangerous in 1/3 ratio, while 73 % of them view the mental ward as the most fearsome part of a hospital and 73 % agree with the statement referring to the unpredictability of mental patients.

We supposed that a medical education would influence positively the attitudes toward mental patient in this item group. If this were true then physicians might be expected to respond positively with significantly greater frequency, not only than the laymen as a whole but also than the subgroup with higher education. The results have not confirmed this supposition. We could only find significant differences in the responses given to items No. 27 and 19. It appears that in this item group the professionals have no such special feature which would lead to any significant attitude alteration.

Table I. Potential Danger of the Mentally Ill (percentage)

Items		Professionals N=106			Laymen N=530			Higher education N=206			Lower education N=424		
	score	5 or 4	2 or 1	3	5 or 4	2 or 1	3	5 or 4	2 or 1	3	5 or 4	2 or 1	3
Anyone who lives among mental patients sooner or later becomes mentally ill himself (8)	Agree		6	8		18	17		10	14		26	17
	Disagree	86			65			76			57		
Regardless of what people may say, mental patients are always dangerous (6)	Agree		10	8		28	13		15	9		35	14
	Disagree	82			59			76			51		
Those who have once been mental patients are no more dangerous than the average person (23)	Agree	43		18	41		27	43		25	41		26
	Disagree		39			32			32			33	
The mental ward is the most fearsome part of a hospital (27)	Agree		20	6		60	14		42	17		72	11
	Disagree	74			26			41			17		
Mental patients unpredictable and you never know what they will do next (19)	Agree		47	15		71	16		66	17		73	15
	Disagree	38			13			17			12		

The Social Acceptability of Former Mental Patients

The questionnaire also contained a scale of social distance. Items No. 7, 9, 11, 16, and 18 postulate various degrees of social intimacy between the respondent and the former mental patient (Table II). One of the main findings of the study is that the attitudes of the respondents are the most negative in this scale. The general tendency is for the respondent's attitude to become more negative the closer the social relationship postulated between him and the former mental patient. The majority of the respondents would steer clear of closer social relationships with former mental patients.

The responses of professionals and laymen differed significantly only in item No. 11. In all the other items the incidence of negative attitudes in both groups increases similarly. As a matter of fact the reactions of the physicians in items No. 7 and 11 were somewhat more negative than those of the laymen. Examined from the point of view of education, the responses of the subgroups, with the exception of item No. 7, were significantly different. The tendency is, however, for the responses of the subgroup with higher education to be more positive than others only in statements expressing a less close relationship.

Comparison of the responses given by physicians and those of the subgroup with higher education revealed a significant difference only in one item (No. 9).

Possibility of Rehabilitation

Items No. 5, 10, 20, 21, 22, and 29 were intended to explore attitudes concerning the possibility of rehabilitation of mental patients (Table III).

A comparison between professionals and laymen shows that the responses – with the exception of item No. 5 – differ significantly from one another. In the first three items the professionals' attitude is more positive than that of the laymen, while in the second three items this tendency does not prevail. According to the majority of doctors, mental patients are willing and able to work and mental illness is just an illness like any other. This positive attitude, however, significantly alters in

Table II. Social Acceptability of Former Mental Patients (percentage)

Items		Professionals $N=106$			Laymen $N=530$			Higher education $N=206$			Lower education $N=424$		
	score	5 or 4	2 or 1	3	5 or 4	2 or 1	3	5 or 4	2 or 1	3	5 or 4	2 or 1	3
I would be willing to have a former mental patient as a neighbor (11)	Agree	68		19	48		23	60		18	40		25
	Disagree		13			29			22			35	
I would be willing to work together with a former mental patient (16)	Agree	57		22	49		21	57		21	44		24
	Disagree		21			30			22			32	
I would let a former mental patient teach my children (18)	Agree	24		24	19		21	26		22	17		20
	Disagree		52			60			52			63	
Most women who were once patients in a mental hospital could be trusted as baby sitters (9)	Agree	13		21	18		29	16		35	19		26
	Disagree		66			53			49			55	
I would give my consent to a member of my family to marry someone who had once been a mental hospital patient (7)	Agree	9		22	15		20	16		23	16		19
	Disagree		69			65			61			65	

Table III. Possibility of Rehabilitation (percentage)

Items		Professionals $N=106$			Laymen $N=530$			Higher education $N=206$			Lower education $N=424$		
	score	5 or 4	2 or 1	3	5 or 4	2 or 1	3	5 or 4	2 or 1	3	5 or 4	2 or 1	3
Most mental patients are willing to work (22)	Agree	75		22	55		30	63		25	51		31
	Disagree		3			15			12			18	
Many mental patients are able to do a job which requires high qualifications in spite of the fact, that in some respects they are rather confused (29)	Agree	81		11	56		24	67		21	47		28
	Disagere		8			20			12			25	
Mental disorder is an illness like any other (20)	Agree	76		4	47		20	53		21	46		20
	Disagree		20			33			26			34	
Mental patients discharged from hospital could usually find their place in everyday life again quite easily if this only depended on them (10)	Agree	44		20	50		28	59		19	47		31
	Disagree		36			22			22			22	
A district nurse who has been a mental hospital patient for a time could return to her job after wards (21)	Agree	36		17	31		31	32		28	30		34
	Disagree		47			38			40			36	
An ex-mental patient could hold a social position with higher re- [illegible]	Agree	18		22	23		26	23		28	26		24
	Disagree		60			51			49			50	

Table IV. Prognosis (percentage)

Items		Professionals $N=106$			Laymen $N=530$			Higher education $N=206$			Lower education $N=424$		
	score	5 or 4	2 or 1	3	5 or 4	2 or 1	3	5 or 4	2 or 1	3	5 or 4	2 or 1	3
If somebody becomes mentally ill it is just like losing him altogether (14)	Agree		7	7		26	15		15	11		34	17
	Disagree	86			59			74			49		
If somebody becomes mentally ill, he remains so throughout his life (33)	Agree		14	15		14	27		7	22		20	30
	Disagree	71			59			71			50		
Those who enter mental hospitals as patients rarely leave it (15)	Agree		4	8		17	33		9	31		24	30
	Disagree	88			50			60			46		
It is no use treating mental patients for their recovery is only virtual (12)	Agree		13	16		20	26		13	24		25	28
	Disagree	71			54			63			47		
Those people who have once been inmates in a mental hospital are never their old selves (26)	Agree		22	17		39	25		29	23		47	25
	Disagree	61			36			48			28		

a negative direction in those items which express the ability of a former mental patient to readjust to society or to hold a social position with higher responsibilities. It is noticeable that 25% of the physicians does not agree with the statement that mental illness is an illness like any other. In another item, not included in this study one quarter of the physicians also agreed with the statement that seriously ill mental patients are no longer real human beings.

With regard to the educational factor, the responses, with the exception of items No. 5 and 21, are significantly different. The attitude of respondents with lower education is considerably more negative in the first four items than that of those with higher one. In the last two items, however, this differences disappear. Those with higher education respond in the same negative way as those with lower education.

It is interesting to note the significant differences between the responses of physicians and persons with higher education apart from items No. 5 and 21.

Prognosis

Statements No. 12, 14, 15, 26 and 33 express stereotypes concerning the outcome of mental illness. Table IV shows the distribution of responses given to these items.

Considerable differences between the responses given by doctors and laymen can be observed in every item. (Differences of responses are significant in every statement.) The lay group gives positive answers a good deal less frequently than the professional group.

According to the educational variable, the differences between the attitudes of subgroups are especially sharp ($p<0.01$). 34% of those with lower education consider the becoming of mentally ill a feeling of total loss. 47% of them do not believe in the possibility of complete recovery. One quarter of this subgroup expresses a kind of therapeutic nihilism.

Comparing the responses of physicians with those of the subgroup with higher education, one can only find significant difference in items No. 14 and 15. In these statements the physicians' attitudes are considerably more positive.

SOME CONCLUSIONS

On the basis of the results obtained, it seems that the effects of a medical education in modifying attitudes are highly dubious. The responses of physicians concerning the potential danger of mental patients, the prognoses regarding mental illnes and some aspects of the possibility of rehabilitation are similar to the responses given by laymen with higher education. In these item groups the responses of the professionals express cultural differences in general rather than the result of a speical professional training. It can be assumed that more positive reactions on the part of both professionals and persons with higher education primarily reflect a higher level of knowledge which may often suppress the supposedly present negative emotions. Moreover physicians and persons with higher education tend to believe in the power of science – especially in connection with prognosis of mental illness – than people with lower education who display a fatalistic attitude.

These differences between physicians and persons with higher education and between both and persons with lower education almost completly disappear as regards attitudes towards former mental patients. The former mental patient is unacceptable in public positions of high responsibility and in closer social relationships. The respondents' standpoint is refusal, or at least social restriction. The basis of this may be a commonly shared cultural belief – transmitted to the ex-mental patient, too – by which mental illness and the mentally ill mean a threat to community, especially to the family. The borderline of social tolerance towards former mental patients is drawn to exclude the family, on the one hand and public positions requiring higher qualification and involving responsibility on the other.

BIBLIOGRAPHY

Jacob Cohen and E. L. Struening, 'Opinions about Mental Illness in the Personnel of two Large Mental Hospitals', *Journal of Abnormal and Social Psychology* **5** (1962) 349–360.

Stanley King, *Perceptions of Illness and Medical Practice*, Russel Sage Foundation, New York, 1962, Part Two (*Disease and its Interpretation*).

Rensis Likert, 'A Technique for the Measurement of Attitudes', *Archives of Psychology* (1932) 1–55.

Rensis Likert, Sydney Roslow and Gardner Murphy, 'A Simple and Reliable Method of Scoring the Thurstone Attitude Scales', *Journal of Social Psychology* 5 (1934) 228–238.

Maclean, 'Community Attitudes to Mental Illness in Edinburgh', *British Journal of Preventive and Social Medicine* (1969) 45–52.

David Mechanic, *Medical Sociology, A Selective View*, The Free Press, New York 1968.

Jum C. Nunnally, jr., *Popular Conceptions of Mental Health, Their Development and Change*, Holt, Reinhart and Winston, Inc., New York 1961.

Marvin E. Shaw and Jack M. Wright, *Scales for the Measurement of Attitudes*, McGraw-Hill, Inc., New York 1967.

Sidney Siegel, *Nonparametric Statistics of the Behavioral Sciences*, McGraw-Hill, Inc., New York 1956.

REFERENCES

[1] Research into this field is especially intensive in North America (see the references in King's book and Maclean's publication). Concerning the socialist countries we have information about Dr. Bizon's research conducted in Warsaw.

[2] In the samples from Pécs and Bóly intellectuals are somewhat over represented. The explanation of this is that the Third District of Pécs includes a recently built housing estate with a disproportionately high number of white-collar workers. In the case of Bóly, this over representation is due to economic circumstances. There is a large agricultural cooperative and a state farm which employ a large number of qualified personnel.

[3] The significance of any observed association in this study was ascertained by means of a χ^2 test (with a 5 percent probability level assumed as the minimum necessary to determine significance).

[4] See the comprehensive analysis of the results in: T. Tahin, I. Kiss, B. Kézdi, G. Kóczán, K. Ozsváth and J. Pörczi, 'Investigation of Attitudes toward Mental Disease', *Szociológia* 3 (1972) 383–407 (in Hungarian).

[5] The subgroup with higher education includes respondents with high school or university degrees or college diploma.

[6] See the analysis of some aspects of relatives' behavior in: J. Pörczi, K. Ozsváth, G. Kóczán, T. Tahin, I. Kiss and B. Kézdi, 'Attitudes towards Mental Illness', *Orvosi Hetilap* 113 (1972) 3059–3065 (in Hungarian).

SOCIAL DIFFERENTIATION OF MEDICAL BEHAVIOUR AMONG WARSAW INHABITANTS. RESEARCH ASSUMPTIONS AND PRELIMINARY RESULTS

ANNA TITKOW

Institute of Philosophy and Sociology, Polish Academy of Sciences, Warsaw, Poland

This report concerns a study of a random sample of 1,165 adult inhabitants of Warsaw, embracing persons between the ages of 18 and 69. This investigation of the social differentiation of medical behaviour among Warsaw inhabitants is a preparatory study for a similar investigation on a national scale.

THE PROBLEMS UNDER INVESTIGATION

The amount of information regarding the relations between the various conditions on the one side and medical attitudes and behaviour of people on the other, is modest in comparison with other spheres of the social sciences. [1]

This situation is undergoing changes, as the result of a recent tendency to view illness and health as a sphere of social behaviour which is conditioned not only by illness, medical institutions and health education, but also by factors connected with social stratification, culture and psychology. [2] This approach involves the study of behaviour patterns related to illness as defined either by physicians or by the sufferers themselves whether formulated in medical terms or not. [3]

The word 'behaviour' may be interpreted in several ways: in the light of the approach outlined above, the most useful definition of medical behaviour would seem to be the kind of individual activities which are connected with health and illness.[4] We assume that such behaviour is the result of free choice on the part of the individual concerned. Such an assumption, which is obvious in the social sciences, requires emphasis in relation to this sphere of social behaviour, which is, as is well known, strongly influenced by biological variables.

By supplementing studies of health and illness (which until recently were based principally on the intensity of pathological changes) with information concerning how the patient feels and how he fulfils his social roles, the behavioural aspects of illness are brought to light.[5] This in turn makes it possible to regard medical behaviour as an indicator of social phenomena and processes. This was the approach adopted in our study of the social differentiations of medical behaviour among Warsaw inhabitants.

Aims of the Investigation

1. There exists a numerous group of Polish sociologists currently concerned with drawing up a set of questions and hypotheses concerning the following problems: do there exist differences in style and standard of living in Polish society (i.e. differences in needs and ways of satisfying these needs), and if so, how great are they? We assume that medical behaviour is included among the set of phenomena which we define by means of the concept of style and standard of living. This is why we wish to ascertain not only the differentiation between particular spheres of medical behaviour, but also to determine whether the differentiation observed corresponds to the division of the investigated population into socio-occupational groups. Our findings are of interest as a correlate of a broader social phenomenon observed in Polish society, namely the process of obliteration of differences between strata and the simultaneous emergence of new elements of differentiation of a cultural character.

2. We trust that this research will be useful in the formulation of social policy. We wish to determine how state health care services are distributed among the investigated population. Possibly it will be necessary to change the way in which the health service is organized at present.

We wish to determine whether the institutions of the state health service as seen by the public fulfil their intended roles.

3. We wish to create a typology of ways in which sick roles are fulfilled.

Assumptions and Basic Definitions

1. We have accepted a functional definition of illness, according to which the individual by either continuing or ceasing to fulfil roles which he has hitherto filled himself decides whether he is ill or not. Supplementing this definition is the sufferer's own recollection of the diagnosis of his illness, which acts as a control variable. The illness is coded according to categories established by physicians and contained in the international classification of diseases. In terms of social role theory, the functional definition of illness describes the behaviour of an ill person and does not have any normative element.

2. Illness is treated as a dynamic event which has two stages. The first stage is the adoption of the sick role (ceasing or limiting the activities of previous roles), and the second is the adoption of the role of a user of medical services, whether state, cooperative or private.

3. This study [6] was preceded by an analysis of the literature on medical behaviour, which enabled us to choose social classes and strata as the variable which would constitute a framework for the assessment of the correlations between other variables and medical behaviour; [7] in this way we were able to study the interconnections between variables concerning medical behaviour against a wider social background than that constituted by a population suffering from a given disease.

4. This investigation of social differentiation in the medical behaviour of Warsaw inhabitants is based on the assumption that in order to be able to predict human behaviour, one must place it in its motivational context, that is, one must consider it as one of a whole set of attitudes, in this case the attitudes towards the fact of being sick and in need of medical attention. A consequence of accepting this assumption was the adoption of a definition of an attitude as an analytical and interpretative category having three components: (1) a disposition to behave in a particular way, (2) evaluative and emotional dispositions and (3) cognitions concerning the object of the attitude. [8] Such a decision seemed necessary in undertaking an investigation which was to be a part of a larger research

project aimed at predicting medical behaviour in Polish society and defining needs in this area. Because of the above methodological assumptions, the main dependent variable 'the attitude to being ill' has three dimensions: one evaluative-emotional, one behavioural and one concerning the medical knowledge of the respondents. All these types of variables together compose a complex of phenomena which we define as medical behaviour.

5. Independent variables include both demographic and such social variables as education and social position (including both present status and intergeneration mobility). The secondary consequences of membership in a defined socio-occupational group were also taken into account, namely: financial status as defined by income, material situation and, as an additional consideration, the way leisure time was made use of and share in the social consumption fund.[9]

Basic Hypotheses

1. Our first hypothesis is that there is a differentiation in the investigated population as concerns particular components of the attitude to being ill and this differentiation is correlated with stratification variables.

2. Our second hypothesis is that this correlation will be stronger if we conduct an analysis against the background of sets of independent variables.

3. Our third hypothesis is that there exist different types of sick role fulfilment. The elements used to distinguish these types are the variables which constitute the behavioural and emotional-evaluative component.

4. The fourth hypothesis holds that among the stratification categories there exist greater differences in medical behaviour if, instead of taking individual elements of the attitude to being ill, we employ previously distinguished types of fulfilment of the sick role (compare hypothesis 3).

SOME PRELIMINARY RESULTS

The investigated population differs as to educational level, socio-occupational position, level of income, material standards and share in the social consumption fund.[10] The last is insufficiently effective in reducing the inequalities associated with the various socio-occupational positions of Warsaw's inhabitants. An exception is the state health service, which forms a part of the social consumption fund. 99% of Warsaw inhabitants are entitled to free health care and 96% make use of this aid in concrete situations.

Medical Biographies of Warsaw Inhabitants

The population investigated in this study consisted of a random sample including both sick and healthy persons. On the basis of our previous experiences in medical sociology, we decided to base ourselves on the respondents' own assessment of their state of health. As a result information was obtained on the respondents' state of health over a given period of time. The diseases were coded according to the international classification.

The medical biographies of the Warsaw inhabitants were constructed from a sociological viewpoint. An analysis of the findings revealed two points of interest. It turned out that the investigated population was comparatively little differentiated with respect to the declared diseases. Particular diseases occurred in more or less similar proportions in the educational categories distinguished.

We have asked our respondents which of the various diseases they had suffered from were the graver. It turned out that there was a similarity between the distribution of all diseases suffered by respondents over a two-year period and the distribution of these particular diseases which were singled out by the respondents as of a graver nature. These results are important from the methodological point of view. The similarity of these two distribution patterns enables us to explain the differences in medical behaviour in terms of social variables. The next observation concerns more general questions such as the validity of applying 'non-medical' indicators of medical biography. Nowadays hospitalization is sometimes regarded as a good indicator of a society's state of health.[11] Our findings suggest that this is not sufficient. As it turns out, information on hospitalization can be misleading for it pertains both to the accessibility of hospitals and to the degree of the population's susceptibility to illness. They must therefore be supplemented by more unequivocal indicators as, for instance, the average number of days spent in the hospital.

The Medical Behaviour of Warsaw Inhabitants

1. The Functioning of Various Definitions of Health and Illness

In naming the diseases from which they suffered or had suffered, respondents made use of the medical terms for these diseases. We were interested in establishing whether the medical and functional definitions of illness covered the same groups of respondents. We asked them whether they considered themselves incapable of functioning normally, of doing their jobs or fulfilling their household duties. We treated the answers as indicators of the tendency to regard oneself as ill. When symptoms of illness appear, respondents of a lower educational level more often declared themselves incapable of fulfilling their job or household obligations. This finding justifies the assumption that this group is either characterized by a weaker tolerance of disease symptoms or by a greater tendency to complain.

An arrangement of the socio-occupational categories according to the percentage of those who consider themselves ill shows the following ascending order of sequence: technicians, office workers, skilled workers, persons with higher education, artisans, unskilled workers, service workers, and those who are not employed. This order may be interpreted by the hypothesis that the more complex the vocational role the weaker is the disposition to consider' oneself ill. An analysis of this disposition among the groups of respondents who declared similar diseases justifies the assertion that there is no complete identity between those who are 'clinically' ill and those who regard themselves as being ill.

The group under study may be subsumed under three definitions regarding state of health. The first is based on the clinical determination of illness as given by the respondents using medical terms.[12] The second is synonymous with the respondents' tendency to assume the sick role. The third corresponds to the severe limitation of the vocational and domestic roles previously fulfilled. 66.9% of all respondents gave the name of their most important disease. Of these, 59.5% were of the opinion that they had been sufficiently ill to justify a limitation of their normal activities, and 23.9% had actually done so. It should be noted that those most liable to assume the sick role were respondents of the lowest educational level, whereas those who were most resistant were respondents with secondary education. There is a significant similarity between the group representing the lowest educational level and that composed of those with higher education as concerns a divergence between the medical and functional determination of illness. Thus, 81% of respondents in the group with the lowest educational level and 78% in the group with higher education did not severely limit their vocational and domestic obligations, although their claims to be ill were confirmed by their doctors.

We asked our respondents what caused them to consider themselves ill. There seems to be no great differentiation among groups with different educational levels as concerns tolerance of troublesome symptoms and resistance to the negative influence of sickness on vocational obligations. Moreover, a very low proportion – 4.4% – gave positive answers in relation to the latter.

The distribution of such a variable as the time interval between the onset of symptoms and the moment when a person regards himself as ill, allows us to note the following divergencies in the sphere of habits associated with illness. The most similar proportions of respondents considering themselves ill the moment symptoms appeared were in the groups with the lowest and highest education respectively. We may venture the hypothesis that different cultural elements leading to similar behaviour were operating here. The situation is similar with the data regarding the promptness with which the respondents sought professional medical aid. In the group of persons with higher education and in the group of persons non-gainfully employed, the results were the same: 42% visited a doctor immediately upon the appearance of disease symptoms.

The fact that in all socio-occupational groups the proportion of those who did not visit a doctor while suffering from illnesses is the same, is an important and interesting finding. This proportion both for the sample as a whole and for each socio-economic group represented in it amounts to 4%.

To be ill may thus mean:

a) treating oneself as being ill without going to a doctor,

b) visiting a doctor for the purpose of diagnosis and therapy,

c) considering oneself sufficiently ill to justify limiting the fulfilment of one's usual social roles,

d) assuming the sick role in the sense of severely limiting one's obligations.

It is necessary to stress the dual function of the respondent's vocational role. The inability to fulfil this role plays an insignificant part in the complex of causes inclining people to consider themselves ill. At the same time, by applying this criterion we are able to sort out those people who are more severely ill, i.e. those who are unable to perform the tasks assigned them. Visiting a doctor and regarding oneself as ill pertain to a considerably larger group than does withdrawal from fulfilling one's normal social roles.

2. The Manner of Utilizing Health Service Institutions as an Element of the Sick Role

A comparison of the plaçes where respondents usually undergo treatment, where they seek aid first and where they undergo treatment when they cannot or do not wish to limit themselves to only one professional consultation, indicates certain constant dispositions to choose a certain form of medical help. This fixed picture of the different ways of utilizing professional assistance reflects the participation of the various sectors of the health service: state, cooperative or private in the general pool of health services. We noted the marked dominance of the state service in meeting the health needs of Warsaw's inhabitants. On the average, only 5% of the respondents went to private doctors, while 2% took advantage of the services of medical cooperatives. A comparison of the findings concerning the utilization of the various sectors of the health service in 1961 and 1972 (when our research was conducted) supplemented our information on the stability of the manner of utilizing medical care. The comparison shows no essential changes in the manner of utilizing medical institutions, except for one which is undoubtedly advantageous. This is the decline in the number of respondents who do not visit doctors at all; which may attest either to the greater accessibility of medical care or to the growing needs for health care.

It is assumed in the state health service that all those entitled to benefit from it have an equal right to attend more than one physician, if the kind of ailment or the needs of the patient require it. Our data show the greatest difference between persons with elementary and higher than elementary education. The lowest proportion of respondents who visited more than one doctor is to be found in the group with only elementary education (which was also the oldest of the education groups). It may be interpreted in terms of psychological distance from health service institutions. This distance may create greater reluctance among this category to utilize the health serivce in accordance with their needs and even to reduce their needs in this respect.

We may say that the above differences in the manner of using medical care are caused by subjective factors. But the way in which health needs are satisfied also depend on the activities of health service institutions. It is a commonly held opinion that patients with higher social status obtain medicines imported from abroad with greater ease and frequency. We are not concerned here with the relative merits of Polish and foreign medicines. The use of these medicines is of interest to us only as a correlate of the respondents' socio-occupational status. The material gathered bore out the opinion concerning the non-equal distribution of imported medicines. Differentiation was noted in favour of respondents with higher education in relation both to the fact of using such medicines and to the way they were obtained.

The basic health needs of our group of Warsaw inhabitants appear to be met. The percentage of respondents outside the range of the state health service is very low (1%). However, these needs are satisfied in different ways. The higher the educational level the greater the tendency to use alternative forms of medical assistance. Thus respondents with higher education more often utilize the services of all three sectors of the health service and make fuller use of the opportunities afforded by the state health service. An example of the first situation is the way in which child health facilities are used. We asked the respondents which medical institution cared for their children. 92% named the state health service. Respondents who also attended private physicians consisted primarily of those with higher education. From the point of view of social policy it is very important to organize a system of medical care which embraces childern. Our findings establish that this goal has been virtually attained.

The group of respondents utilizing alternative forms of medical care is fairly small, but it may be of interest in analyzing the quality of the services available to different groups in Polish society.

The next example of differences in the provision made for health needs is the way in which advantage is taken of hospitals. In Poland hospitals are owned and run by the state. Their services, which are guaranteed to all citizens entitled to social security, are in principle distributed on a territorial basis. Our data show that this principle is observed differently in various socio-occupational groups. In our sample regional hospitals were utilized by 32% of persons with higher education and by 66% of the group of unskilled workers. [13]

The Attitudes Associated with Receiving Medical Care [14]

Here we proceeded from the assumption that the existence of a free, universally accessible health service does not eliminate the possibility of distortions in the manner in which its benefits are utilized. Our definition of the attitude to utilizing professional medical care was related to the factors which may hinder people from using the health service. We presented our respondents with a list of reasons why people delay visiting a doctor as long as possible. We asked them which reasons operated in their case. The reasons given may be grouped into three types, as follows:

1) those associated with the respondents' vocational and family roles,
2) those associated with the respondents' general attitude to medicine, i.e. their degree of willingness to make use of medical institutions, degree of confidence in doctors and medicine,
3) those associated with the subject's assessment of the accessibility of state health service institutions.

No essential differences were observed among the educational groups as regards factors constituting subjective obstacles to utilizing medical care. But there was a difference in the impact of particular factors on the delay in taking advantage of medical care. The strongest influence was exerted by the factor we describe as 'the anti-institutional attitude to medicine'. It is composed of such elements as: tolerance of symptoms, confidence in the possibility of successful treatment at home, reluctance to turn to doctors with trivial complaints, embarrassment before physicians and a proneness to regard treatment as more troublesome than the disease.

As we know, two spheres of phenomena compete in moulding the individual's medical behaviour. One of them is built into the cultural characteristics of the group; the other is created and promoted by the representatives of official medicine.[15] Our sample of Warsaw inhabitants confirmed this general rule. As indicated, the anti-institutional attitude to medicine constitutes the greatest cause of delay in taking advantage of medical aid. At the same time findings regarding the intensity with which medical institutions are utilized point to the competing influences of medicine and of cultural factors.

The literature concerning the utilization of health service institutions devotes much space to the role of the experience acquired by patients using the services provided by these institutions. These experiences are considered either as negative or as positive stimulators of medical behaviour. The complex of factors shaping a person's attitude to making use of the services of professional medicine is at least to a certain extent moulded by the experience acquired from his contact with health service institutions.

The respondents' demands upon medical institutions rise with their educational level. Most of the complaints in all educational groups pertain to the organizational aspects of the outpatient service: the length of time spent waiting for admission to a doctor and in what conditions, the possibility of consulting a specialist, the amount of time and professional attention devoted to the patients, the registration personnel's manner in dealing with patients, the way laboratory tests are conducted, the cooperation between specialists in different fields. Patient-doctor relations were regarded as requiring least change of all aspects of functioning of medical institutions. We base this conclusion on the respondents' assessment of the physicians' attitude to those of the patient's troubles arising out of his illness, their general manner towards the patient and also the behaviour of the auxiliary personnel.

The opinions of beneficiaries of the state health service may concern not only the functioning of this institution.

We were interested in discovering whether in the social consciousness the state health service institutions provide equally good services for all those who are supposed to benefit from them, and consequently gathered such information as would serve as an indicator of the degree to which people felt they enjoyed equal opportunities in the satisfaction of their health needs. It appeared that the higher the educational level, the greater the number of persons saying that not all those who are entitled to make use of state medical services have the same opportunity of receiving effective treatment. Thus 19% of the group with only elementary education held this opinion, as compared to 52% of the group with higher education.

SUMMING UP

The dependent variables appearing in this investigation may be arranged according to their capacity to differentiate the group under study. The following is such an arrangement in ascending order of capacity to differentiate:

1) access to state health service benefits; nearly all the investigated population (99%) was covered by health insurance;
2) utilization of professional medical services; 96% of those respondents who fell ill made use of such services;
3) utilization of state health service; in the out-patient service the state sector dominates over the others – private and cooperative;
4) adoption of the sick-role; in all socio-occupational and educational groups divergencies were observed between the cilnical and functional definitions of illness;
5) attitudes towards taking advantage of professional medical care; the role of particular factors in shaping such attitudes varied and different attitudes were observed among particular social categories;
6) forms of satisfaction of health needs in the in- and out-patient services (members of the group with higher education more often employed the services of more than one physician, use imported medicines and attend different kinds of hospitals);
7) evaluation of the functioning of the out-patient service – criticism increases with the educational level;
8) assessment of the degree of equality or non-equality of opportunies for successful treatment for all those who are medically insured (respondents with higher education make fullest use of the health service in all its sectors and at the same time see the greatest discrepancies in these opportunities).

It turns out that the way in which the basic out-patient services are made use of is similar in all educational groups. In in-patient medical service a differentiation is observed in the manner and degree in which hospitals are made use of; and, as concerns out-patient services, there is a differentiation in the course of the therapy.

Besides in the manner of satisfying health needs, we observed divergencies in the evaluation of opportunities for effective therapy. Respondents with higher education made more intensive use of the health service, and at the same time their perception of such divergencies was keener.

The way in which the sick-role is fulfilled and the attitudes towards seeking medical aid may be regarded as indicators in analyzing the similarities and differences between educational and socio-occupational groups. We can say that in medical behaviour we are confronted with a new type of differentiation. Differentiation in habits associated with illness is not always associated with stratification variables.

The variations observed in the behaviour associated with illness incline us to seek types of sick-roles which may differentiate a population without reference to stratification.

We confirmed that 'being ill' may designate different things. The fulfilment of a 'sick-role' is the strongest criterion of the existence of illness.

REFERENCES

1 A. Malewski (ed.), *Zagadnienia psychologii społecznej* (*Problems of Social Psychology*), PWN, Warszawa 1962.

2 These topics are covered in: A. Titkow, *Zachowania medyczne. Systematyzacja problematyki* (*Medical Behaviour. Systematization of the Issues*). This work was written in the Social Structures Study Group, Institute of Philosophy and Sociology, Section for Social Health Problems, Warszawa 1973.

3 E. Freidson, 'The Sociology of Medicine. A Trend Report and Bibliography', *Current Sociology* X/XI (1961–62).

4 The term 'illness behaviour' would appear to be too narrow to express the area of interest to us.

5 M. Sokołowska, *Zdrowie a społeczeństwo. Zarys wybranych problemów* (*Health and Society. Survey of Selected Topics*). This work was written in the Social Struc-

tures Study Group, Institute of Philosophy and Sociology, Section for Social Health Problems, Polish Academy of Sciences, 1972.

[6] See Note 2.

[7] Social classes are categories which are culturally no less differentiated than ethnic groups. The use of this category enables us to discover the essential mechanisms influencing the behaviour of individuals, including medical behaviour. This is not only a question of financial standing, which is a direct result of the socio-occupational position occupied. Several studies have shown that above a certain moderate level, rises in income influence medical behaviour to a very slight degree. In addition, the free medical care available in some countries compensates for differences in material circumstances. However the secondary consequences of an individual's social position are important (position here is used in a broader sense than that represented by financial circumstances). As secondary consequences we should consider access to certain social resources, e.g. social services or sources of information, and also the individual's own evaluation of his social position and its socio-psychological consequences. These hypotheses were formulated concerning the links between the secondary consequences of occupying a defined socio-occupational position; for example the evaluation mentioned above is held to influence ways of using sources of information and social services.

[8] "The attitude of a certain person towards a certain object or category of objects, or towards a certain situation or class of situations is the sum of the relatively permanent evaluating-emotional inclinations which are directed by him towards this object and his relatively permanent conceptions as to the properties of this object together with his relatively permanent inclinations to behave in a certain way towards the object or situation." S. Nowak, 'Pojęcie postawy w teoriach i stosowanych badaniach społecznych', in: *Teorie postaw* ('The Concept of Attitude in Theory and Applied Social Studies', in: *Theories of Attitudes*), PWN, Warszawa 1973, p. 23.

[9] By 'social consumption fund' we understand the total of resources and services with which citizens are provided by the state and social institutions free of charge or at a subsidized rate. What we were interested in was whether and to what degree the social consumption fund affects the existing differences in the respective living standards of particular social groups and strata.

[10] See Note 9.

[11] See M. Sokołowska and J. Bejnarowicz, 'Socjolog a pojęcie stanu zdrowia' ('The Sociologist and the Concept of State of Health'), *Studia Socjologiczne* 3 (1973).

[12] If the respondent could not give the proper name of a given disease, the interviewer asked him for a description of the symptoms and the treatment used. The answers were coded by a physician.

[13] It is a common opinion that the hospitals to which patients are directed according to their place of residance, provide services of inferior quality, and that it is difficult to be admitted to the university clinics. In order to avoid the localization

principle in hospital admittance it is necessary according to this opinion, to undertake special endeavours and especially to be in a position to contact the relevant physician.

[14] By 'attitude' we understand here factors of an emotional-evaluative character which hamper people in seeking profesional medical care.

[15] E. Freidson, 'Client Control and Medical Practice', *American Journal of Sociology* LXV (1960).

II. THE TRANSFORMATION OF MEDICAL INTERVENTION

ETHICAL AND EXISTENTIAL DEVELOPMENTS IN CONTEMPORANEOUS AMERICAN MEDICINE: THEIR IMPLICATIONS FOR CULTURE AND SOCIETY*

RENÉE C. FOX

Department of Sociology, University of Pennsylvania, Philadelphia, Pa., U.S.A.

Contemporaneous Western medicine is often depicted as a vast body of scientific knowledge, technical skills, medicaments and machinery wielded by physician-led teams of hospital-based professionals and paraprofessionals, garbed in uniforms of starched white, surgical green and auxiliary pink or blue. Underlying this image is the conception that medicine is shaped primarily by scientific and technological advances, and that its major impetus derives from a highly organized collective effort vigorously to preserve life, by attaining progressive mastery over illness and preventable death.

However commonplace and accurate this notion of modern medicine may be in some regards, it is distorted and obsolete in others. It does not take into account a new and important set of developments in present-day medicine that seem to be gaining momentum. Over the course of the past fifteen years, in a number of European and American societies, concerned interest in ethical and existential issues related to biomedical progress and to the delivery of medical care has become both more manifest and legitimate in medical circles, and in other professional and organized lay groups, as well. This is a phenomenon that merits sociological attention for it suggests that a serious re-examination of certain basic cultural assumptions on which modern medicine is premised may be taking place.

This paper will identify some of the forms in which these moral and metaphysical problems are currently being raised in the medical sector of American (U.S.A.) society. It will also essay an interpretive analysis of the broader socio-cultural implications of the more general re-evaluative process that we believe is occurring in this fashion.

> Recent advances in biology and medicine make it increasingly clear that we are rapidly acquiring greater powers to modify and perhaps control the capacities and activities of men by direct intervention into and manipulation of their bodies and minds. Certain means are already in use or at hand – for example, organ transplantation, prenatal diagnosis of genetic defects, and electrical stimulation of the brain. Others await the solution of relatively minor technical problems... still others depend upon further basic research...
>
> While holding forth the promise of continued improvements in medicine's abilities to cure disease and alleviate suffering, these developments also pose profound questions and troublesome problems. There are questions about who shall benefit from and who shall pay for the use of new technologies... There will be questions about the use and abuse of power... There will be questions about our duties to future generations and about the limits on what we can and cannot do to the unborn... We shall face questions concerning the desirable limits of the voluntary manipulation of our own bodies and minds... We shall face questions about the impact of biomedical technology on our social institutions... We shall face serious questions of law and legal institutions... (and) problems of public policy...
>
> ...as serious and vexing as these piactical problems may be, there is yet another matter more profound. The biomedical technologies work directly on man's biological nature, including those aspects long regarded (as) most distinctively human... The impact on our ideas of free will, birth, and death, and the good life is likely to be even more staggering than any actual manipulation performed with the new technologies. These are matters of great moment and we urgently need to take counsel from some of our best minds...

The statement quoted above was not made by a physician, a scientist, or a philosopher. It was delivered by the Honorable Walter F. Mondale of Minnesota, a member of the United States Senate. He made these remarks from the floor of the Senate in 1971, as he introduced a bill to establish a National Advisory Commission on Health Science and Society. The measure was intended to provide for "study and evaluation of the ethical, social and legal implications of advances in biomedical research and technology". What is particularly significant about the Mondale proposal (which was unanimously passed as a resolution by the Senate) is that it demonstrates that involvement with the issues it cites is not confined to medical and academic milieux. Rather, these matters have entered political and public domains in American society.

The specific advances in biology and medicine to which Mondale alludes are those most generally invoked in the various contexts where such ethical, existential and social questions are pondered. Actual and anticipated developments in genetic engineering and counselling, life support systems, birth technology, population control, the implantation of human, animal and artificial organs, as well as in the modification and control of human thought and behavior are principal foci of concern. Within this framework, special attention is concentrated on the implications of amniocentesis (a procedure for detecting certain genetic disorders *in utero*),[1] *in vitro* fertilization, the prospect of cloning (the asexual reproduction of an unlimited number of genetically identical individuals from a single parent), organ transplantation, the use of the artificial kidney machine, the development of an artificial heart, the modalities of the intensive care unit, the practice of psychosurgery, and the introduction of psychotropic drugs. Cross-cutting the consideration being given to these general and concrete areas of biomedical development, there is marked preoccupation with the ethicality of human experimentation under various conditions, with the proper definition of death and the human treatment of the dying, and with the presumed right of every individual and group to health and adequate health care. Certain moral and metaphysical themes recur in the discussions of all these aspects of the so-called new biology and medicine. Problems of uncertainty, meaning, of the quality of life and death, of scarcity, equity and distributive justice, of freedom and coersion, dignity and degradation, solidarity and societal community, and of the vigor with which one ought to intervene in the human condition are repeatedly mentioned.

The media and agencies through which these concerns are expressed are manifold. Articles and editorials on these topics not only appear frequently in medical and scientific journals,[2] but also in popular magazines and daily newspapers. In the course of the week of July 8 to July 15, 1973,[3] for example, *The New York Times* published the following relevant items: two bulletin-type articles on the performance of two new heart transplants; two articles on recent cases of 'euthanasia' or 'mercy killing' that raise questions about the 'right to die' and 'death with dignity'; a long article reporting and analyzing a decision rendered by the Wayne County Circuit Court in Michigan that experimental psychosurgery may not be performed on persons confined against their will in state institutions, even when such a person's consent for this surgery is formally obtained; two feature articles with photographs, and an editorial on the ethical and legal implications of a case under investigation by three Federal agencies and a Senate subcommittee, in which it is alleged that two mentally retarded Black girls, ages 12 and 14, were sterilized by a federally funded family planning clinic in Montgomery, Alabama, without either their informed consent or that of their parents; another article with byline, announcing that based on comparable cases, the American Civil Liberties Union was filing a suit in Federal District Court, seeking to void as unconstitutional a North Carolina law allowing sterilization of 'mentally defective' persons; a substantial article summarizing a report published in a journal of biomedical ethics concerning five experiments on human beings funded by grants from divisions of the Public Health Service that raise "disturbing ethical questions"; an article by one of the paper's major medical writers on the "complex and not always obvious issues of medical research ethics" that have surfaced in a "recent spate" of stories of "abuse, real or potential", evoking "newly critical looks at medical ethics (by) Government and private citizens and new proposals for more effective controls"; and, finally, an article by the same writer on the redesigning of a national blood policy that is now underway in the United States with the goal of achieving and all-volunteer donor system in the next two years.

The number of books that have been published on such subjects and themes in the past ten years is impressive.[4] Leading the list, in saliency and frequency, is a group of books on death and dying.[5] The most famous of these, writen by a psychiatrist, Dr. Elizabeth

Kübler-Ross, and published in 1969, had sold over 100,000 copies in the paperback edition alone by the end of 1972. Presenting first-hand case materials based on her intensive work with incurably ill and dying patients, Dr. Kübler-Ross delineates what she considers to be the five psychological stages through which a dying person characteristically evolves. She both explicitly and implicitly affirms that persons passing through these 'final stages of life', can be our 'teacher(s)', helping medical professionals, and all of us, not to "shy away from the 'hopelessly' sick", as she feels we are inclined to do in American society. Those who 'get closer' to the dying, she asserts, will not only "help them during their final hours... they will learn much about the functioning of the human mind, the unique human aspects of our existence, and will emerge from the experience enriched... perhaps with fewer anxieties about their own finality".[6] Less directly, Dr Kübler-Ross' book also evokes questions about the rationality and humanity of our medical and cultural propensity to do everything possible to 'save' and prolong life. If there is a phenomenon akin to a 'death and dying movement' occurring in the United States, as we believe there may be, then Elizabeth Kübler-Ross is one of its charismatic leaders.[7]

Another important collection of books that has appeared in the last few years is devoted to the ethics and legal aspects of biomedical research on human subjects.[8] In all these books, the problem of the rights and adequate protection of subjects looms large, as does the question of how best to establish surveillance and social control over the activities of investigators, without unduly impeding research. A great deal of consideration is given to the necessity and difficulties of obtaining truly informed and voluntary consent from subjects. Special attention is focussed on candidates for research who are already subject to particular kinds of dependence, disability or constraint, such as children, persons who are mentally retarded or mentally ill, prisoners, the poor and the minimally educated. The question of what constitutes the most just allocation of limited and costly experimental therapies is debated in these works, along with the issue of when a society may expose some of its members to risk or harm, in order to seek benefits for them, for others, or for the society as a whole. Each of these volumes cites and examines problematic instances of human experimentation that are known to have taken place.

Two other types of relevant books are being published in significant numbers: those dealing with ethical and existential aspects of specific biomedical developments, and those that treat a broad range of such moral and metaphysical issues as they apply to numerous medical phenomena. Examples of the former include: *Abortion: Law, Choice and Morality* by Daniel Callahan, *Physical Control of the Mind* by José Delgado, *Mankind Evolving* (a work on genetics) by Theodosius Dobzhansky, *Behavior Control* by Perry London, *Give and Take* (on tissue transplantation) by Francis D. Moore, *Contraception* by John T. Noonan, Jr., and *The Gift Relationship* (a comparative study of blood donation systems in Great Britain and the United States) by Richard M. Titmuss. Some instances of the more general type of work are: *Who Shall Live?* prepared by H. J. Cadbury *et al.* for the American Friends Service Committee, *Updating Life and Death: Essays in Ehtics and Medicine*, edited by Donald R. Cutler, *A God Within* by René Dubos, *The American Health Empire: Power, Profits and Politics* by Barbara and John Ehrenreich, *Moral Responsibility: Situation Ethics at Work* by Joseph Fletcher, *Biology and the Future of Man* by Philip Handler, *In Critical Condition: The Crisis in America's Health Care* by Edward M. Kennedy, *Life, Death and the Doctor* by Louis Lasagna, *Human Aspects of Biomedical Innovation*, edited by Everett Mendelsohn and colleagues, *Chance and Necessity* by Jacques Monod (translated from the original French edition), *Fabricated Man* and also *The Patient as a Person* by Paul Ramsey, *The Biological Time Bomb* by Gordon Taylor, and *Ethical Issues in Medicine*, edited by E. Fuller Torrey.[9]

A number of social patterns applicable to this flow of articles and books are worthy of note. To begin with, the authors of these works come from a broad spectrum of fields, including journalism, politics, the law, the clergy, philosophy, ethics, theology, social science, social work, nursing and psychiatry, as well as medicine and biology. Secondly, a considerable amount of the research and reflection on which these writings are based has been sponsored or supported by established private foundations like the Ford, Robert Wood Johnson, Joseph P. Kennedy, Jr., Rockefeller and Russel Sage Foundations, by scholarly bodies, such as the American Academy of Arts and Sciences, the New York Academy of Sciences, the United States National Academy of Sciences, and by some government agencies, notably, several branches of the National Institutes of Health and the National Endowment for the Humanities.

What is perhaps more striking is the fact that the interest and work that these publications reflect have brought into being a network of new organizations whose principal *raison d'être* is to deal with these matters. Among the most prominent in the United States are the Institute of Society, Ethics and the Life Sciences in Hastings-on-the-Hudson, New York, the Society for Health and Human Values in Philadelphia, the Foundation of Thanatology in New York City, the Euthanasia Society of America and the Euthanasia Educational Fund, both in New York City, the Committee on the Life Sciences and Social Policy of the National Research Council, a division of the National Academy of Sciences in Washington, D.C., and the Joseph and Rose Kennedy Institute for the Study of Human Reproduction and Bioethics, located at Georgetown University in Washington. With the exception of the two euthanasia societies, these groups, and others like them, have all been founded since 1969.[10]

Mention has been made of the pending creation of a National Advisory Commission on Health Science and Society in the United States Congress, for which Senator Walter Mondale has been lobbying. In addition, the Health Subcommittees both of the Senate and the House of Representatives have been transformed by their respective chairmen, Senator Edward M. Kennedy of Massachusetts and Representative Paul G. Rogers of Florida, into groups that are actively engaged in conducting investigations and hearings on medical issues of social, ethical and existential import, in raising public consciousness about these matters, and in proposing legislation and other control mechanisms bearing upon them. It is of some consequence to observe that the medico-moral concerns to which Mondale, Kennedy and Rogers are addressing themselves have sufficient public resonance to enhance the political following and prestige of these men in the eyes of their local and national constituencies. The most important piece of legislation that has thus far resulted from their activities is the National Research Act (H.R. 7724) which was passed by both houses of Congress, and signed into law by President Nixon on July 12, 1974. Title II of this act established a temporary two-year National Commission for the Protection of Human Subjects of Biomedical and Behavioral Research. The commission, an advisory body to the Department of Health, Education, and Welfare (HEW), is composed of eleven members who were named by HEW Secretary Caspar Weinberger on September 10, 1974. Their task is to study a number of ethical issues set forth in the law. These include fetal research, the problem of obtaining informed voluntary consent for investigations in which children, prisoners, or persons who are mentally ill or retarded are asked to participate as subjects, and the ethics of psychosurgery. When the two-year life span of the commission is ended, a permanent council to deal with these matters will come into being.

Their growing numbers and diverse backgrounds notwithstanding, the scholars, scientists, medical and legal practitioners, authors, foundation officials, organization members and legislators seriously involved in considering ethical and existential aspects of biomedicine can be said to constitute a closely knit 'social circle'. Not only do they belong to overlapping groups and read each other's work attentively, but they participate in many of the same formal meetings, meet informally, communicate with one another through correspondence and by telephone, call upon one another as consultants, and recommend each other for relevant assignments and honors.[11]

The new institutional forms that are being summoned forth by these developments in contemporaneous medicine extend beyond the establishment of pertinent contemplative and action-oriented groups. Another kind of emergent phenomenon is the gradual formation of 'bioethics', an incipient new discipline. Its contours are still not clear. In the words of Daniel Callahan, "Most of its practitioners have wandered into the field from somewhere else, more or less inventing it as they go. Its vague and problematic status in philosophy and theology is matched by its even more shaky standing in the life sciences".[12] Callahan goes on to advocate that if bioethics is to develop into a full and accepted field, it should be interdisciplinary and problem- and case-focussed in the following regards:

> ...so designed, and its practitioners so trained that it will directly – at whatever cost to disciplinary elegance – serve those physicians and biologists whose position demands that they make practical decisions. This requires, ideally, a number of ingredients as part of the training... of the bioethicist: sociological understanding of the medical and biological communities; psycho-

> logical understanding of the kinds of needs felt by researchers and clinicians, patients and physicians, and the varieties of pressures to which they are subject; historical understanding of the sources of regnant value theories and common practices; requisite scientific training; awareness of and facility with the usual methods of ethical analysis as understood in the philosophical and theological communities... and personal exposure to the kinds of ethical problems which arise in medicine and biology.[13]

Although bioethics is still a tentative field, and its definition and legitimacy are under discussion, a comprehensive *Encyclopedia of Bioethics* is already being prepared. Its editor (Warren T. Reich, a former theology professor at Catholic University) and his staff are based at the Kennedy Institute of Georgetown University. Their advisory editors are drawn from multiple university, foundation and government milieux. And the project is financed by the Kennedy Foundation and the National Endowment for the Humanities.[14]

Quite apart from the prognosis for bioethics as a discipline, a new conception of medical ethics seems to be unfolding in the medical profession. Increasingly, medical ethics is being viewed less exclusively as a code of professional etiquette. It is coming to be regarded as a component virtually of all medical decision-making and to include the questions of how such decisions should be made and who should participate in them, as well as what ideally ought to be done in given cases. Even the conservative American Medical Association has expanded its ethical program to encompass these broader considerations, along with the dilemmas posed by recent biomedical advances.

But it is in medical schools that one sees the most significant activity in this regard. In 1970, for example, under the aegis of Drs. Robert M. Veatch and Willard Gaylin, both members of the Institute of Society, Ethics and the Life Sciences, the Columbia College of Physicians and Surgeons launched an experimental Medical Ethics Program.[15] This Program included lectures, seminars, clinical case conferences, dinner-discussion meetings and intensive workshops for students in every stage of medical school training. An internship in medical ethics for several fourth-year students was also created; an interdisciplinary seminar on 'the new biology and the law' that brought medical students together with students from Columbia Law School and the Union Theological

Seminary was organized; and sessions on medical ethics for interested faculty and clinical staff were arranged. This Program has had wide repercussions. For, its staff has made a survey of the teaching of medical ethics in medical schools throughout the country, has developed bibliographies and case studies that are available upon request, has acted as consultants to other medical schools, and, in June 1972, organized a National Conference on the Teaching of Medical Ethics. Although their survey revealed that in the curricula of most medical schools medical ethical issues are presented largely on an informal and somewhat *ad hoc* basis, the response that the Medical Ethics Program staff has experienced "suggests a rapidly developing interest in the (formal) teaching of medical ethics".[16] By October 1971, they had already been consulted by 29 American medical schools, in addition to faculty in biology, philosophy, religion, law and social science departments and about 150 representatives from medical school faculties attended the National Conference on the Teaching of Medical Ethics.

In our view, one of the most significant patterns that Veatch and Gaylin report is that their whole undertaking was initiated by medical students:

> Early in 1970 a group of students, upon hearing a lecture pointing out the ethical implications of the judgments made in the practice of psychiatry, approached the curriculum committee of the school and members of the Institute of Society, Ethics and the Life Sciences and asked that a full program be established, one which would make ethical and social perspectives an integral part of their medical education...[17]

This is consistent with what we believe to be a fundamental shift in the outlook of American medical students. It has been remarked that medical students of the late 1960's and early 1970's appear to be more socially concerned than their predecessors. They are especially outspoken about the inadequacies and inequities in the nation's system of health care delivery, about the responsibility that they feel the established medical profession bears for the existence of these deficiencies and injustices, and about their own determination to play an active role as physicians in eliminating them. How deep these concerns and commitments of the 'new' medical student go, and how enduring they will prove to be is a matter of some debate not only medical educators, but also among students themselves (who are inclined to be self-critical in this, as well as in other matters). Whatever their long-term import, these medical student tendencies are sufficiently notable to have elicited continuing discussion about whether they are 'authentic' or 'largely rhetorical', and whether or not they will persist under the impact of students' medical educational experiences and the demands that their subsequent medical careers will make upon them.[18] Accompanying the ostensible social consciousness of present-day medical students, and integrally related to it, is their manifest interest in ethical and existential aspects of medicine. Along with their concern about a more just allocation of material and immaterial medical resources in American society, one of the areas in which students' moral and metaphysical interests are most apparent is that of 'death and dying'. Their orientation is distinctly different from the attitudes towards death and the ambiance surrounding in that predominated in American medical schools twenty years ago. In a recent article, we have portrayed the contrast as follows:[19]

> ...In the medical school climate of the 1950's... faculty virtually never raised questions with students like 'what is death?', 'why death?' or 'in what deeper senses, if any, does death differ from life?' Even in situations conducive to such querying – notably, the anatomy laboratory, the autopsy, or in the face of students' early confrontation with terminally ill patients – instructors rarely initiated such discussions. And if a student made a timorous effort to do so, he was likely to be silenced by classmates and faculty alike with the quip, 'that's too philosophical'. Decoded, this meant 'the matters of which you speak are not sufficiently rational, objective, scientific or pragmatic to fall within the proper domain of medicine, or of truly professional behavior'. It was also characteristic of this decade that (medical students and their teachers) were more inclined to speak euphemistically about the death of a patient – 'he (she) expired', 'passed on', or 'was transferred to Ward X' – than straightforwardly to state that death had occurred. In sharp contrast to such medical attitudes in the 1950's (at least in academic milieux where new physicians were being trained and scientific research emphasized), the late 1960's and early 1970's appear very 'philosophical', indeed...

In addition to new organizations, new intellectual disciplines and new perspectives on the part of medical students and educators, certain spokesmen for medical practitioners, some legislators and sectors of the lay public, the ethical and existential refocussing of medicine has been accompanied by three other institutional responses. These consist of new guidelines, or codes, several moratoria, and a number of legal decisions and statutes.

Perhaps the most momentous guideline issued thus far is the new criterion for judging a person dead that was formulated and proposed by Harvard Medical School's Ad Hoc Committee to Examine the Definition of Brain Death, chaired by Dr. Henry K. Beecher.[20] (The Committee consisted of nine physicians, a lawyer, an historian of science and a theologian). The Harvard Report opened with the statement that their "primary purpose (was) to define irreversible coma as a new criterion for death", and that there were two reasons why there was "a need for a definition":

> (1) Improvements in resuscitative and supportive measures have led to increased efforts to save those who are desperately injured. Sometimes these efforts have only partial success so that the result is an individual whose heart continues to beat but whose brain is irreversibly damaged. The burden is great on patients who suffer permanent loss of intellect, on their families, on the hospitals, and on those in need of hospital beds already occupied by these comatose patients. (2) Obsolete criteria for the definition of death can lead to controversy in obtaining organs for transplantation.

From there, the Report went on to identify and describe in detail the major characteristics of a state of irreversible coma, which indicates a "*permanently* (italicized in the Report) nonfunctioning brain". These are: "unreceptivity and unresponsivity (to) externally applied stimuli and inner needs"; "no spontaneous muscular movements or spontaneous respiration"; and "the absence of elicitable responses". A flat or isoelectric electroencephalogram is held to be "of great confirmatory value". Furthermore, it is advocated that all the tests involved in these various determinations (which not only assess higher brain functions, but brain stem and spinal cord acitvity and spontaneous respiration, as well) should be "repeated at least 24 hours later with no change". In effect, the Committee has recommended that the traditional method used by physicians for ascertaining and pronouncing death – the total cessation of all vital signs, that is, heart beat and respiration – be replaced by criteria for 'cerebral death' or 'brain death'. Although this proposal has evoked a certain amount of commentary and some disquietude both in lay and professional circles, by and large, it has been well received, particularly in the medical community. "It is remarkable", comments Dr. David D. Rutstein of Harvard Medical School, with concern, that "a revolution in our cultural concept of death... this major ethical change... has occurred right before our eyes, and that this change is more and more widely accepted with little public discussion of its significance. This new definition... raises more questions that it answers".[21]

A second important set of guidelines that have been set forth are those "relating to moral and ethical aspects of clinical investigation", established in 1966 by the National Institutes of Health (NIH) and Public Health Service (PHS).[22] More specifically, this policy statement mandated that all clinical research involving human subjects supported by the NIH or PHS should be submitted to peer review by a committee of colleagues from the principal investigator's institution. That review should address itself to the rights and welfare of the human subjects involved, to the appropriateness of methods used to secure their informed consent, and to the risk-benefit ratio that the research entails. In 1971, these requirements were extended to all research on human subjects supported by any agency of the Department of Health, Education and Welfare (HEW), the parent organization of the NIH and PHS. It is expected that over the next two years, the federal commission on ethics created by the National Research Act will supplement these general guidelines with more specific recommendations concerning psychosurgery, as well as clinical research on the fetus, the abortus, children, prisoners, and on the institutionalized mentally disabled. In principle, the commission has no regulatory authority, and its guidelines apply only to research funded by HEW. But its *de facto* influence on HEW and also on other agencies is expected to be considerable. For, the act requires that whenever the commision submits a recommendations to the Secretary of HEW, within 60 days, the must publish it in the *Federal Register* for comment. No more than 180 days later, the Secretary must act upon the recommendation, and if he decides to reject it, he must give his reasons for doing so, in writing. Although legally, the commission's deliberations are only relevant to research funded by HEW, many members of Congress are eager to have guidelines developed that are broadly applicable to other governmental organizations. And the commision has been asked to devise a mechanism to make the rules pertaining to human experimentation uniform.

In addition to guidelines advocating a new operational definition of death published by a physician-led interdisciplinary university group, and those setting up a peer review system promulgated by the foremost government agency sponsoring biomedical research, a third type of policy statement has been set forth. This concerns a formal determination of where, on the experiment-therapy spectrum a therapeutic innovation can be said to fall at a given phase in its development, and how and when, in the light of its status, it ought (or ought not) be utilized. The best example of this sort of guideline are the statements on human cardiac transplantation issued by several different medical associations and government-affiliated medical groups.[23] The overall judgment on heart transplants that emerges from these position papers is that, "The procedure of total cardiac replacement is so formidable and uncertainties about the duration of life after replacement are so great that physicians may be expected to be conservative about recommending it for an individual patient". It cannot "as yet be regarded as an accepted or of therapy, or even an heroic one. It must be clearly viewed for what it is, a scientific exploration of the unknown, only the very first step of which is the actual feat of transplanting an organ". For this reason, it is maintained, "it may be reasonably assumed that imminent death will be the basic criterion for total cardiac replacement, at least in the near future". The "primary justification" for heart transplants at this time is deemed to be the "new knowledge of benefit to others in our society" that may come from it. In light of this view, and in recognition of the fact that "theologians, lawyers and other public-spirited persons, as well as physicians are discussing with deep concern the many new questions raised by the transplantation of vital organs", specific recommendations are made about the proper treatment of donors and recipients, the types of medical center qualified to undertake the operation, and the appropriate reporting of a transplantation both in medical journals and the mass media.

This period of 'deep concern' about the issues raised by human experimentation and by biomedical advances like the increasing ability to maintain certain signs of life artificially, or to transplant human organs has also generated moratoria of several kinds. The first of these is what we have called clinical moratoria: the suspension of the use of a still experimental medical or surgical procedure on patients.[24] This type of moratorium usually occurs in the stage of development of a new treatment when the uncertainties and risks associated with it are very high and become starkly apparent. Often, the patient mortality rate seems unbearable or unjustifiable. Pressure for such a moratorium can come from physician-investigators' own reactions to the situation and/or from 'external' sources (from their colleagues, the institution in which they work, patients and their families, organizations sponsoring their research and, less frequently, from the courts).

One important instance of such a moratorium (that we have personally had an opportunity to study) is the virtual cessation of human heart transplants.[25] As compared with 1968, for example, which was heralded by the mass media as the 'Year of the Transplant', because 105 cardiac transplantations were performed throughout the world in that year alone, 1973 was a time when only an occasional heart transplant was done. The very high mortality rate of the persons who have undergone this procedure and their relatively short period of survival have been primary factors in the demise of the operation. The pressures that resulted in this moratorium came principally from within the medical profession itself, from prospective donors, recipients and their families, and from the mass media's continual publishing of heart transplant 'box scores'.

We have already identified another, more recent moratorium enacted into state law this July in a Michigan Circuit Court. Here, three judges rendered a unanimous opinion against the experimental performance of psychosurgery on persons involuntarily confined to state institutions. The judges based their opinion on the fact that brain surgery to attempt the correction of behavioral abnormalities like murderous aggression is "clearly experimental, poses substantial danger to research subjects, and carries substantial unknown risks", such as the blunting of emotions, the deadening of memory, the reduction of affect and limitation of ability to generate new ideas. Furthermore, the judges reasoned, there is "no persuasive showing" that, in its present stage of development, this neurosurgical procedure would have its intended beneficial effects.

In addition to the "unfavorable risk-benefit ratio" involved, it was concluded that the procedure ought not to be performed in the kind of case under consideration, because an involuntarily confined mental patient, living in an "inherently coercive atmosphere", has been intrinsically deprived of the basic conditions that are requisite to voluntary consent.

This ruling is related to another type of moratorium that is being considered: the halting of medical experimentation on certain categories of persons. In this case, what is being contemplated is calling a moratorium on research conducted on 'captives' of the State – prisoners, as well as involuntarily committed mental patients – in order to provide optimal conditions for reevaluating the circumstances, if any, under which such research might be justified. The major impetus for this moratorium is coming from the Senate Health Subcommittee, while a serious review of research on prisoners, mentally ill and mentally retarded persons and on children is underway at the National Institutes of Health as part of their general inquiry into ethical guidelines for clinical research.

The federal commission on ethics created by the National Research Act has also been asked to examine this question.

A last genre of moratorium that is pending in the National Institutes of Health is one that advocates forbidding a kind of experimentation with fetuses that has not yet been attempted by medical scientists working in the United States: 'in vitro' fertilization, entailing the implantation into a woman's uterine cavity of human egg cells that have been fertilized by human sperm in the test tube. The intent of this moratorium is to prevent the advance of this line of biomedical research from the animal to the human level of experimentation, in order to avert the social, moral and metaphysical problems that it is anticipated would ensue from the successful application of a 'new method for making babies'.[28]

A final indicator of the degree to which not only the American medical profession, but the society at large has been deliberating ethical and existential issues associated with biomedicine is some of the legislation concerned with life and death matters that has been drafted in the last few years. The Kansas Death Statute, the Uniform Anatomical Gift Act and the United States Supreme Court decision on the Texas abortion case of *Roe versus Wade* represent three such major pieces of legislation.

In 1970, the State of Kansas adopted 'An Act relating to and defining death', which was the first attempt legislatively to reformulate the standards for determining death.[29] The Kansas statute sets forth and grants equal validity to two "alternative definitions of death": the traditional notion that a person is "medically and legally dead" if a physician determines "there is the absence of spontaneous respiratory and cardiac function and... attempts at resuscitation are considered hopeless"; and the new, irreversible coma criterion of death, which turns on the absence of spontaneous brain function if during "reasonable attempts" either to maintain or restore spontaneous circulatory or respiratory function, "it appears that further attempts at resuscitation or supportive maintenance will not succeed". The statute has received a great deal of attention. It has served as a model for similar legislation enacted in the state of Maryland in 1972, as well as for statutes now under consideration in a number of other jurisdictions. It has also been vigorously criticized for its dualistic approach to death, for the fact that it implies that a special definition of death, 'brain death', has been developed to facilitate cadaveric organ transplantation, and because it mixes the question "when is the patient dead"? with "when may the doctor turn off the respirator"? and "when may a patient be allowed to die"?.[30]

The Uniform Anatomical Gift Act is a statute designed to insure the provision of a more adequate supply of cadaver organs for transplantation than has been possible under traditional American law.[31] In this Common Law heritage, courts have ruled that in order for the next of kin adequately to discharge his (her) responsibility for proper burial of the deceased, that relative has the right to receive the body in the same condition as it was at the time that death occurred. Furthermore, in keeping with Judeo-Christian views on the sacredness of the body and respect for the dead, the body of a deceased person is not to be regarded as an item of commerce, to be bought, sold or used to pay off debts. Courts expressed these premises by stating that there are no "property rights" in the body of the deceased. From this, there developed the ruling that a person could not direct the manner of his burial, because the body is not property and therefore not part of his estate.

In recent years, partly as a consequence of advances in the transplantation of corneal and other tissues, these views have come under increasing criticism. In the 1950's, donation statutes were enacted in several states which allowed an individual to determine what was to be done with his remains and to authorize donation for medical purposes. However, "most statutes failed to recognize the unique time requirements for organ and tissue removal and frequently viewed the act of donation as merely an extension of the testamentary disposition of property".[32] The Uniform Anatomical Gift Act is the product of a three-year investigation into the matter of cadaver organ procurement that was conducted by a Special Committee of the National Conference of Commissioners on Uniform State Laws. The study was initiated in 1965. On July 30, 1968 the Act was approved by the Commission. It was endorsed by the American Bar Association on August 7 of the same year, and subsequently received support from virtually every relevant medical organization.

Blair and Alfred Sadler who played a major role in drafting the Uniform Anatomical Gift Act, summarize its key provisions as follows:

> Under the Uniform Act, a person of sound mind and 18 years of age or more may give all or part of his body for any purpose later specified in the Act, the gift to take effect after death. In the absence of a contrary statement by the deceased before death, the next of kin (in a specified order of priority) are authorized to donate all or part of the body of the deceased. The individual's interests are paramount to the next of kin's. Consequently, if a physician obtains adequate consent from an individual via the card mechanism (a donor card), he need not consult the next of kin for this purpose. The consent mechanism is greatly simplified under the Act and includes any written instrument such as a card carried on the donor's person, signed by the donor, and witnessed by two people. Consent by the next of kin can be obtained by an unwitnessed document or by recorded telegraphic or telephonic message.[33]

The Act forms the basis of new laws that have now been adopted in 51 jurisdictions, including the District of Columbia. It has "enjoyed unprecedented success", for, "never in the 78-year history of the National Conference of Commissioners on Uniform State Laws has a uniform act been so widely adopted during the first three years of consideration by state legislatures".[34] When one considers the existentially fundamental and sacrosanct nature of what this Act has legislatively influenced or altered, the ease and rapidity with which it has been widely accepted is all the more remarkable. Like the Kansas Statute, it represents a basic change in conceptions of death and of the human body. It also places the desires and commitments of the individual with respect to his body at death above those held by members of his family (including inhibiting traditional religious sentiments that this relatives may hold in this connection). The Act not only makes it easily possible for many individuals to make a sacrificial gift of life-in-death, but it also implicitly encourages them to do so. And it legally sanctions a new and ultimate way of expressing the Judeo-Christian injunction to be "our brothers' (and our) strangers' keepers".[35]

The Supreme Court abortion decision handed down on January 22, 1973 has been called one of the most controversial decisions of this century. Its core rulings are as follows:

> 1. A state criminal abortion statute of the current Texas type, that excepts from criminality only a *life saving* (italics in text) procedure on behalf of the mother without regard to pregnancy stage and without recognition of the other interests involved, is violative of the Due Process Clause of the Fourteenth Amendment.
>
> (a) For the stage prior to approximately the end of the first trimester, the abortion decision and its effectuation must be left to the medical judgment of the pregnant woman's attending physician.
>
> (b) For the stage subsequent to approximately the end of the first trimester, the State, in promoting its interest in the health of the mother, may, if it chooses, regulate the abortion procedure in ways that are reasonably related to maternal health.
>
> (c) For the stage subsequent to viability the State, in promoting its interest in the potentiality of human life, may, if it chooses, regulate, and even proscribe, abortion except where it is necessary, in appropriate medical judgment, for the preservation of the life or health of the mother.

The full legal and moral implications of this decision are too complex to discuss here. But several aspects of the ruling should at least be singled out, because they bear so directly on the matters we are considering. To begin with, although ostensibly the Court's decision grants a woman what it deems a 'right' to abortion, it not only regulates this right, but also equivocates about it. For, while affirming the right, throughout its exposition, the Court recurrently declares that abortion is "inherently and primarily, a medical decision" to be "left to the medical judgment of the pregnant women's attending physician". Furthermore, after the first six months of pregnancy, the life of the fetus, termed here "the potentiality of human life", is given precedence over all other considerations short of the "preservation of the life or health of the mother" herself. In these ways, the Court has adhered to the conviction about the sanctify of life and the importance of safeguarding it, that is so strongly upheld in the traditional legal, as well as value system of American society.

The definition of health developed by the Court is a broad one. It has been extended to include "the stigma of unwed motherhood", "the distress for all concerned associated with the unwanted child", and an unspecified complex of conditions referred to as "the full setting of the case". The fact that such psychological and social considerations have been incorporated into this legal conception of health can be expected to have influence that extends beyond the abortion situation.

From our perspective, the dimension of the Court's decision that is the most significant and debatable is its implicitly expressed point of view on when human life begins. In his majority opinion, Associate Justice Harry A. Blackmun disclaims that the Court has done so. "We need not resolve the difficult question of when life begins", he states. "When those trained in the respective disciplines of medicine, philosophy, and theology are unable to arrive at any consensus, the judiciary, at this point in the development of man's knowledge, is not in a position to speculate as to the answer". However, in fact, the Court's decision does more than speculate. It says by implication that life does not begin during the first two trimesters. And it suggests that it begins in "the stage subsequent to viability" when it mandates the State, "if it chooses", not only to regulate, but to "even proscribe" abortion thereafter. The Court's position on the point at which personhood comes into being is more blurred. It reaffirms that "the word 'person', as used in the Fourteenth Amendment, does not include 'the unborn'"; but it does not distinguish the commencement of human life from the inception of personhood.

What emerges fi om the overview sketched out in these pages is a picture of a contemperaneous system of medicine that has reached a stage of development characterized by diffuse ethical and existential self-consciousness. This state of awareness involves the searching out of ways in which certain moral principles and metaphysical assumptions on which American society is traditionally based have been imperfectly realized, or violated. It also entails a reaffirmation of these premises and the initiation of various forms of social action intended to modify the medical system, so that it will more fully actualize its stated ideals. Among the major values and beliefs that are being reasserted are the right of every individual to some modicum of integrity, dignity, autonomy and fulfillment; the right of all men, women and children, independently of their personal endowment or social status, to have equal access to conditions, like the alleviation of illness-induced suffering that are indispensable to their personal and collective humanity; and the right freely to give of one's self to others in life-enhancing ways.

In other regards, this ethical and existential *prise de conscience* in American medicine is accompanied by what appear to be major shifts in fundamental conceptions about health and illness, life and death. Increasingly, health is being defined as a universal human right, rather than as a privilege, a sign of grace, or an aleatory consequence of good fortune. Both health and illness are coming to be viewed in a more societal and less individualistic framework. Along with the absence of adequate medical care, lack of good health and affliction with illness are now more frequently attributed to society-borne stresses, deprivations and injustices than they were in the past. A discernable modification in the absolute nature of the cultural commandment to preserve life is also occurring. While the sacredness of human life and its preservation continue to be affirmed, the new operational definition of death, the assertion, however qualified, of the right to abortion and the mounting insistence both on "the right to die" and on "death with dignity" all suggest that medicine is moving from an ethic based on the unconditional "sanctity of life" to one premised on the "quality of life".[36] Furthermore, the reconceptualization of death as 'brain death' and the Supreme Court decision on abortion are important crystallized expressions of the point that American society has now reached, in what seems to be a gradual movement towards revised definitions of viable life, personhood and 'humanness'.

Finally, numerous of the phenomena that we have identified and discussed suggest that there is a peaking of doubt over the unconditional virtue of still another important value-component of American medicine. The debates over how much ought to be done to maintain the life of terminally ill or dying patients, for example, the moratorium on experimentation with *in vitro* fertilization, the apprehension about what the consequences of prospective developments in genetic engineering and behaviour control may prove to be, all constitute challenges to the eneretic, often aggressive meliorism for which American medicine is known. This blend of activism and meliorism rests on the assumption that out of unrestrictedly vigorous efforts to advance and apply biomedical knowledge and technique will come indisputable gains in human capacities, health and longevity, and in the alleviation of suffering. That conviction is now being thrown into question by many biologists and physicians, as well as by members of other professions, of government agencies and of the general public. There is palpable skepticism about whether we have the "ultimate wisdom", to deal with the fact that "recent advances in biology and medicine suggest... we may be rapidly acquiring the power to modify and control the capacities and activities of men by direct intervention and manipulation of their bodies and minds":

> If we can recognize that biomedical advances carry significant social costs, we may be willing to adopt a less permissive, more critical stance toward new developments. We need to reexamine our prejudice not only that all biomedical innovation is progress, but also that it is inevitable. Precedent certainly favors the view that what can be done will be done, but is this necessarily so? Ought we not to be suspicious when technologists speak of coming developments as automatic, not subject to human control? Is there not something contradictory in the notion that we have the power to control all the untoward consequences of a technology, but lack the power to determine whether it should be developed in the first place?...[37]

Although the danger of excessively deterring medical progress is continuously reiterated, the present trend is clearly in the direction of greater regulation of actual and incipient biomedical developments. The origins of this tendency are complex, but one of the important factors contributing to it is the growing belief that heroic medical scientific and technical efforts to improve 'man's estate' are not unequivocally admirable or good, and that some of their consequences may be seriously harmfull to collective as well as individual human existence.

The data presented suggest that modern American medicine is entering a new evolutionary stage. Organized concern about ethical and existential matters has become one of its salient features. The prominence and legitimacy of medicine's interest in these issues, and the involvement of many non-medical groups in them indicate that a new rapprochement is taking place in the profession and the society. The overweening emphasis on scientific and technological phenomena that has characterized modern medicine, and its insistence on separating these so-called objective considerations form more 'subjective' and 'philosophical' orientations toward health and illness, life and death seem to be giving way to a closer integration between the two dimensions. Some of the ethical and existential issues under consideration in medicine entail reaffirmations of ultimate values in American culture and society. Others involve either a modulation or a broader generalization of such basic values. In two critical respects, the ethical and existential reorientation that is occurring implies a sharper break with cultural tradition, and seems to presage more radical sociocultural change. We refer here to the major shifts away from some of the principles on which the ethic of the sanctity of life and the ethic of progress are founded.

It is tempting to assume that these value shifts and changes are predominantly, if not exclusively caused by recent biomedical developments. And, indeed, in the relevant literature, this allegation is frequently made. However, such an interpretation does not take note of the fact that in many other domains of American society, there is increasing preoccupation with the same questions of values, beliefs and meaning that have been raised in the medical sector. Concern about the quality, dignity and meaningfulness of life, about 'assaults' on nature and the human condition, about distributive justice, equity, universalism, solidarity, community and the "theme of the gift",[38] have also been prominent, for example, in the civil rights, peace, anti-poverty, ecology and women's movements visible on the American scene.[39] In our perspective, these are but some of the phenomena which suggest that the ethical and existential developments in contemporaneous medicine examined in this paper may be part of a broader process of change that is carrying American society into a new stage of modernity.

REFERENCES

* This is the original paper prepared for presentation at the Conference on Medical Sociology sponsored by the Polish Academy of Sciences and endorsed by the Research Committee on the Sociology of Medicine of the International Sociological Association, Warsaw (Jabłonna), Poland, August 20–25, 1973.

A somewhat altered version of this paper was published in the Milbank Memorial Fund Quarterly *Health and Society* **52** (1974) 445–473. It has been changed primarily to report certain bioethical developments which have occurred since 1973.

[1] This technique involves the insertion of a hollow needle through the abdominal and uterine walls of a pregnant woman into the amniotic sac, and withdrawing fluid and cells shed by the fetus.

[2] In *Research on Human Subjects* (New York, Russell Sage Foundation, 1973), Bernard Barber and co-authors comment that, "the recent increase of concern in the biomedical research community... (about) the possible or actual abuse of the subjects of medical experimentation and medical innovation... can be seen perhaps most clearly in the dramatic rise of medical journal articles devoted to facets of this problem" (p. 2). Barber and his colleagues report that in a survey they made of articles listed in *Index Medicus* over the period 1950 to 1969, those that dealt with the ethics of biomedical research on human subjects increased "in both the absolute number and the proportion of articles in this area... The figure begins to get large in 1966" (pp. 2–3).

[3] This is the week when I happened to be writing this section of my paper. In that sense, it was chosen randomly.

[4] For an excellent review-essay of the scope and content of the burgeoning literature on ethical and existential aspects of medicine published during the decade 1960–70, see J. R. Elkinton, 'The Literature of Ethical Problems in Medicine' (Parts 1, 2 and 3), *Annals of Internal Medicine* **73**, Nos. 3, 4 and 5, November, 1970, pp. 495–498, 662–666 and 863–870.

[5] Among the major works on death and dying that have appeared are: Herbert Bailey, *A Matter of Life and Death*, New York (G. P. Putnam's Sons, 1958); Orville G. Brim, Jr., *et al.*, eds., *The Dying Patient*, New York (Russell Sage Foundation, 1970); Robert Fulton, ed., *Death and Identity*, New York (John Wiley and Sons, Inc., 1965); Barney G. Glaser and Anselm L. Strauss, *Awareness of Dying*, Chicago (Aldine Publishing Company, 1968); Barney G. Glaser and Anselm L. Strauss, *Time for Dying*, Chicago (Aldine Publishing Company, 1968); David Hendin, *Death as a Fact of Life*, New York (W. W. Norton and Company, Inc., 1973); John Hinton, *Dying*, Baltimore (Penguin Books, 1967); Elizabeth Kübler-Ross,

On Death and Dying, New York (The Macmillan Company, 1969); Ignace Lepp, *Death and its Mysteries*, New York (The Macmillan Company, 1968); Leonard Pearson, ed., *Death and Dying*, Cleveland (The Press of Case Western Reserve University, 1969); Virginia Peterson, *A Matter of Life and Death*, New York (Atheneum Press, 1961); Edwin S. Schneidman, ed., *Essays in Self-Destruction*, New York (Science House, 1967); Edwin S. Schneidman, ed., *Death and the College Student*, New York (Behavioral Publication, 1972); Bernard Schoenberg, *et al.*, *Loss and Grief: Psychological Management in Medical Practice*, New York (Columbia University Press, 1970); David Sudnow, *Passing On*, Englewood Cliffs, N. J. (Prentice-Hall, 1967); Robert H. Williams, ed., *To Live and to Die*, New York (Springer Verlag, 1973); Martha Wolfenstein and Gilbert Kliman, eds., *Children and the Death of a President*, New York (Doubleday and Company, Inc., 1965).

[6] Elizabeth Kübler-Ross, *On Death and Dying*, Preface (no page given).

[7] Professor Diana Crane (who is also a member of the Department of Sociology of the University of Pennsylvania) and I are planning a paper on this phenomenon, tentatively entitled, 'The Death and Dying Movement: A New Kind of Social Movement?'.

[8] Prominent recent books on human experimentation include: Bernard Barber, *et al.*, *Research on Human Subjects*, New York (Russell Sage Foundation, 1973); Henry K. Beecher, *Research and the Individual*, Boston (Little, Brown and Company, 1970); Paul A. Freund, ed., *Experimentation with Human Subjects*, New York (George Braziller, 1970); Jay Katz (with the assistance of Alexander M. Capron), *Experimentation with Human Beings*, New York (Russell Sage Foundation, 1972); Irving Ladimer and Roger W. Newman, eds., *Clinical Investigation in Medicine*, Boston (Boston University Law-Medicine Research Institute, 1963); Irving Ladimer. ed., 'New Dimensions in Legal and Ethical Concepts for Human Research', *Annals of the New York Academy of Sciences* **169** (1970); M. H. Papworth, *Human Guinea Pigs*, London (Routledge and Kegan Paul, 1967) and Boston (Beacon Press, 1967); G. E. W. Wolstenholme and M. O. Connor, eds., *Ethics in Medical Progress*, Boston (Little, Brown and Company, 1966).

[9] The full references to the works cited in the text are as follows: Daniel Callahan, *Abortion*, New York (The Macmillan Company, 1970); José Delgado, *Physical Control of the Mind*, New York (Harper and Row, 1969); Theodosius Dobzhansky, *Mankind Evolving*, New Haven, Conn. (Yale University Press, 1962); Perry London, *Behavior Control*, New York (Harper and Row, 1969); Francis D. Moore, *Give and Take*, Garden City, N. Y. (Doubleday Anchor Books, 1965); a more recent edition of this book, entitled *Transplant: The Give and Take of Tissue Transplanation* was published by Simon and Schuster, New York, 1972; John T. Noonan, Jr., *Contraception*, Cambridge, Mass. (The Belknap Press of Harvard University, 1965); Richard M. Titmuss, *The Gift Relationship: From Human Blood to Social Policy*, New York (Pantheon Books, 1971); H. J. Cadbury, *et al.*, eds. (for the American Friends' Service Committee) *Who Shall Live?*, New York (Hill and Wang, 1970); Donald R. Cutler, ed., *Updating Life and Death*, Boston (Beacon Press, 1968); René Dubos, *A God Within*, New York (Charles Scribner's Sons, 1972);

Barbara and John Ehrenreich, *The American Health Empire* (a report from the Health Policy Advisory Center), New York (Random House, 1970); Joseph Fletcher, *Moral Responsibility*, Philadelphia (The Westminster Press, 1967); Philip Handler, *Biology and the Future of Man*, New York (Oxford University Press, 1970); Edward M. Kennedy, *In Critical Condition*, New York (Simon and Schuster, 1972); Louis Lasagna, *Life, Death and the Doctor*, New York (Alfred A. Knopf, 1968); Everett Mendelsohn, Judith P. Swazey and Irene Taviss, eds., *Human Aspects of Biomedical Innovation*, Cambridge, Mass. (Harvard University Press, 1971); Jacques Monod, *Chance and Necessity*, New York (Alfred A. Knopf, 1971); Paul Ramsey, *Fabricated Man*, New Haven, Conn. (Yale University Press, 1970); Paul Ramsey, *The Patient as a Person*, New Haven, Conn. (Yale University Press, 1970); Gordon Taylor, *The Biological Time Bomb*, Cleveland (World Publishing Co., 1968); E. Fuller Torrey, ed., *Ethical Issues in Medicine*, Boston (Little, Brown and Co., 1968).

[10] In the international sphere, there are some comparable developments. For example, the Council for International Organizations of Medical Science (CIOMS), a nongovernmental agency created in 1949 by the World Health Organization and Unesco to re-establish scientific communications after World War II, has now turned its primary attention to interdisciplinary conferences and publications on such as, the "protection of human rights in the light of scientific and technological progress in biology and medicine". (Round Table Conference scheduled to be held in Geneva, November 14–16, 1973). Furthermore, the CIOMS has recommended that a new international entity be established to explore the "moral and social issues" raised by new and forthcoming developments in biomedicine.

[11] A systematic study of the sociometry of this circle, its patterns of communication, and their consequences for intellectual growth and policy formation in this area, such as Diana Crane carried out in two scientific communities would be illuminating. See her book, *Invisible Colleges*, Chicago (University of Chicago Press, 1972).

[12] Daniel Callahan, 'Bioethics as a Discipline', *The Hasting Center Studies* 1 (1973) 68.

[13] D. Callahan, 'Bioethics as a Discipline', p. 73.

[14] An interesting history and sociology of science kind of question that might be posed here is whether there is any precedent or principle that would lead one to assume that the preparation of such an encyclopedia will help to establish a field that only potentially exists. For, normally, one would expect an encyclopedia to appear when a field is firmly rooted and recognized, with a sufficiently well-defined body of theory, methodology and empirical data to be articulated.

[15] For a more detailed discussion of this Program see: Robert M. Veatch and Willard Gaylin, 'Teaching Medical Ethics: An Experimental Program', *The Journal of Medical Education* 47 (1972) 779–785.

[16] R. M. Veatch and W. Gaylin, 'Teaching Medical Ethics', p. 785.

[17] R. M. Veatch and W. Gaylin, 'Teaching Medical Ethics', p. 783.

[18] Studies of the social backgrounds of men and women currently entering medical

school, of the attitudes, values, sentiments and life experiences that led them to opt for medicine, and of the socio-psychological as well as cognitive learning that they undergo in the course of medical school, house officer training and their early years of practice are very much needed. Whereas several such major studies of medical socialization were carried out in the 1950's, for reasons that merit investigation, no such studies that are comparable in depth and scope have been attempted more recently. My own comments about medical student attitudes and interests set forth in this paper are based upon the data I gathered as chief field worker for a study of the education and socialization of medical students conducted in the mid-1950's by the Columbia University Bureau of Applied Social Research. *The Student Physician*, edited by Robert K. Merton *et al.*, Cambridge, Mass. (Harvard University Press, 1957), was a product of that investigation. My observations on medical students in the late 1960's and early 1970's are less extensive and systematic. They grow out of my role as a sociologist in the Departments of Psychiatry and Medicine of the University of Pennsylvania, and from the numerous opportunities that I have to visit other medical schools as a consequence of my continuing research and teaching in the sociology of medicine.

[19] Talcott Parsons, Renée C. Fox and Victor M. Lidz, 'The 'Gift of Life' and its Reciprocation', *Social Research* **39** (1972) 367–415.

[20] See, Ad Hoc Committee of the Harvard Medical School to Examine the Definition of Brain Death, 'A Definition of Irreversible Coma', *Journal of the American Medical Association* **205** (1968) 85–88.

[21] David D. Rutstein, 'The Ethical Design of Human Experiments', in: *Experimentation with Human Subjects* (Paul A. Freund, ed.), New York (George Braziller, 1970), p. 386.

[22] For a detailed account of the development of these regulations and those instituted in the same period by the Food and Drug Administration, see William J. Curran, 'Governmental Regulation of the Use of Human Subjects in Medical Research', in: *Experimentation with Human Subjects* (Paul A. Freund, ed.), pp. 402–454.

[23] See, 'Cardiac Transplantation in Man: Statement Prepared by the Board of Medicine of the National Academy of Sciences', *Journal of the American Medical Association* **24** (1968) 805–806; 'Cardiac and Other Organ Transplantation in the Setting of Transplant Science as a National Effort', in: *American College of Cardiology's Fifth Bethesda Conference, September 28–29, 1968, American Journal of Cardiology* **22** (1968) 896–912; *Cardiac Replacement.* A Report by the Ad Hoc Task Force, National Heart Institute, Washington, D. C. (U.S. Government Printing Office, October 1969); 'Ethical Guidelines for Organ Transplantation', American Medical Association Judicial Council, *Journal of the American Medical Association* **205** (1968) 341–342. For a fuller discussion of these statements see: Renée C. Fox and Judith P. Swazey, *The Courage To Fail: A Social View of Organ Transplants and Dialysis* (Chapter 3, 'The Experiment-Therapy Dilemma'), (University of Chicago Press, 1974).

[24] See Judith P. Swazey and Renée C. Fox, 'The Clinical Moratorium: A Case

Study of Mitral Valve Surgery', in: *Experimentation with Human Subjects* (Paul A. Freund, ed.), pp. 315–357.

[25] See Renée C. Fox and Judith P. Swazey, 'The Heart Transplant Moratorium', Chapter 6 of *The Courage To Fail.*

[26] Supreme Court of the United States, *Roe et al.* v. *Wade*, District Attorney of Dallas County, Appeal from the United States District Court for the Northern District of Texas, No. 70–18. Argued December 13, 1971; reargued October 11, 1972; decided January 22, 1973. We will comment on some of the implications of this decision in the next section of the paper.

[27] Leon R. Kass, 'Making Babies – the New Biology and the 'Old' Morality', *The Public Interest* **26** (1972) 32.

[28] L. R. Kass, 'Making Babies', p. 19.

[29] Law of Mar. 17, 1970, ch. 378 (1970) Kan. Laws 994 (codified at KAN. STAT. ANN. § 77–202 (Supp. 1971).

[30] See Alexander Morgan Capron and Leon R. Kass, 'A Statutory Definition of the Standards for Determining Human Death: An Appraisal and a Proposal', *University of Pennsylvania Law Review* **121** (1972), especially pp. 104–111.

[31] For the account of the legal background of the Uniform Anatomical Gift Act and its provisions that follows, I am inedbted to the writings of Blair L. Sadler and Alfred M. Sadler, Jr., especially their co-authored article, 'Providing Cadaver Organs: Three Legal Alternatives', *The Hastings Center Studies* **1** (1973) 14–26.

[32] B. L. Sadler and A. M. Sadler, Jr., 'Providing Cadaver Organs', p. 16.

[33] B. L. Sadler and A. M. Sadler, Jr., 'Providing Cadaver Organs', p. 25.

[34] *Ibid.*

[35] Richard M. Titmuss, *The Gift Relationship: From Human Blood to Social Policy*, New York (Pantheon Books, 1971), *in passim.*

[36] This opinion was offered by the ethical scholar, Joseph Fletcher, in the course of a keynote address that he delivered at the National Conference on the Teaching of Medical Ethics, held at the Tarrytown Conference Center, Tarrytown, New York, on June 1–3, 1972. The conference was co-sponsored by the Institute of Society, Ethics and the Life Sciences and the Columbia University College of Physicians and Surgeons.

[37] Leon R. Kass, 'The New Biology: What Price Relieving Man's Estate?' *Science* **174** (1971) 779, 786.

[38] Marcel Mauss, *The Gift*, trans. by Ian Cunnison, Glencoe, Ill. (The Free Press, 1954), p. 66.

[39] Many of the participants in these social movements have been young people, relatively affluent and well-educated. Once again, this raises the question whether or not the 'new' youth will prove to be effective agents of change. It also suggests the intriguing hypothesis that one of the prerequisites for widerspread collective involvement in the kinds of moral and metaphysical issues dealt with here is a sufficient level of prosperity and fulfillment to free whole groups in a society from primordial anxieties about food, shelter, employment and the like.

THE DILEMMAS OF GENETICS

IGNACY WALD

Department of Genetics, Psychoneurogical Institute, Warsaw, Poland

Of all the branches of science in which research has made progress in recent years, an area of research which has exercised a profound influence not only on the understanding of biological laws, but also on scientific thinking as a whole, is that of genetics. The discovery of the biological role of nucleic acids, the uncovering of the structure of genetic information and its role in regulating life processes – these are discoveries the importance of which can hardly be overestimated. These achievements do not only have theoretical significance, as they afford a more precise understanding of genetical determination of a whole range of traits, including pathological traits, create a basis for effective medical and preventive intervention in many diseases, and also outline the possibilities – still rather remote, perhaps – of genetical engineering, i.e. of controlled programming of the traits of an individual.

In this situation it is natural to seek examination of a problem which has long faced the biological and social sciences, namely the problem of the interdependence between the biological and social aspects of man. These are not new problems in the history of science, having been surfacing throughout its course in the form of controversy between the concepts of preformation and epigenesis, nature and nurture, and finally, on the relative roles of biological and social factors in the development of man. The development of modern science has indicated that many of these alternatives were either erroneous or inadequate, that the solution does not lie in contrasting heredity and environment but rather in the analysing the mutual interaction of hereditary and environmental factors, or, to be more accurate, in the analysis of the relative weight of the genetic and environmental elements and their interdependence in the general interaction of the organism.

In modern science the variation between genetic and social problems appears in manifold forms, on various levels of abstraction, and in various fields of research and practical activity. Thus, on the one hand we have the question of social influence upon the genetic structure of organisms or populations, and on the other the social implications of genetic processes and changes in the genetic structure. Especially the latter problem is attracting growing interest in connection with our increasing knowledge of genetically determined defects, the development of genetic counselling, and changes in the selective value of individual traits as a result of therapeutic advances.

These problems have been of interest to both scientific and public opinion, the latter in connection with the discussion concerning genetic or biological influence on social structure, stratification, mobility and development, and the possible use of genetic control for improper purposes. Obviously this discussion involves various problems: on the one hand there are differences in the systems of values applied and the difficulties in choosing among the various conceptions, on the other hand, however, there is a striving to achieve an objective appraisal of the processes involved and their possible lines of development.

For scientists the question amounts to the genetic problems of the development of general health of the population and the development of medicine. This aspect is of much greater interest to us today, so we shall try to concentrate on the main medical connotations of genetics.

The growth of interest in these problems has various causes:

1) The progress od medicine is reducing the health hazard of contagious diseases in developed countries, while at the same time their place is being taken by – apart from traumas – degenerative constitutional diseases in which genetic factors play a distinct role. According to many authors, genetically conditioned diseases, or diseases with a clear genetic component account for 25 to 40 per cent of all cases treated by the health service. In most cases these are chronic diseases – which inincreases the ratio between prevalence and incidence, and requires protracted medical treatment.

2) The development of technology and the changes it has brought in the natural environment have aroused us to examining the potential threat of these processes to man's genetic equipment and to the very future of homo sapiens.

3) The range of therapeutic and preventive possibilities in the treatment of genetically conditioned diseases is growing, and as a result more and more energy is being channelled into this field of treatment.

4) The expansion of preventive and therapeutic possibilities leads to the question of the possible effects a change of intensity and direction od natural selection may have on the genetic and phenotype structure of future generations.

Let us attempt then, on the basis of a consideration of these two sets of problems to show what our current knowledge contributes to their illumination with regard to:

1) the genetic and environmental determination of mental retardation,

2) the interrelationships between natural selection and the development of medicine.

MENTAL RETARDATION

Mental retardation refers to significantly subaverage level of mental efficiency, which arises during an individual's developmental period (usually before the age of 15) and affects maturation, learning capability and social adaptation. It follows from definition that mental retardation is not a specific nosological entity, but rather a heterogeneous category of residual states after various diseases and forms of retarded development.

Mental retardation is an important social problem both because of its high prevalence, and because of the burden the mentally retarded constitute for their families and society.

If we take mental retardation to mean a mental level below two standard deviations from the mean (which in the majority of intelligence scales means approximately 70), then we shall find that in the majority of developed countries mental retardation effects about 3% of school-age children. Thus mental retardation is the most widely prevalent group of handicap which is often of lifelong duration. In this heterogeneous group we may distinguish two broad sub-categories: that of low-grade retardation (intelligence quotient under 50) affecting about 0.4% of the child population, and that of mild retardation (intelligence quiotent between 50 and 70) affecting about 2.6% of the child population.

Epidemiological studies of the total population usually show that the mutual proportions between these two subcategories undergo considerable change. The size of the more retarded group usually remains stable, while a considerable part of the less retarded group is 'absorbed' by the general population and under favourable conditions functions more or less normally.

These two groups differ in various important respects:

1) damage to the central nervous system is, as a rule, diagnosed in the case of the more retarded group, while so-called organic neurological signs are relatively rare in the case of the mildly retarded group.

2) in the low-grade group it is much easier to diagnose the causative factor of the disorder. In part, these are disorders of a genetic character, such as hereditary diseases or chromosomal anomalies and in part exogeneous disorders such as intrauterine infections or infections contracted in early childhood, poisoning, perinatal problems injuries etc. In the mild group, on the other hand, the identification of the causative factor is very difficult, and it is generally accepted that the disorder is of multifactorial origin.

3) there are considerable differences in the levels of correlation between the intelligence quotients of children and parents in the two groups: in the low-grade group the correlation between the mental levels of children and parents approximates to 0, while in the mild group the correlation approaches 0.5, which corresponds to the relationship within the general population.

4) the social distribution in these two groups is different; while there is generally no connection between the social situation of the parents and the presence of the disorder in the more retarded group, recent epidemiological studies have revealed that over 95% of cases of milder retardation are noted in families belonging to 'lower' social strata.

The interpretation of the above data poses serious difficulties. For many years, the view prevailed among researchers that mild retardation was genetically determined mostly multifactorially and was part of the normal spread of intelligence, the variation of which was also conditioned to a large extent by multiple genetic factors. This interpretation concurred both with the above-mentioned correlations, and with the agreement between the epidemiologically observed and the expected – on the basis of normal distribution of intelligence – proportion of the mildly retarded in the population. This led to the conclusion that the social situation of families with mild retardation could be the effect of their genetically determined lower mental efficiency. This thesis served as a basis for the concern, voiced particularly frequently at the beginning of this century, that the improvement of general living conditions and the development of education, social welfare and care for the mentally retarded, could lead to a decrease in the intelligence level of the general population. These fears proved unfounded, since longitudinal surveys of the intelligence of children, conducted in several countries, did not show a decrease but actually a slight rise in the scores. As has been demonstrated by Penrose, a genetic model of mild mental retardation does not imply a lowering of the mental efficiency of the population. Due to gene segregation, the 'low intelligence' group produces offspring of varied mental level, and since the severely retarded usually do not reproduce, a genetic balance is achieved in which the higher fertility of persons with slightly lowered mental efficiency is compensated by the lack of fertility among the very retarded.

Recent studies have indicated that the situation is more complex than might be concluded from the estimates of the early fifties and late sixties, and that the role of environmental factors in conditioning mild mental retardation may be higher than was supposed. The basic argument supporting this thesis is the research conducted by Heber in the so-called Milwaukee project. The author studied the offspring of mothers on social welfare in Milwauke and found that 75 % of children with mental retardation (mild) had mothers with an intelligence quotient under 80. This finding supported the genetic conception described above. But in the next stage of his investigation the author carefully selected an experimental group, in which children a few days old were subjected to systematic care and stimulation. A control group was also set up of children who stayed under ordinary social welfare conditions. After six years of observation, it was found that the intelligence quotient in the experimental group averaged 122, while in the control group the mean was about 90 %.

Heber's findings require confirmation on the basis of wider material. Nevertheless they do indicate that the environmental part of the variance connected with the mental level of mildly retarded persons is indeed greater than was supposed. The findings also open the way for preventive action against this widespread form of disablement, and serve to emphasize the importance of early and systematic environmental stimulation in human development.

The above-mentioned studies show that psychological-genetic and social research combined can lead to highly significant theoretical and practical results.

In recent years we have witnessed another type of use of genetical research in combating severe mental retardation. The possibility of early diagnosis of such metabolic diseases as phenylketonuria, galactosemia, maple syrup urine disease, and others together with the possibility of early dietary treatment, make it possible to ensure the normal mental development of children affected with these diseases. It might appear that the problem is not of great social significance since the diseases involved are rare. But when account is taken of the fact that for example in Poland the frequency of the phenylketonuria gene equals about 1/83, that one person in 42 is a carrier of this disease, and that patients with phenylketonuris in 1965 made up 3% of all persons treated in Polish institutions for the mentally retarded, the true social significance of the problem will be realized.

Further possiblilities of preventive treatment with regard to mental retardation are connected with the diagnosis of diseases leading to mental retardation in the early stages of pregnancy. These possibilities cover such disorders as chromosomal anomalies (of which the most frequent is the Down syndrome, which occurs once in every 700 births) and many metabolic diseases, which lead to mental retardation. The wide scale introduction of this type of preventive treatment could decrease the incidence of low-grade mental retardation by about 10%.

The development of this type of treatment naturally poses a number of social problems and raises questions concerning social policy. Various questions arise in connection with the attitudes and social situation of families covered by this type of treatment, with the estimation of the social costs of this type of treatment in comparison with traditional methods, and finally with the evaluation of the long-range genetic consequence of this type of activity. I shall be returning to the latter question later.

Mental retardation is an interesting illustration of the complex interplay between genetic and environmental factors, both as regards the problems of causation and of prevention.

GENETICS AND THE PROGRESS OF CIVILIZATION AND MEDICINE

Let us now pass on to a more general problem, namely the problem of the genetic effects of the progress of civilization and medicine. Like all problems of long-range forecasting, it is very difficult of solution, and history has taught us that the worst forecasts are sometimes the ones made by experts. Nevertheless considering the great public interest in this question, let us attempt to present the current view of the majority of geneticists on this topic. It is a common opinion that keeping alive ever increasing numbers of sick persons leads to the deterioration of the genetic composition of the population. A further implication of this thesis is the conclusion that there is a contradiction between the treatment of an individual patient by a doctor and the dysgenic effect of this treatment on the population. It would appear that such views are at least incomplete. After all, one should realize that the development of civilization and medicine not only has dysgenic consequences (by increasing the number of harmful genes in the population), but also a eugenic effect (in the sense of reducing the proportion of harmful genes in the population). First, I shall consider the dysgenic effects.

There exist data to support the assertion that over the past thirty years there has been a rise in the incidence of diabetes, a disease largely determined by genetic factors. Part of the rise can probably be explained by increased detectability and demographic shifts. Nevertheless it may be supposed that there is a genuine rise in its incidence. But it is very doubtful that this higher incidences could be primarily explained by the rising number of genes over these thirty years. In fact, most of the data available indicates that the higher incidence could be caused to a considerable extent by dietary changes which lead to more frequent manifestation of the disease in susceptible persons.

The survival and procreation of individuals carrying pathological genes can lead to the increase of frequency of disease genes in the population. But it is an extraordinarily slow process. As an example, one might take phenylketonuria, a disease which has a simpler genetic determination than diabetes, since it is passed on as a simple recessive trait. The frequency of this disease among the Polish population is 1 case per 7000 persons. The introduction of the low-phenylatanine diet makes possible a normal development for persons affected with the disease. Till recently, the relative fitness of the affected (i.e. number of offspring in relation to the average number of offspring in the population) equalled 0. Let us imagine that all affected persons attain the normal level of fitness and have as many children as the average individual. In such a situation, it would require 100 generations – or 3,000 years – to double the number of genes in the population (which would lead to one case of phenylketonuria in 1750 births). This illustrates how slow genetic changes are in comparison with environmental changes. Thus it makes little sense to propose a limitation of medical treatment because of the possible genetic consequences. Let us also note that a whole range of ailments, such as myopia for example, are also genetically determined. One could suppose here that the widespread use of eye-glasses is the price humanity has to pay for decreased natural selection as regards shortsightedness. But most people would surely agree that it is not a high price to pay.

Now let us turn to the second matter, which is that the progress of civilization also has eugenic effects (in the sense of reducing the number of harmful genes). As an example, one might quote here Allison's discovery of balanced polymorphism of the gene of sickle-cell anemia. This is a genetically determined disease in which the haemoglobin has an abnormal structure. Individuals with one gene of this disease are clinically healthy, and their red blood corpuscles only look abnormal under the microscope. Persons with two genes of this disease suffer from acute anemia and in most cases die before puberty. The disease is prevalent among blacks, especially in certain parts of Africa. It has been found that the area where the disease is most prevalent also showed the highest frequency of tropical malaria. Further studies have shown that carriers of the sickle-cell gene have higher resistance to tropical malaria than persons without the pathological gene. And so malaria was the factor maintaining the high frequency of haemoglobinopathy. It follows that the overcoming of malaria would help reduce the frequency of the haemoglobinopathy gene.

There are grounds to suspect that balanced polymorphism is not a rare mechanism in maintaining genetic balance in the population, and the use of this mechanism could constitute one of the eugenic effects of the progress of civilization.

Genetic counselling, depending on the methods used and the diseases it concerns, can have dysgenic as well as eugenic effects. In any case, its influence on the frequency of a gene is negligible and very slow. It would appear therefore that among the many threats to the human race, the danger stemming from medical genetics is minimal.

The last question which I would like to consider, is the possibility of implementing genetical research to improve the genetic composition of the population, not by decreasing the number of harmful genes, but by increasing the proportionate number of 'good' genes (as distinct from genetics, which deals with the laws governing heredity, the practical activity directed at improving the genetic composition of the population is called eugenics; the relationship of genetics and eugenics may be compared to the relationship between sociology and social work). This field is sometimes called positive eugenics. The supporters of positive eugenics have for years been promoting, as the basic remedy for the defects which afflict the human race, intensified procreation on the part of particularly valuable individuals, which would increase the number of good genes in the population. A most admirable idea, but its realization is difficult for two reasons:

1) The majority of socially valuable traits, such as – let us say – intelligence and positive character features, though partially determined biologically, are not inherited in such a simple way as, say blood groups or other biochemical indicators. These traits have a complex, multifactorial determination both genetical and environmental. It would be difficult to expect, therefore, that the use of breeding methods would yield direct results, especially since selection with regard to one trait might well mean the deterioration in other traits.

2) The second, even greater difficulty, lies in the fact that genetics, and probably not only genetics, does not have at its disposal the knowledge of which traits are good and which are bad (if we exclude clearly pathological traits).

As an example of the difficulties involved here we may quote the fact that one of the leading advocates of using the sperm of outstanding individuals for mass artificial insemination, the Nobel prize-winner Herman Muller, in two editions of his work on the subject included two different lists of people whom he suggested as suitable donors. It appears that at present genetics not only does not possess adequate knowledge of the laws determining socially valuable traits, but also lacks an adequate system of social values or any knowledge of their possible requirements which the environment may put before the human race in the future. On the other hand, our present genetical knowledge points to the advisability of maintaining in the evolution of the human kind the present level of variation, which has considerable genetical value. But it is known, however, that socially important traits are determined to a high extent by environmental factors, and the use of environmental (or eugenic) effects has considerably broader prospects for success. This is indicated by the astounding speed of cultural evolution, which stems from biological evolution, but is governed by its own autonomous laws. This does not mean, of course, that sociology and social policy should not interest themselves in the progress of genetics. On the contrary – the development of this field and a closer study of genetical processes at all levels of organization of life are also of profound social significance.

SOME NOTES ON THE EPIDEMIOLOGICAL AND ECOLOGICAL MODELS*

MERVYN W. SUSSER

Division of Epidemiology, Columbia University School of Public Health, New York, N.Y., U.S.A.

In medicine and public health during the second half of the nineteenth century, the development of powerful new concepts on specific agents of disease and immunity led to a narrowing of the focus of study. For many investigators of the early era of microbiology, the physical environment became all important in the search for the specific agents that caused specific diseases; the proliferation of eponyms was symptomatic of this feverish search. The environment tended to be seen as a source, or a wehicle, of specific agents rather than as a shaping force with many interacting elements.

Epidemiologists of the time emphasized infectious diseases, often to the exclusion of all other diseases from their interests, and they were zealous in the search for new infectious agents. Their professional responsibilities for the prevention and control of disease, however, obliged epidemiologists also to investigate the environmental sources of infectious agents and modes of transmission of infection. Although concern with infection gave many epidemiologists a onesided view of the determinants of health disorders, this view could not exclude the environment. Their work demanded a broad concept of disease that synthesized the triad of agent, host, and environment.

A single, well-documented condition best illustrates the use and limitations of these three elements in a causal analysis. Schistosomiasis, or bilharzia, will serve the purpose.[1] We turn first to the agent. The life cycles of the flatworms *Schistosoma mansoni* and *Schistosoma haematobium* alternate between man and certain species of snails (see Exhibit 1).

Man is the primary host in which *S. mansoni* and *S. haematobium* undergo their adult and sexual life; they embed themselves in no other mammal. Each subspecies of schistosome also has an intermediary host and seeks out various snail species as hosts of predilection. The free-living forms that alternately infect humans and snails can exist only in water. Thus, the life cycle of the schistosome could not have

Exhibit 1. Life cycle of schistosoma

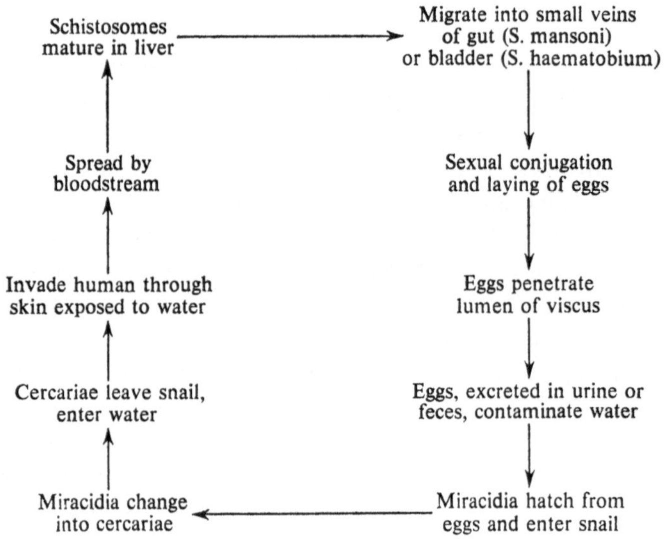

evolved if man had not habitually dwelt, bathed, and excreted in the vicinity of pools or slow-running streams infested by snails. Human beings are part of the ecology of the schistosome, and human ways of life made their infection by the schistosome possible. This epidemiological model can be represented as a simple causal sequence of events between agent, host, and envirnment. (See Exhibit 2,1.)

The necessary environment of the intermediate forms of the schistosome is quiet waters. The snails that are host to these intermediate forms also need or prefer a special environment. The human host of the schistosome can survive in most environments, but man prefers some environments to others, and he changes the environment to suit himself. Man developed tools, family life, and the social organization of group society; he came to live in increasingly dense aggregates of people. These developments in turn modified the relations between the schistosome and its human hosts.

Exhibit 2. Schistosomiasis: epidemiological and ecological models

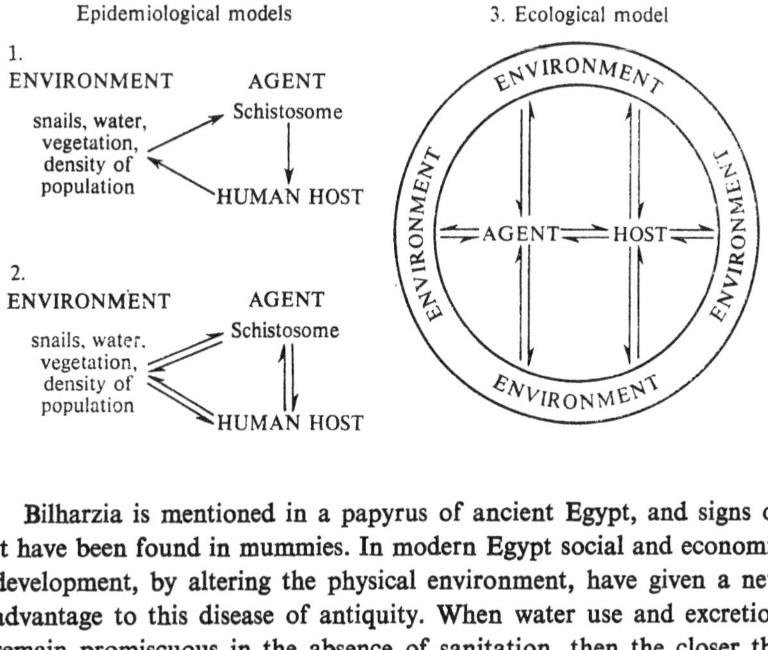

Bilharzia is mentioned in a papyrus of ancient Egypt, and signs of it have been found in mummies. In modern Egypt social and economic development, by altering the physical environment, have given a new advantage to this disease of antiquity. When water use and excretion remain promiscuous in the absence of sanitation, then the closer the settlement to water and the denser it is, the heavier the rate of infection in a population. The traditional form of irrigation in Egypt was to collect the flood waters of the Nile in basins, to water the fields from the basins once a year, and to allow the land to dry out in the off season. Nowadays the waters of the Nile are collected in huge reservoirs, and water is released gradually over the whole year through a network of canals. This perennial system of irrigation makes better use of the land, produces more food, and creates a favorable environment for the people, so that more of them survive to live there. At the same time, the irrigation system creates an environment permanently damp and full of vegetable matter that is favorable to snails and cercariae. In this new environment created by economic development, habits of water use and excretion remained the same as the population grew, and the prevalence of bilharzia rose. In the areas where the traditional form of irrigation is practiced, the rate of infection is about 6 per cent among the population. In areas watered from the reservoirs, it is often 60 per cent [29].

Even in this example, chosen for its simplicity, there are more complex relations between agent, host, and environment. The environment, and in this instance the prevalence of the agent itself, can alter the response of the host to the agent. Many Egyptian adults show little reaction to bilharzia infection, and it seems that they acquire a degree of resistance from frequent exposure in their youth. Persons newly exposed to the parasite do not show such resistance and have more severe reactions. When Napoleon's troops were billeted in the Nile delta during his Egyptian campaign, they apparently suffered marked reactions to bilharzia, as did British troops in Egypt in World Wars I and II. Thus immunity to an infecting agent varies in populations with opportunities for exposure, with previous experience of infection, and with age at first exposure. Resistance to infection probably varies also with other factors unrelated to the agent, such as nutrition.

The epidemiology of bilharzia is further complicated by the fact that, while the reactions of the human host to infection are modified by the pervasiveness of the agent in the environment, the host population in turn influences the pervasiveness of the agent by its role in distributing it. The host population exposes snails to infection through promiscuous excretion, eliminates snails or the vegetation on which they depend, or alters its own habits of excretion and bathing.

The simple sequential causal model (Exhibit 2,1) has developed into a model in which the triad of agent, host, and environment are engaged in processes of reciprocal interaction (Exhibit 2,2). A complex ecological model[2] (Exhibit 2,3) is a still better representation of reality: agent and host are engaged in continuing interactions with an enveloping environment.

ABSTRACTING VARIABLES FROM ECOLOGICAL MODELS

In the ecological model, the interrelationships are appropriately described by terms like 'web', 'network', or 'configuration'. Nearly all the interactions between factors in the particular system we have examined are reciprocal and multiple. In this situation, the terms 'agent', 'host', and 'environment', and the associated concepts, can be used to describe ecological relationships. They are not precise enough to describe causal relationships.

The triad of agent, host, and environment helped epidemiologists to focus on different classes of factors, especially with communicable disease, and so to tease out their relations. But when the elements of all three components interact, analysis in terms of cause becomes clumsy. The activity and survival of both host and agent depend on environment, are altered by it, and in turn alter the environment. Before a disease becomes manifest, with a characteristic distribution in a population, many elements of the triad interact with each other in manifold fashion.

Current genetic models [5] have developed in a way remarkably similar to epidemiological models. Few characteristics are now attributed to single genes, as they were in the simple and elegant Mendelian model. For instance, the heritable components of a characteristic that has a continuous distribution, say IQ or blood pressure, are assumed to be polygenic and to result from a number of genes at several loci on the chromosome. Each gene may be polymorphic, in that each gene may express itself in different forms and each form in different degrees. These many forms of expression allow for a subtle and complex interaction of heredity with the environment. The interaction produces change and diversity in the characteristics and health disorders of populations.

Thus current genetics, in common with epidemiology, uses models of multiple causality. Even where the heritable component of a particular characteristic appears to be large, the models are compatible with dramatic changes in the frequency of the characteristic produced by change in the environment. The current rates of occurrence of tuberculosis and rheumatic fever, diseases for which a genetic element seems established, have dwindled to a small fraction of the rates that existed a half-century ago. The scale and rate of these changes indicate that they are environmental in origin. Current genetic models allow for such interaction of genetic forms with environmental forces.

To handle these complexities, the variables must be conceived in a way that makes them accessible to being counted, qualified, and manipulated. For this purpose, we shall try to develop a set of concepts and a terminology that simplify the multiple interactions and reciprocities discernible in any ecological system. The variables must be at once more general and abstract in conception than the classic triad of agent, host, and environment and more specific and limited by definitions when applied. The terminology must describe any specific element in any segment of the system we choose to examine, and yet it must not limit thinking to one or another of the three broad components in the system under examination.

MacMahon *et al.* [15] used the terms 'experiential' and 'manifestational' variables: experiential variables describe the experiences or hypothetical causes to which the population under study is exposed; manifestational variables describe the manifestations or supposed effects under study in the population. Another set of terms, still more general, refers to independent and dependent variables:

For our purposes, and *independent variable* is a variable the value of which is independent of the dependent variable (or manifestation) within the defined area of relationships under study; that is, the independent variable is not influenced by the manifestation but may cause it or contribute to its variation.

For our purposes, a *dependent variable* is a variable the value of which is dependent on the effect of other variables in the defined area of relationships under study; that is, the dependent variable is a manifestation or outcome whose variation we seek to explain or account for by the influence of independent variables.

USES OF MODELS

Ecological systems can be simplified in terms of these variables. The system is reduced to a model comprised of related variables. The function of such models is either to predict or to represent. Both functions help develop and clarify statements about causal relationships.

Consider first the *predictive* function; this is perhaps the most widespread use of explicit model building. Such models begin with the relations between variables known to exist in present and past trends. From these relations future trends can be extrapolated and predicted within estimated margins of error. These predictions will always be somewhat shaky: the assumption is made that known relations will remain constant and hold in the future and that past trends will continue. In other words, present circumstances are assumed to have future consequences. Population models provide familiar examples. The variables included are most usually fertility rates (birth rates specific for the age groups of fecund women), age distributions of fecund women, and age-specific death rates. Predictions of future populations differ according to the initial assumptions concerning the trends of the variables included in the model.

Predictive models are an essential aid to planning. Planning is a process that aims to devise rational responses to estimated future needs. A rational response implies that one makes particular choices among courses of action in the expectation that what follows from the choice can to some degree be predicted. Planning proceeds, therefore, by predicting the effects of various interventions. Predictions are necessarily founded on assumptions about causal relationships. Thus, for his special purposes, the planner needs predictive models from which to estimate the outcomes he can expect from one or another type of response to a situation. In terms of variables, the planner assigns alternative values to the various independent variables included in the system, and he then assesses the effects of these alternatives on the dependent variables [16]. For example, one multivariate model aims to predict fecundity or, more precisely, the susceptibility of populations of women to becoming pregnant. The digital computer is used to simulate the state of fecundity of various populations as determined by age, fertility rates, prevailing pregnancies, and lactation. Different levels of susceptibility to pregnancy can then be taken into account when ways of controlling fertility are quantitatively assessed [22].

We turn now to the *representational* function of mathematical models; Lazarsfeld emphasized this aspect under the description 'linguistic functions' [11]. The purpose of these models is to represent existing or postulated relationships in simplified form. The representations serve at least three subfunctions: organizing, mediating, and analyzing.

The *organizing* function of models is illustrated to some extent in the previous discussion of epidemiological and ecological models. Such models organize and synthesize a complex of related factors into coherent forms. (See Exhibit 2).

The *mediating* function of models is less familiar. The model reveals the common ground between formulations that appear distinct or even disparate at first sight, but here the disparity is merely the result of a parochial view. The ecological model for schistosomiasis developed in the preceding discussion has such a mediating function. The model mediates between the traditional epidemiological formulation of agent, host, and environment and the multivariate formulations that quantify the relationships among the many variables of the ecological system (see pp. 178 ff).

An example of explicitly mathematical models that have mediating functions for epidemiologists are those used by economists for the analysis of time trends and 'business cycles'. One approach to studying the health effects of air pollution, for instance, is to relate the time trends of sickness and death to those of pollutants in the ambient air. These trends must also take into account the periodic fluctuations with season and with other time cycles, and they are best represented by just such models as economists have devised for entirely different purposes [24, 10, 27]. The model serves like a synapse to connect the separate concerns of econometrists and epidemiologists with facets of the same phenomenon.

The *analyzing* (explanatory) function involves models that pose alternatives among the possible relations between variables. Exhibit 1 provided models in which the same manifestations, or dependent variables, were conceived as the outcome of quite different causal sequences. These alternative pathways help reveal the gaps in knowledge and point the way to the studies needed to fill these gaps.

Models of alternative pathways have a central role in the disciplined procedures of scientific method. Scientific method is founded on cycles of inductive inference. General explanations are inferred by induction from particular facts and associations. The scientific procedure is then to test the consistency of these explanations, hypotheses, and theories in particular situations specially devised. An ideal test will be crucial, that is, the outcome will eliminate one or more of the competing hypotheses. Within this series of steps, analytical models are constructed to represent alternate explanatory hypotheses, which can be subjected to crucial test.

In epidemiology, models have fulfilled all these functions of prediction and planning and of representation and explanation. Their use began with an effort to predict the onset and course of epidemics. In the second report of the Registrar General of England and Wales, published in 1840, William Farr first developed the beginnings of a predictive model for a communicable disease epidemic [6]. He had recognized regularities in the smallpox epidemics of the 1830s. By calculating frequency curves for these past outbreaks, he estimated the deaths to be expected. From these studies he generalized to other epidemics. Thus, in a letter to the press during the 1866 outbreak of the rinderpest among cattle, he used a mathematical model to refute a parliamentary prediction that the epidemic was bound to grow and end in catastrophe [21]. His refutation turned out to be correct in broad terms, although not in detail.

Farr's work was taken up again only in the twentieth century. Hamer, in his model of 1906, tried to represent and 'explain' the waxing and waning of epidemics [7]. The model was based on the number of infected persons in a population, on the number susceptible to infection, and on the frequency of contacts between them. These variables still underlie the sophisticated current models of infectious disease epidemics [21, 1, 8]. At the same time Brownlee tried to use epidemic models for the analytical purpose of discovering the natural laws governing epidemics. He first constructed curves of the waxing and waning of epidemics from the records of many past epidemics. These curves did not entirely accord with those derived from Hamer's hypotheses, in that observed epidemics subsided more quickly than expected. To fit the observed epidemic curves, therefore, Brownlee proposed a modified biological hypothesis that explained the waning of an epidemic by a postulated reduction in the 'infectivity' of the microorganism [2]. Although his hypothesis has not been sustained, Brownlee was a pioneer in the analytical use of mathematical models.

Among the most extensive and successful applications of models for planning, that is, for selecting among alternative modes of action, has been the effort to eradicate malaria sponsored by the World Health Organization. Ronald Ross, who in 1897 made the dramatic discovery that mosquitos were the vectors of the malaria parasite, published work on epidemic models of malaria as early as 1908. His prime interest was to test plans for prevention of the disease and, in particular, an attack on the mosquito vectors which he advocated as the rational course. Ross's model suggested that there was a critical density of mosquito vectors. Above the critical density, the incidence of the disease rose, while below that density incidence dwindled. His interest was also analytical [20].

> ...all epidemiology, concerned as it is with the variation of disease from time to time or from place to place, must be considered mathematically, however many variables are implicated, if it is to be considered scientifically at all. To say that a disease depends upon certain factors is not to say much, until we can also form an estimate as to how largely each factor influences the whole result. And the mathematical method of treatment is really nothing but the application of careful reasoning to the problem at issue.

Ross described his model as a "Theory of Happenings". He chose this title to convey the generality of the model; he was aware of its mediating potential for other disciplines such as economics and sociology.

Much later MacDonald, to back up his advocacy of eradication programs, also turned to the study of epidemiological models of the dynamics of malaria [14]. MacDonald ascribed to his model the function that it "...support technical knowledge and experience in the field by design techniques, which can present the probable result of any suggested course of action or any number of variants on it. By doing this, the epidemiologist can refine his ideas and can have a guided method of choice between alternative lines of action, and with it a yardstick of expected results to guide evaluation month by month, so that the earliest signs of deviation can be identified" [12].

An array of independent variables was developed for inclusion in the malaria model. With regard to the vector, these included the man-biting habit, density of population, and expectation of life for mosquitos. With regard to the human host, the variables included the recovery rate from malaria in man and the number of secondary cases of malaria that arise from a single primary case. The dependent variable was the prevalence of parasites in the blood of the human population at risk.

MacDonald's models suggested that the eradication of malaria within a limited time period was feasible.

Alternative methods of blocking the cycle of malaria transmission, such as attacks on larval or adult anophelene mosquitos to control the vector, or mass treatment of human populations, were tested by the model. In nearly all circumstances, attack on adult mosquitos was the most effective single measure [12].[3] The predictions of the model have been tested, and to a degree validated, by the World Health Organization eradication program. The central thrust of these programs in most areas has been to destroy adult mosquitos by spraying their resting places with long-acting residual insecticides.

MacDonald later extended his planning models to the study of schistosomiasis [13]. His model will serve to illustrate how complex ecological relations, set out in Exhibit 6 in the case of schistosomiasis, can be reduced to a system of variables that can be handled and analyzed by epidemiologists. In this schistosomiasis model, MacDonald introduced four main sets of variables:

1. A fertility factor measured the over-all output of eggs by the schistosome infecting the human host. The chance of the worms sexually pairing and producing eggs depends on the worm load in the body systems of the human host and on the longevity of the worms.
2. A contamination factor measured the number of schistosome eggs introduced into the local water. This factor depends on the number of excreted eggs carried into the water (determined by the excretory habits and methods of sanitation of the human hosts).
3. A snail factor measured the output of cercariae by infected snails. This factor depends mainly on the density of the susceptible snail population in the water contaminated by schistosome eggs. Snail density determines the chances of a snail being infected by the miracidia generated by the eggs, as well as the number of cercariae excreted by the snails into the water.
4. An exposure factor measured the chance of cercariae excreted by the snails infecting the human host. This factor depends on the number and extent of the contacts with infected water made by potential hosts.

MacDonald used his model to predict the effectiveness of several approaches to eradication of the disease in a community. As Ross

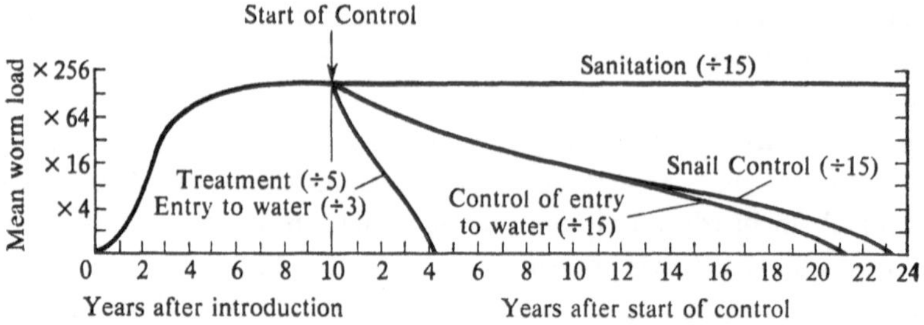

Exhibit 3. The rise and fall of a helminth infection. Model of effects of four schistosomiasis control programs introduced after the infection has risen above the break point, viz., reduction of contamination; reduction in number of snails; reduction of exposure; and treatment with complementary lessening of exposure or of snails. The four types of controls are all of apparently similar value in that each reduces one of the factors involved to one-fifteenth its original value. *Source*: Mac Donald [13].

"A following set of programmes... completes these observations by testing over a long period, 20 years, the effects of equal reduction in contamination, snails, exposure, and worm longevity by treatment, supported by reduction of exposure, to a degree at which some of them at least would be expected to produce ultimate eradication. The effect of reduced contamination to one 15,000th of excreta reaching water, which represents a very high standard of sanitation, is virtually negligible over the entire period. The effects of snail control and control of exposure in the form of entry to water are virtually identical during most of the period of fall, though during the later stages control of exposure is somewhat more effective, resulting in a slightly earlier disappearance of the infection. Ultimate disappearance following either of these methods is delayed for over 20 years, throughout all of which effective measures would have to be carried out, and even improvement to a level approaching perfection would only slightly reduce the time involved, to 14 or 15 years, owing to the long mean length of life postulated for the worms, 3 years. By contrast, the combination of systematic treatment with either reduction of exposure or snail control produces a rapid result, the final effects of which are visible between 4 and 5 years after the start."

had found with the anophelene malaria vector, he too found that there was a critical number of worms in a given environment, a 'break point', above which numbers would increase until they reached a stable infection level and below which numbers would decrease and disappear. Exhibit 3 illustrates the effects of four different control programs on the prevalence of the human host population. The model predicted that sanitation alone would prove ineffectual. Less surprisingly, the model predicted that the most effective approach would prove to be a combination of measures intensively applied at a local level. The technological development that would bring the most rapid benefits at least cost, according to the model, was the improvement of mass therapeutic methods. Although the predictions of this model have not been tested and validated, as have those of the malaria models, predictions seem to be in rough accord with past experience of preventive programs.[4]

Whereas the successes of malaria eradication programs have encouraged model builders, the failures of the programs have instructed them. Even the largest and most serious of all the programs, in India, has controlled malaria but not eradicated it from the land. The failures are of two main types. On the biological side, the models cannot be universal. The processes of transmission are not everywhere the same, and as a result programs that work in Ceylon do not work in Gambia and Ethiopia. On the mathematical side, the models are too simple to encompass all the relevant variables. Significant biological variables, for instance immunity, vector resistance, and human migration, are not included. Significant social and political contexts, which were critical for the execution of programs, could not have been quantified even if their effects had been anticipated. For models that try to represent causal sequences, moreover, the time dimension is especially significant. Processes evolve through time, and adequate models must simulate the continuing unfolding of interacting events [19]. Such simulation had to await the advent of electronic computers.

Here there is no need to argue the merits of particular models. Our concern is only to show that the concept of abstract variables with general properties is a heuristic one for epidemiologists.

BIBLIOGRAPHY

[1] N. T. J. Bailey, *The Mathematical Theory of Epidemics* (Hafner, New York 1957).

[2] J. Brownlee, 'Statistical Studies in Immunity: The Theory of an Epidemic', *Proc. Roy. Soc. Edinburgh* **26** (1906) 484–521.

[3] J. Cassel and H. A. Tyroler, 'Epidemiological Studies of Culture Change', *Arch. Environ. Health* **3** (1961) 25–33.

[4] B. P. Dohrenwend and B. S. Dohrenwend, *Social Status and Psychological Disorder: A Causal Inquiry* (Wiley–Interscience, New York 1969).

[5] J. H. Edwards, 'Familial Predisposition in Man', in: C. E. Ford and H. Harris (eds.), *New Aspects of Human Genetics, British Medical Bulletin* **25** (1969) 58–64.

[6] M. Greenwood, *Medical Statistics from Graunt to Farr* (Cambridge University Press, Cambridge 1948).

[7] W. H. Hamer, 'Epidemic Disease in England. The Evidence of Variability and Presistency of Type' (Milroy Lectures), *Lancet* **1** (1906) 733–39.

[8] J. S. Horn, *Away with All Pests* (Monthly Review Publications, New York 1969), pp. 94–106.

[9] J. O. Irvin, 'The Place of Mathematics in Medical and Biological Statistics', *J. R. Statist.* **A 126** (1963) 1–41.

[10] J. Johnson, *Econometric Methods* (McGraw-Hill, New York 1963).

[11] P. F. Lazarsfeld, 'Evidence and Interference in Social Research', Deadalus **LXXVII** (1958) 90–130.

[12] G. MacDonald, *The Epidemiology and Control of Malaria* (Oxford University Press, London 1957).

[13] G. MacDonald, 'The Dynamics of Helminth Infections, with Special Reference to Schistosomes', *Trans. Roy. Soc. Trop. Med. Hyg.* **59** (1965) 489–506.

[14] G. MacDonald, C. B. Cuellar and C. V. Foll, 'The Dynamics of Malaria', *Bull. W. H. O.* **38** (1968) 743–55.

[15] B. MacMahon, T. F. Pugh and J. Ipsen, Epidemiologic Methods (Little and Brown, Boston 1960).

[16] V. Navarro and R. D. Parker, 'Models in Health Services Planning', in: W. W. Holland (ed.), *Data Handling in Epidemiology* (Oxford University Press, London 1970), pp. 181–98.

[17] J. V. Neel and W. J. Schull, *Effects of Exposure to the Atomic Bomb on Pregnancy Termination in Hiroshima and Nagasaki* (National Research Council, Washington D. C. 1956).

[18] D. D. Reid, 'Sickness and Stress in Operational Flying', *Brit. J. Soc. Med.* **2** (1948) 123–31.

[19] M. W. Riley and E. E. Nelson, 'Research on Stability and Change in Social Systems', in: B. Barber and A. Inkeles (eds.), *Stability and Social Change: A Volume in Honor of Talcott Parsons* (Little Brown, Boston), pp. 407–79.

[20] Sir. R. Ross, *The Prevention of Malaria*, 2nd ed. (E. P. Dutton, New York 1910).

[21] R. E. Serfling, 'Historical Review of Epidemic Theory', *Human Biology* **24** (1952) 145–66.

[22] M. C. Sheps and J. A. Menken, 'A Model for Studying Birth Rates Given Time Dependent Changes in Reproductive Parameters', *Biometrics* **27** (1971) 325–43.

[23] R. Shyrock, *Development of Modern Medicine: An Interpretation of the Social and Scientific Factors Involved* (Knopf, New York 1947).

[24] C. C. Spicer, 'Some Empirical Studies in Epidemiology', *Proc. Fifth Berkeley Symp. Math. Statist. Probab.* **4** (1967) 207–15.

[25] Z. A. Stein and M. W. Susser, 'The Social Dimensions of a Symptom', *Soc. Sci. Med.* **1** (1961) 183–201.
[26] M. Susser, *Community Psychiatry: Epidemiologic and Social Themes* (Random House, New York 1968).
[27] A. H. Thomas, 'Short Term Effects of Air Pollution on Mortality in New York City', *Environmental Science and Technology* **4** (1970) 589–97.
[28] Tien-Hsi Cheng, 'Schistosomiasis in Mainland China: A Review of Research and Control Programs since 1949', *Amer. J. Trop. Med. and Hyg.* **20** (1971) 26–53.
[29] C. Wilcocks, *Aspects of Medical Investigations in Africa* (Oxford University Press, London 1962).
[30] W. Winkelstein, S. Kantor, E. W. Davis, C. S. Maneri and W. E. Mosher, 'The Relationship of Air Pollution and Economic Status to Total Mortality and Selected Respiratory System Mortality in Men', *Arch. Environ. Health*, part 1, **14** (1967) 162–71, part 2, **16** (1968) 401–405.

REFERENCES

* This material presented at the Warsaw Conference on the Sociology of Medicine in August 1973 involves Chapter 3 of the book *Causal Thinking in the Health Sciences* by M. Susser, Oxford University Press, 1973, and it is reprinted by permission of the author and publisher.

[1] There are many cases in New York City, all imported from elsewhere. That schistosomiasis should appear in New York, the epitome of megalopolis, is a commentary in itself on the intimate relations between social forces and the distribution of disease.

[2] The main distinction between epidemiology and ecology is that while epidemiology is centered on the state of health of man, ecology embraces the interrelations of all living things. Epidemiology could be described as human ecology, or that large part of human ecology relating to states of health.

[3] This modified Ross's conclusion of a half-century before, that larval mosquitos should be attacked in their breeding grounds. The intervention advocated by MacDonald depended on the discovery of residual insecticides, particularly DDT, and was not available to Ross.

[4] In China the story seems to be a different one. The disease caused by *Schistosoma japonicum* is reported to be serious and even devastating. Eradication is known to be complicated, and various approaches are being used. Mass treatment is being undertaken; night soil is collected and stored until the heat generated kills the excreted ova; and snails are destroyed by filling in old canals or burying the snails on the banks. The attack is carried out by the technique of the 'human sea', by which many thousands of people are mobilized in communal effort. Several country districts are reported to have been cleared by these means, with dramatic improvement in the people's health [8], [28].

TEAM WORK IN HEALTH CARE IN THE U.S.: A SOCIOLOGICAL PERSPECTIVE

SAAD Z. NAGI

Mershon Center, The Ohio State University, Columbus, Ohio, U.S.A.

Reactions to team work whether in health care, science and research, or in other areas are seldom neutral. While some see in it a panacea that will help solve many stubborn organizational problems, others condemn it on a variety of grounds. To borrow Homan's expression, it seems that team approaches are viewed as matters of morals rather than matters of strategy. In spite of those strong attitudes, or perhaps because of them, literature on this topic remains more descriptive and prescriptive than analytical. The attempt in this paper will be to clarify the place of team work in health care, to review the thrusts of current studies and the important findings, and to point out some neglected dimensions that warrant research attention.

THE PLACE OF TEAM WORK IN HEALTH CARE

Impetus to the development of team approaches to the delivery of health care, and concern over their performance have been tied to a number of trends. To begin with, health care has experienced a marked increase in specialization and division of labor. For the most part, this trend has been the product of a phenomenal expansion in health-related knowledge and technology. The modal practice for a physician in many societies, and certainly in the U.S., has changed from a general one to one of specialization in certain systems or pathologies, and often to more narrow specialization within these (Somers and Somers, 1961). Modern diagnoses call for a varied number of laboratory, radiologic, psychometric, and other tests. Interdependence in present day surgery is built around an array of health personnel.

Another relevant trend has been one of an expanding scope for the concept of 'health', and a corresponding increase in the domain of activities encompassed under the rubric of health care. This trend stems from a better understanding of the tendency of human problems to cluster, and a recognition that health concerns can be addressed with greater effectiveness when considered within the context of other problems. Diverse health professionals are brought into closer working relationships with others dealing with such problems as poverty, unemployment, housing, delinquency and other forms of deviance.

Specialization with its associated fragmentation of services, and the interdependence of health workers and others dealing with related problems underlie the many attempts toward 'coordination' and 'integration' of services. Specialization, beneficial in many ways, is destined to continue and increase in the face of expanding knowledge and technology. The most obvious way to overcome its negative side effects lies in the notion of bringing together the opinions and approaches of specialists to bear upon a problem that cuts across their specialties. Team work in health care is an operational manifestation of this notion. This is not to say that teams represent a new phenomenon in the field, nor that they necessarily have been or are comprised of differing specialties. Earlier and present collaboration among general practitioners is known in the form of group practices or in consultation with each other over complex cases. However, much of the current team work represents multiple specialties and often multiple professions. At any rate, primary concern in this paper is with these latter types of teams.

Another important factor in the significance of team approaches in health care delivery stems from certain aspects of the manpower situation. While the supply of physicians has not kept pace with rising demands for health services, there has been a phenomenal proliferation of health professions. In the absence of long range and effective manpower policies in this field, the development of new professions has been highly unsystematic. Discussions of these policies revolve around such issues as realigning the boundaries of professional domains and the articulation of roles among the various professions. These lines of thought are generally predicated on the assumption that many of the functions presently performed by the highly trained health professionals, such as physicians who are in short supply, could be delegated to others with lesser training requirements. In fact, some would contend that the problem is not one of shortage of physicians, but of coordinating roles in the delivery system. Here again, the team concept arises as a mechanism for such coordination.

Beyond the traditional physician-nurse teams and others consisting of specialists from different areas of medicine itself, the last three decades have witnessed a phenomenal increase in the numbers and types of team formations in health care. In institutions for the mentally ill or retarded, therapeutic teams have included combinations of psychiatrists, other physicians, psychologists, psychiatric social workers, nurses, occupational therapists, and others. Rehabilitation service centers and long term facilities for the physically impaired are organized around teams that include some of the specialists mentioned above in addition to others in physical therapy, prosthetics, and vocational rehabilitation. Ambulatory facilities such as in programs of maternal and child health provide services through primary teams that include pediatricians, psychologists, nurses, social workers, nutritionists, and often laymen who may perform outreach functions. Patients have also been included as part of the collective therapeutic process usually referred to as therapeutic communities. Different health care programs may also designate liaison members who in effect become teams to work on the integration of these programs.

A common characteristic shared by these teams is the direct face-to-face interaction among members in the course of performing services. Concern with team work, however, goes beyond these face-to-face formations to the problems of articulating the roles and functions of health care providers within the larger institutional or community contexts. The problems are not unrelated but emphasis in this paper is upon the primary face-to-face teams.

PROMINENT THEMES IN THE LITERATURE

Much of the analytical literature on team work is about interdisciplinary research and other forms of collaboration in scientific activities. This literature will be drawn upon whenever useful in clarifying issues related to health care teams. Although research and analysis of teams have been primarily structural in perspective, some analysts have placed their emphasis on social psychological factors such as 'good interpersonal relations among team members' and 'being able to work together'. One study of research teams concludes that "collaborators must have strong common values, confidence in each other's ability, and certainty in each other's interests to contribute to a common goal" (Eaton, 1951). Other investigators refer to the need for 'leadership skills' on the part of some members, and 'membership skills' on the part of all (e.g., Rubin and Beckhard, 1972). Most analyses, however, are organized around structural variables and processes that will be summarized in the following paragraphs.

Status, Power, Authority, and Influence

The dominance of the medical profession in health care activities has been well explained. As Freidson (1970) points out, "in spite of... struggling" segments "within the ranks of those holding the M.D. degree and in the face of non-medical occupations struggling for access to the task of healing, the profession (Medicine) still preserves a common identity and sustains a superordinate position". Such dominance manifests itself in the structure of authority and decision making which seem to vary according to the settings. Surgical wards were reported to be more structured than medical wards where decision making was generally by consensus (Coser, 1958). And, as would be expected, authority within surgical teams in operating rooms is highly structured (Wilson, 1966). Earlier studies on stratification among staff members in hospitals show that fuller and clearer communication to and about patients was more characteristic of wards with low than with high stratification (Seeman and Evans, 1961). Evidence also indicates that some hospital staffs neither accept the status positions they are assigned nor the system that assigns such hierarchies (Lentz, 1950). Although these findings represent hospital wards, the generalizability of the propositions to team work seems plausible. Corroborative evidence of the superiority-inferiority problem and its negative influence on collaboration comes from studies of team work in science (Hagstrom, 1967). It is not clear, however, as to what degree physicians are involved in the struggle for status and authority in health care teams. It might be argued that their dominance is more widely accepted, and that such struggles are more intense among the other professions still seeking a place in the hierarchy (Zander *et al.*, 1957).

The class and status positions of patients in relation to the health professionals, and the influence of these factors on the services patients receive, have been largely assumed rather than verified. The issue is important to the performance of 'therapeutic communities' where patients become part of larger teams. In connection with public health activities, Simmons (1966) points out that class and status considerations have significance to the functioning of the teams by influencing interpersonal relations within the health teams and between the teams and the public. One conclusion drawn from this work is that optimal therapeutic relationships evolve when professionals and patients are from similar class backgrounds. In part, this proposition underlies the employment of indigenous groups as outreach personnel in many health care and other services dealing with low income families. The assumption is that similarity in status would help facilitate communication.

Roles and Professional Domains

A considerable amount of the literature in this area is concerned with the roles of the various health professions including time and motion studies (e.g., Bergman *et al.*, 1966). The utility of such literature to the analysis of team work is limited in that it does not address the articulation of roles of different professions. However, these accounts are instructive to the extent that they show the ambiguities of roles in certain professions and the overlap among them that can become a source of difficulty in organizing team work. In this connection, it is important also to note that roles performed by persons from the same profession vary in different settings.

Although some writers may question the need for physicians in certain types of health delivery teams (e.g., Wise, 1970); most discussions of division of labor assume the centrality of the physician's role. Several demonstrations report the expansion of physicians' practices and capabilities to serve more people by the addition of one type of health profession or another (e.g., Silver, 1963; Rogers *et al.*, 1968). Underlying some of these demonstrations is an attempt to show that some of the traditional functions of the physicians can be performed by others, such as nurses, social workers, etc. Data on this issue, however, is still vague and bears little fruit for action. Lacking is information about the specifics of the physician's role, the legal boundaries of the role, the specifics of what other professions can undertake, whether or not such change would require alterations in existing laws, and the consequences of changes in roles and tasks to the quantity and quality of health care delivered. Difficulties in realigning the boundaries of professional domains are greatly compounded by potential economic and other status consequences associated with roles which lie at the heart of inter-professional struggles.

A related theme in the literature concerns the articulation of roles. Differing but complementary roles and orientations were found to contribute to cohesion (Turk, 1963). Specialization is seen as a deterrent to the members of a given profession against meddling into the professional domain of the others. Several analysts speak of the necessity of a clear division of labor as a condition for the effectiveness of team work in health care as well as in other collaborative endeavors (e.g., Svarstad, 1970; Beckhard, 1972; Rubin and Beckhard, 1972; George *et al.*, 1971; Horowitz, 1970). Developments in this direction are predicated on at least four elements: (a) clarity and specificity of roles; (b) specialization and minimal overlap; (c) complementarity of roles in working toward a collective goal; and (d) shared understanding and acceptance of role definitions by members of the teams. Specialization and understanding of the roles of others may seem to be contradictory requirements. However, the significance is in the degree, and some understanding of the roles of other team members is neccessary for the articulation of one's own activities with those of others. Such articulation constitutes the difference between integrated team work and the collection of activities of independent professionals who are disparate in education and modes of services. It is one thing to identify such elements in the articulation of roles, but a far more difficult task to provide relevant hard information useful for organizing teams. As has already been mentioned, the literature is replete with assertions of prerequisites for effectiveness but exhibits serious gaps in systematic analyses of these topics. It is important to mention that the lack of clarity in accounts of roles and their specification cannot be merely considered as a limitation of studies and research, but as a reflection of ambiguities in the roles themselves.

Decision Making and Communication

Two aspects of team decision making warrant attention. *First,* is the structure of decision making which relates closely to the structure of roles and authority. Two models of decision-making structures are depicted in the literature – the 'hierarchal' and the 'egalitarian'. The merits and demerits of these models are argued in the main on ideological grounds with limited and often no empirical verification (e.g., Lewis, 1969; Crombie, 1970). Reported also are feeble attempts to integrate the two models by simply specifying some personal characteristics of leaders, and prescribing flexibility in roles and openness in communications (Lewis, 1969). Most teams operate within the framework of larger organizations. The authority structure within parent organizations and the constraints they impose on the teams can be expected to influence the team's structure for decision making. Organizational constraints are equally, if not more, important in the decision making structure of *inter*-organizational teams. When members of such teams represent independent organizations, each usually becomes endowed with a veto power over unacceptable decisions. The resulting structure varies from the two models mentioned above.

The *second* aspect of decision making is a substantive one, that is, what agreements and disagreements take place among team members in regard to the substance of decisions. Difficulties in this respect stem from differences in perceptions, concepts, methods, and treatment modalities. The issue is one of barriers in communication. Blocks and distortions in communication have been reported in several studies (e.g., Frank, 1961; Brodsky, 1968). Team members from varying professional backgrounds were shown to differ in their perceptions and evaluation of patients and their conditions (e.g., Weissman, 1969). It should be noted, however, that these studies usually derive data from case studies of individual teams, and therefore influences evolving from differences in professional orientations are not sifted from differences in other characteristics of team members. To unravel the relative weights of these two sources of influence would require an experimental design that incorporates a number of professions and a number of persons from each profession.

In addition to the influence of substantive variations among the health care fields, communication among team members can be further complicated because of differing orientations in regard to the importance of services versus inquiry. Even within the same field some training institutions emphasize services while others may emphasize research and insistence upon verification. The two orientations entail many points of conflict (Nagi, 1965). Consistent with a service stance is a belief in techniques and modalities being applied to patients, while an orientation toward inquiry means that information is always held in a tentative status. Furthermore, commitment to services orients health practitioners to the uniquenesses of patients, while commitment to inquiry focuses attention on patterns. Although differing orientations along these lines might impede substantive communication, their influence on the social cohesion of teams might not be necessarily negative (e.g., Turk, 1963). The conditions under which differing orientations affect communication and cohesion and the direction and degree of effect, are empirical questions still largely unexplored.

Another issue in communication that remains obscure concerns the direction of information flow across fields and its relation to the relative status of the various professions and their centrality in the teams' operations. Even when the members of a team lack in knowledge about each other's fields at the beginning, learning is bound to take place as the team continues. The question is: Which fields are members of a team more likely to learn about? It is submitted that the flow of information will be influenced by the relative status of the professional hierarchy, and will tend to move from the higher to the lower ones. At the risk of oversimplification, it can be said that the flow of information depends upon: (a) the readiness of those who possess the information to transmit it; (b) the readiness of the ones to be informed to seek or at least receive it; and (c) a variety of conditions related to means and contexts of information transfer. The direction of flow hypothesized here is not necessarily predicated on the readiness of members of the higher status fields as transmitters of information about their fields, but primarily on the receptivity of members of the lower status fields to such information. One consequence of this pattern of information flow, if empirically true, is that the articulation of roles in teams comes about primarily as a result of accommodations of the lower status fields to those of higher status. This limits the possibilities of re-examining the roles and realigning the boundaries of the higher status fields and professions.

NEGLECTED DIMENSIONS

The foregoing discussion is neither intended to be an exhaustive account of available literature, nor of possible topics around which the material can be organized. However, it conveys the important themes explored and the quality of work reported. It is largely atheoretical, and with very few exceptions, has not benefited from theoretical developments in such related areas and topics as small groups, decision making, exchange, coalition formation, and the like. Most of the studies represent descriptive case studies and results of simple demonstrations carried out and reported apparently with little or no awareness of these theoretical traditions. Furthermore, the literature exhibits conspicuous gaps of which the following are important examples.

The Effectiveness of Teams

Among the primary, if not the most significant, objectives of team work and other approaches to the delivery of health care is enhancing the quality as well as the quantity of services. Most of the studies, however, concentrate on the dynamics of team relations with such phenomena as cohesion, communication, and patterns of decision making being the most common dependent variables. Often, these variables are presented as measures for the effectiveness of teams. Several factors might have contributed to the lack of studies that test the effectiveness of teams in terms of the quality of care they provide. Difficulties in measuring the quality of care are well documented (e.g., Donabedian, 1966; Kessner *et al.*, 1971; Birk *et al.*, 1971). And, problems of access to data might have constituted another barrier to the assessment of quality of care. Such studies are usually threatening to teams and therefore are resisted. For many advocates of the team approach, positive influence is considered as self-evident and needs no further verification. Even if the superiority of team approaches over individual and sequential service arrangements is to be accepted on face validity, which in my opinion remains an open empirical question, comparative studies of teams are needed to determine the relative effectiveness of varying types and formations.

Patients' Reactions

It seems that not only members of a team would need to know about each others' fields, in order to coordinate their roles and functions, but that optimum services would require that patients in many types of practice settings have some understanding of the roles of the different professionals. In rehabilitation, psychotherapy, and preventive health practices, the cooperation, if not the participation, of patients and clients is essential for the effectiveness of such services. In view of the increasing specialization and proliferation of the health professions, it is important to assess the knowledge of patients, clients, and the public at large about these professions and to determine the relations of levels of knowledge in response to therapy. Participation in a social process implies complementarity of roles including those of patients as well as those who act on their behalf. Obviously, the issue is not that patients need to become specialists in the various health fields. Rather, the question concerns the type and amount of knowledge about a professional role prerequisite to appropriate interaction and response on the part of patients. Although the question is applicable to individual practices as well, it is particularly important to teams in which there is overlap in the domains and roles of professional members.

Gate-Keeping Decisions

Differences among the professions in points of view, skills, and social positions are as manifested in gate-keeping decisions as in any other aspects of team operations. Gate-keeping decisions control the admission or rejection of applicants for services. Two patterns for the processes of gate-keeping decisions have evolved, each of which entails serious limitations, thus creating the elements of a double-bind. The *first* pattern is to assign gate-keeping decisions to the representative of a given field who becomes a 'coordinator'. Gate-keeping decisions under this arrangement may extend beyond the admission and rejection of applicants, to influencing the referral to other team members for services. In effect, coordinators become gate-keepers in relation to the other fields. Members of the other professions are brought into contact with the client when the coordinator detects a problem that requires their services. The limitation inherent in this model lies in the ability of the person with a given professional background to recognize problems that fall within the domains of other professions. Team approaches are based upon the assumption that clients' problems are complex and involve facets that can be better understood and ameliorated through specialized knowledge and skills possessed by various professions. To illustrate, can a social worker make differential diagnoses of physical conditions? Or, can a nurse take the place of a psychologist or a social worker in identifying emotional or social problems? Aside from these technical considerations, monopoly over gate-keeping powers by given professions fosters resentment on the part of others.

The *second* pattern of decision making in interprofessional teams accords greater recognition to specialization and appeals more to democratic principles. Representatives of each profession on the team are given the opportunity to interview or examine the patient and to determine the presence or absence of problems within their domains. The limitation of this model lies in the possible tendency for members of the teams to overdiagnose as a means for protecting their professional domains and demonstrating the significance of their services to the teams. In this way, the model tends to serve the interests of the team members rather than those of the patients.

Manpower and Training

As has already been mentioned, division of labor, coordination of roles, and other factors in optimizing team performance require some familiarity on the part of members with the substance and methods of each other's fields. It is important also that students of health services learn about future roles in team work during their training. Such requirements can have much bearing upon the types of curricula, experiences, and training settings that would contribute to effective team work in health care. Principles of anticipatory socialization would strongly suggest that new recruits should be sensitized to team work during their professional training. These approaches are not prevalent in present curricula especially those of medical colleges. New products of these colleges know little about many of the health professions and less on how utilize the skills of these professions in coordination with their own. Experimentation with new curricula and training experiences is greatly needed.

Another aspect of training not systematically addressed in the literature on team work is that of the numbers of people to be trained in the various health fields. The issue is one of manpower needs and production. Manpower policies in most western societies, and certainly in the U.S., are vague and largely inoperative. In the main, reasons for the lack of effective policies in this area are ideological. They relate to individual career choices in contrast to centralized planning and manpower mobilization. In the absence of manpower policies the need for health services personnel and their availability become poorly synchronized. The inelastic supply and demand schedules of trained manpower contribute greatly to putting needs and availability out of phase. This inelasticity results from the long period of time required for the mounting or expanding professional training programs and for training the needed personnel themselves. Once programs are built and students attracted to them, voluntary adjustments to contracting markets also become slow. Therefore, the supply lags behind the increasing demands of expanding health manpower markets. And, once the supply has risen to a high level, the over-production continues out of phase with decreasing needs. Training funds for students and institutions have been used in the U.S. and other countries to stimulate the supply of trained personnel in the health fields. However, extending and withdrawing these funds have not followed well planned policies. In fact, the sudden availability and abrupt termination of such funds have caused considerable dislocations in educational institutions. In the absence of specific information on the types, units, and needs for the services of the various professions in relation to the incidence and prevalence of health problems, manpower policies will always be vague and ill-founded. It is hoped that future research on team work in health care would seriously address these issues.

BIBLIOGRAPHY

Richard Beckhard, 'Organizational Issues in the Team Delivery of Comprehensive Health Care', *Milbank Memorial Fund Quarterly* **3** (1972) 287–316.

A. B. Bergman, S. W. Dassel and R. S. Wedgewood, 'Time-Motion Study of Practicing Pediatricians', *Pediatrics* **38** (1966) 254–63.

Peter Birk, Cynthia Dalton and Thomas Ward, 'Problem Oriented Analysis of Medical Care Episodes – A New Evaluation Model', 99th Annual Meeting (1971), American Public Health Association.

Carroll M., Brodsky, 'Communication and Behavior on a Small Psychiatric Unit', *Comprehensive Psychiatry* **9** (1968) 525–35.

Ruth Laub Coser, 'Authority and Decision-Making in a Hospital: A Comparative Analysis', *American Sociological Review* **23** (1958) 56–63.

D. L. Crombie, M.D., 'Group Dynamics and Domiciliary Health Team', *Journal of the Royal College of General Practitioners* **19** (1970) 66–78.

Avedis Donabedian, 'Evaluating the Quality of Medical Care', *Milbank Memorial Fund Quarterly* **44** (1966) 166–206.

Joseph W. Eaton, 'Social Processes of Professional Teamwork', *American Sociological Review* **16** (1951) 707–13.

Lawrence Frank, 'Interprofessional Communication', *American Journal of Public Health* **51** (1961) 1798–1804.

Eliot Freidson, *Professional Dominance*, Atherton Press, Inc., New York 1970.

Madelon, George, Kazuyoshi Ide and Clara Vamber, 'The Comprehensive Health Team: A Conceptual Model', *Journal of Nursing Administration* **1** (1971) 9–13.

Warren O. Hagstrom, *Competition and Teamwork in Science*, Final Report to the National Science Foundation for Research Grant GS657 to the University of Wisconsin (1967).

John J. Horowitz, 'Dimensions of Rehabilitation Teamwork', *Rehabilitation Record* **10** (1970) 37–40.

David M. Kessner, Rashid L. Bashshur and Carolyn E. Kalk, 'A Methodology for the Evaluation of Ambulatory Health Services: The Development of the Tracer Concept', 99th Annual Meeting (1971), American Public Health Association.

Edith Lentz, 'Morale in a Hospital Business Office', *Human Organization* **9** (1950) 17–21.

Jerry M. Lewis, M.D., 'The Organizational Structure of the Therapeutic Team', *Hospital and Community Psychiatry* **20** (1969) 206–8.

Charles Lowe and D. Alexander, 'Health Care of Poor Children', in: A. L. Schorr (ed.), *Children and Decent People*, Basic Books, New York 1974, p. 153.

Saad Z. Nagi, 'Practitioners as Participants in Research', *Rehabilitation Record* **6** (1965).

Kenneth D. Rogers, Mary Mally and Florence Marcus, 'A General Medical Practice Using Non-Physician Personnel', *Journal of the American Medical Association* **206** (1968) 1763–1767.

Irwin Rubin and Richard Beckhard, 'Factors Influencing the Effectiveness of Health Teams', *Milbank Memorial Fund Quarterly* **3** (1972) 317–35.

Melvin Seeman and John W. Evans, 'Stratification and Hospital Care: I. The Performance of a Medical Intern', *American Sociological Review* **26** (1961a) 67–80.

Melvin Seeman and John W. Evans, 'Stratification and Hospital Care: II. The Objective Criteria of Performance', *American Sociological Review* **26** (1961b) 193–204.

George A. Silver, *Family Medical Care*, Harvard University Press, Cambridge, Mass., 1963.

Ozzie G. Simmons, 'Implications of Social Class for Public Health', in: J. R. Volta and E. S. Deck (eds.), *A Sociological Framework for Patient Care*, John Wiley and Sons, Inc., New York 1966, pp. 35–42.

Herman Miles Somers and Anne Ramsay Somers, *Doctors, Patients and Health Insurance*, The Brookings Institution, Washington, D.C., 1961.

Boni Svarstad, 'Sociological Factors Affecting Medical Team-Work', The Dr. Martin Luther King, Jr., Health Center Fourth Annual Report (1970).

Mathew Tayback, *et. al.*, 'Evaluation Studies on Maternal and Infant Care Projects', Department of Social and Preventive Medicine, University of Maryland School of Medicine (September), 1973, p. 8.

Herman Turk, 'Social Cohesion through Variant Values: Evidence from Medical Role Relations', *American Sociological Review* **28** (1963) 28–37.

Herbert N. Weissman, 'The Psychiatric Team as a Differential Decision Maker with Child Patients', *Psychological Report* **25** (1969) 11–17.

Robert N. Wilson, 'Teamwork in the Operating Room', in: W. R. Scott and E. H. Volkart (eds.), *Medical Care Readings in the Sociology of Medical Institutions*, John Wiley and Sons, Inc., New York 1966.

Harold Wise, 'Patterns of Health Care Delivery', The Dr. Martin Luther King, Jr., Health Center Fourth Annual Report (1970) 5–25.

Alvin Zander, Arthur R. Cohen and Ezra Statland, *Role Relations in the Mental Health Professions*, University of Michigan Press, Ann Arbor 1957.

THERAPEUTIC COMMUNITY AND PSYCHIATRY IN THE COMMUNITY: A COMPARATIVE STUDY OF THE FRENCH AND ANGLO-SAXON LITERATURES*

CLAUDINE HERZLICH

École Pratique des Hautes Études, Centre d'Étude des Mouvements Sociaux, Paris, France

I have chosen to analyse in these few pages the French attempts to reform the mental health care system and the expression these attempts have found in psychiatric and sociological literature. This may be a surprising choice. Indeed, in practice as well as in theory, France is far behind the Anglo-Saxon countries and undoubtedly far behind other European countries in this field. Nevertheless, I preferred to study the problem from this point of view for several reasons. First, because I couldn't possibly cover all the literature – particularly the literature in English – in this field (especially since I am not a specialist on the problems of mental illness and psychiatric institutions). Furthermore, I felt it would be out of place with regard to such a topic, to present material of which my knowledge is but indirect and acquired from books. Finally, discussing less well-known experiences, even if they have limitations, and comparing them with the 'classic' Anglo-Saxon situation, seemed to me interesting in itself.

*   *

*

The very long history of treatment given to the mentally ill, its evolution, its alternating between different forms of permissiveness and repressiveness, are probably familiar to all. In France, the concept of madness and the need to exclude the madman, are brought forth through the ruling ideology during the Enlightenment when such terms as reason and happiness became identified with normality. Psychiatric methods were influenced by the fact of confinement of the mentally ill.[1] Later, Philippe Pinel's unchaining of the patients at the Bicêtre Asylum took on a symbolic value. The revolution in attitudes towards madmen seems to be inseparable from the new conceptions of man expressed at the same time by the French Revolution.

But today French psychiatry is still influenced by traditions of asylum organization of the 19th century. The 1838 legislation recognized the preponderance of the asylum, according to Esquirol's wish, for whom an asylum "is the most powerful agent in the hands of a skillful physician".[2] We can observe here an anticipation of the modern conceptions of a therapeutic environment, but the therapeutic action of 'isolating' the mental patient in a protected environment and the repressive method of 'locking up', were assimilated at the same time. The French movement of 'moral treatment', apparently very much less permissive than its homologues in other countries,[3] completed the synthesis of medical action and social control. It was based on the idea of an absolute 'take over' and a total reconditioning of the patient's life, so that reason, discipline and morality could triumph.[4] With the passing of time, this 'total' attempt watered down gradually to the custody of the mental patient, an undesirable person, while the asylum kept on materially decaying and morally ruining itself.

A reforming reaction similar to that occurring in the Anglo-Saxon countries took place after the Second World War. One fact is directly related to the other. The humanitarian concern was very important: nearly forty thousand (40,000) mental patients died in France during the War because of the disastrous conditions in which they lived. But nevertheless, the War also provided one opportunity of realizing an experience which served as a model for a whole generation of French psychiatrists. During the German occupation, the small hospital of Saint Alban, in the Lozère region, directed by Dr. Tosquelles was organized to allow the survival of patients and staff, and even "developed activities which became a social pole for the region, a cultural centre. Taking part in the 'Résistance' which was operating in the vicinity, serving as illicit shelter for the wounded, the hospital lost its segregating function, unhinged itself and those who work there as well as those with whom it was in contact".[5]

Right after the War, a group of young psychiatrists organized meetings, public proclamations and articles, [6] tried to press for a change in policy regarding mental health and care tried to bring about a transformation of the situation in the hospitals. Their first attempts were mainly meant to bring about a renewal of the mental hospital on a basis similar to the one adopted by the Anglo-Saxon therapeutic communities. This movement will be called '*institutional psychotherapy*'. Its aim was to improve the physical facilities inside the hospital, redefine the social relationships among patients and staff, and establish an open door policy in order to reduce the gap between hospital and community. Later, these basic trends were coloured by *psychoanalytic thinking*. The objective reality of the institution was reinterpreted in psychoanalytic terms. The symbolic values of institutional life were emphasized, as well as the unconscious conflicts expressed in everyday life. But, at the same time, a third trend made its appearance, aimed at *breaking up the hospital*, by transforming it into one of several elements of a flexible care system directly implanted in the 'normal' community.

Despite the numerous attempts to transform the hospital that were made during all these years, the general situation has hardly progressed at all. A sociologist entering a mental hospital in 1972, can write as follows: "A novice who happens to enter a mental hospital is immediately provoked by the apparent aspect of moral and physical misery. The public mental hospital came into existence characterized above all by poor living conditions, patient overcrowding and an obvious shortage of staff (nursing and medical)".[7] As to the institutional routine and the oppressive relationships between patients and staff, the descriptions parallel those of the American State Mental Hospitals, such as the ones published, for example, by I. Belknap [8] and E. Goffman. [9]

Before we analyse the actual content of the attempts at transformation, a brief description of the general trends in the French mental health care system is necessary. Its first characteristic is the prevalence of public institutions (roughly equivalent to city and county hospitals), usually very big (more than half of them have between six hundred and one thousand five hundred beds), which are archaic both in conception and equipment. These hospitals are closely dependent on a central administration, controlled by the state. The local hospital administration, on the other hand, has very little authority and the physician in charge is the only person who has the power to try any kind of transformation or innovation. But there is no lack of conflicts with the central administration, mainly in order to obtain the necessary money and equipment for these attempts. The mental hospital physician, in most cases less well paid, and much less respected than his general hospital colleague, only stays for a short time in each hospital. Consequently, if he has the courage, he will have to start his reform attempts again in each place. In several years, with one physician in charge succeeding another, the same hospital will experience more or less daring attempts and then regress to the asylum routine.

Thus, the French attempts are very different from some well-known American experiments [10] taking place in small private hospitals, where patients are chosen according to their socio-economic stiuation. They are closer, nevertheless, to the British experiences with a public health system. The experience of a therapeutic community must be integrated with the public mental hospital, adapted to its architecture, to its budget and to its staff. The different experiences always share these two realities. Maybe this is one of the reasons why the French literature, more than the American for example, seems to concentrate more upon the resistance provoked by attempts at change and the adoption of 'new methods' as well as it shows better their limits and its failures.

* *

*

The mistrust harboured by the French medical profession towards specialists in other fields (sociologists and psychologists) perhaps explains why until very recently nearly all studies concerning mental hospitals were made exclusively by doctors of medicine. Consequently, it is often very difficult to evaluate these studies: how can one clearly separate the physician's professional bias from an objective description of the reality? The few recent sociological studies do not overlook these criticisms. We have chosen two studies as examples for analysis of the concrete content of those realizations. In both,[11] the authors, as participating observers of the life of the hospital, show an apriori positive attitude. Their criticisms therefore carry all the more weight.

In both cases, the 'new methods' applied in a public mental hospital are quite close to the 'classic' British and American expences, inspired perhaps by an even greater readiness to open the hospital, and reduce the gap between the institution and the 'normal community'.[12] Thus in one case the patients take themselves an active part in the rehabilitation of those leaving the hospital by helping financially or visiting them at home. Here, the gap between patient and non-patient, and the distinction between medical staff and patients are both questioned: the 'patient' who is still in hospital takes part in the therapeutic consolidation of the individual who is 'cured'.

As to the rest, concrete decisions can be classified under the headings used by Rapoport in his study of the Belmont Hospital,[13] in spite of a difference in the vocabulary. 'Democracy': in one of the two case studies, especially the formal democracy concerning decisions (made collectively during different meetings with patients and staff or with different parts of the staff) is considered as the main mover in the change. '*Permissiveness*' officially becomes the basis of the staff's attitude towards the patients. The suppression of a great deal of restrictions and means of control has this very special meaning. One can also put a label of *communalism* employed by Rapoport, upon all arrangements having a drive towards the suppression of gaps between patients and staff (making it impossible for the nurses to have their meals separately, for example) and towards an improvement of communication. The effort to continually analyse each person's attitudes and the conflicts arising with the problems of everyday life, seems similar to the attitude of '*reality confrontation*' extolled at Belmont Hospital.

The functioning of the institution thus transformed shows many parallels with the most classic Anglo-Saxon studies. One can find in the inner life of the hospital the oscillatory patterns between organization and disorganization, between liberalism and repression, between the apparent success and failure of the experiment, as described by Rapoport. The same goes for cases of collective disturbance emphasized both by Caudill and by Stanton and Schwartz.[14] The problem of the 'special case' of a 'symptomatic patient' is of great importance. But the symptom is not interpreted as a result of bad functioning among the staff. It is integrated into a more symbolic conception (the staff's problems are expressed through the patient's conduct) and generalized to all groups interacting with in the hospital: a 'symptomatic resident physician' or a 'symptomatic nurse' may appear as well as a symptomatic patient.[15] This point allows for the articulation of the 'language of the hospital' where the unconscious conflicts among the various interacting groups are expressed.

Yet, whether they are psychiatrists or sociologists, the authors refuse a conception according to which organizational rules, however flexible and permissive, and better communication may in themselves be altogether effective. Maybe because it is more recent, the French literature seems to be slightly more critical than the first Anglo-Saxon 'classics' of what may be called a psychosociological approach of the mental hospital,[16] its dysfunctioning, and the possibilities of the transformation. The fact that this approach was tinged by psychoanalytic thinking was also of great importance.[17] If it did not change the actual content of the innovations, it greatly influenced the function which is nowadays assigned to them: that of being mainly a basis for the expression of phantasms and unconscious conflicts. A great number of psychoanalysts in mental hospitals, also have their own notion, more sophisticated if not more easily provable than that of the first authors, of the therapeutic possibilities of the institution. The 'environment' is not active in itself; efficiency is a result from a permanent analysis involving patients and physicians without distinction, and therefore the institution in itself. This conception is also contrary to that of individual psychotherapeutic treatment which a number of psychiatrists, like Stanton and Schwartz before them, acknowledge as being often difficult and inefficient in the hospital.[18]

The role of the psychiatrist is also distinct from the one he fulfils in the traditional hospital. In the latter, he appears very clearly as the repository of all authority, in addition to representing the 'normal' outside world. The new conceptions, with their insistence upon the therapeutic team,[19] the introduction of new specialists, the separation of the role and person of the psychotherapist from those of the institutional doctor seem to originate from a desire to lessen the power of the doctor. In fact, what we are dealing with here is more a new conception of what that power can be (and it seems very clear to us that some psychiatrists are demanding the establishment ot medical authority over the mental hospital). The psychiatrist, and above all the psychoanalyst, no longer represent, in the 'new style' hospital, the outside authority, but are conceived as being the moving spirit in the life of the institution. He is a 'model for identification'[20] for the staff as well as for the patients, the main support of the collective transference and thus the mediator through whom all therapeutic effect actually passes.

That is why the fact of saying that 'everything' can and must be therapeutic in the new hospital, the fact of insisting upon the idea of a therapeutic team, appeared to some sociologists to be a mask hiding a different reality: the power of medical ideology, or, in psychoanalytic terms, the 'physician's desire'. Some authors detected a basic contradiction in these 'new methods' and, ultimately, one of the reasons for their failure. Considering themselves as liberators the physicians actually impose these new methods on thc staff and the hospital in general. These methods are an expression of the doctor's power, and the democracy of the open hospital is mere semblance. A. Levy's study on the 'paradoxes of liberty in a mental hospital', shows how the most permissive decisions can in reality be turned into oppressive methods. These methods are substitutes for meeting the new demands made on the traditional hospital. The result is the failure of the experiment: a return to custodial practice, to routine, to hierarchy. The conflict between old and new methods also expresses the struggles between the professional groups present in the institution, with their different status and ideologies.

* *

*

In contrast to the efforts at transforming the mental hospital, implanting psychiatry in the community is a trend intended to provide an alternative, to cause a rupture, to bring about a 'reversal of the institutionalisation processes' for practical as well as for theoretical reasons.

The practical reasons are first of all due to the overcrowding of hospitals. "The mental hospitals lack beds, and certainly nothing would have been achieved by this movement, in which psychiatry as a whole has been engaged, if it were not for this outstanding reality: overcrowding."[21] Reducing the amount of time spent on hospital treatment, or even making it unnecessary, become thus principal goals. Furthermore the evolution of mental illness itself is important. The mental patient may now arouse from institutional torpor, thanks to a more active style of therapy. His evolution demands a more varied type of care and allows for a more flexible take over.

On a more theoretical level, tempted by experiences of psychiatry in the community, some physicians start from the often established fact, which occupies a central place in Rapoport's study, of the difference between treatment and rehabilitation. One of them has written: "All those professionally concerned with the care of mental patients can mention many patients 'cured' by the hospital who have a relapse as soon as they go back to their family."[22]

The problem here may be summed up by the fact that the therapeutic community is a 'closed' milieu. It also concerns the ambiguity of the very concept of therapy and recovery in the hospital institution, whether it be modernized or not. Because the 'milieu', the institution, is used as a therapeutic means, it is impossible to determine the patient's health situation otherwise than by judging his good or bad adjustment to the institution. Starting from a redefinition of the milieu community psychiatry may be a means to solve this problem.

Community psychiatry can also be an incentive for the suppression of the distinction between normal and pathological, and of differences between settled categories of psychotics, neurotics and delinquents existing in classic psychiatry. However, it would be erroneous to see in this approach to mental illness, the evasion of the 'medical model'. On the contrary, the community psychiatrist extends his field of practice. First because of the emphasis on prevention and post-recovery, the physician extends the temporal scope of his activity. But also, because the problem is no longer treating a patient but treating a 'suffering set', the "relational network joining the criminal, the victim and society, the madman, his family and the neighbourhood, the absentee, his foreman and the factory, the alcoholic, his wife and the family circle".[23] In this way, the physician feels he can simultaneously influence mental illness and the rejecting attitudes towards it. Thus community practice adopts the assumptions of milieu therapy in an institution. Only the definition of the milieu is changed from the closed milieu of the hospital framework and staff to a milieu intended to be more open through the 'day hospital' or the therapeutic work-shop for example, yet protected and specialized. This extension of the medical approach to all cases of deviance or marginalism which are liable to be questioned owing to their pathological configuration, seems alarming to some authors. "So much the better for the patient", says R. Castel, "if he can thus avoid the most brutal forms of segregation, but too bad for everyone else if no one can avoid the medical or paramedical suspicion."[24]

Ever since 1960, the 'sectorial' (or district area) policy has been the official mental health policy in France. The official doctrine aims at replacing the traditional notion of a 'hospital bed' by a 'place' in a hospital or an extra-hospital care system corresponding to a given geographical area: the sector (or district area). In fact this concept is still centered on the hospital. The physician in charge and the hospital team are in charge of the sector (or district area). Yet, in spite of the legislation, the actual implementation of this policy is only in its infancy and the history of the past twelve years would be mainly the story of the problems and hindrances it has encountered. Some branches of community psychiatry, which are very much developed elsewhere, hardly exist in France, as for example action within the family and through the family which may be considered as the typical example of a 'suffering entirety'.

However, two important projects have been fruitful in their effects. One in Paris, in the 'XIIIth arrondissement',[25] the other, more recently, in the Lyons area. For a long time unique, the Parisian experiment was carried out in special conditions[26] and was for a long time considered as exemplary. It is composed of a group of extra-hospital institutions (mental health clinics, day hospitals, convalescent homes, therapeutic work-shops) each having different roles, but directed by a single team. The continuity of the team, which is composed of various specialists, was essential to the success of the experiment. The Lyons experiment works according to the same model. However, the hospital occupies a central place in the whole organization, especially with regard to the handling of the more serious cases.[27]

Since there are no precise sociological studies on the subject, it is very difficult to judge these experiments. One can see that the 'sector' tries to avoid the falling back upon itself of the therapeutic community, which has often happened in the past. One can only be impressed by the attempt to overcome the absolute gap between the normal and the pathological as well as by the effort to bring psychiatric intervention closer to the patient's home and place of work. However, one can wonder whether the psychiatry in the community does not risk the same kind of difficulties as the practice in the institution. The 'open' milieu recreates, in new forms, specific structures for mental illness. Observations,[28] seem to show that segregative attitudes towards madness can still be found among the staff of a day hospital or a convalescent home. The asylum walls need not always be of concrete.

* *

*

Any analysis of the attempts at renovating psychiatric practice would be insufficient if it is not placed within a larger context. Like in many countries, the whole of the mental health field is now, in France, the subject of the most radical criticism. For psychiatrists, what has been called the 'crisis of psychiatry' reveals a general indictment of the continuing hospital reality.[29] It is also expressed—and here the influence of the Anglo-Saxon and Italian anti-psychiatric literature is evident—by doubts about the possibility of its retransformation. Nor must we ignore the impact this literature has had on the public in general and the often passionate controversies on madness and mental hospital in the press.

Sociologists interested in the problems of mental illness stress the persistence of the segregative function of psychiatric institutions. On the policy-making level they draw attention to the way in which certain isolated experiments conceal unfortunate persistence of the whole system. These problems have been stated by E. Goffman, for example, with regard to the actual character of the psychiatric institution, or, as C. Dufrancatel says, "should not the sociologist mistrust the interpretation of the institution given by the psychiatrist, who presents it as a care institution, in order to confirm the existence of a social control system?"

The efforts at change over the last few decades are but a partial answer to these problems. C. Perrow has pointed out that the introduction of milieu therapy has brought a necessary 'humanizing influence'[30] but has not really changed the actual goals of the mental hospital.

The role of the therapeutic community is not free from ambiguities: by locking up the patient, the traditional hospital reponded directly to the danger he represented for society. The intention behind the 'open' hospital was to renounce this type of primary defense. But it still assumes the same function: to rid society of the mentally ill. R. Castel also notes that "the permissiveness introduced in the mental hospital through psychoanalytical ideology *also* contributes to make an essentially unchanged structure in which the segregative functions are preserved, more acceptable".[31]

The criticism concerning the finality of the institution is inseparable from a redefinition of medical authority and knowledge of mental illness. It may take different forms: from the criticism of the most established aspects of nosography to the denial of any kind of reality to mental illness. M. Foucault's[32] work has been a determining factor: it has shown, according to one of the authors quoted here, "how psychiatry has justified in the past, with the same confidence and the same display of scientific arguments, the greatest variety of practices, from cold showers to hypnosis". But, it would be wrong to cast on a historical past "this contamination of psychiatric concepts by remnants of beliefs, moral attitudes, nonadmitted values".[33] Today's psychiatric jargon is still impregnated with this contamination and psychiatry's pretensions to knowing, treating or curing mental illness are still in a precarious state.

REFERENCES

* Direct reprint requests to: Claudine Herzlich, École Partique des Hautes Études, Centre d'Étude des Mouvements Sociaux, Paris, France.

[1] Cf. M. Foucault, *Folie et déraison, Histoire de la Folie à l'Age Classique*, Plon, Paris, 1961.

[2] E. Esquirol, *Des maladies mentales*, vol. II, Baillière, Paris 1838, p. 398.

[3] Cf. C. Perrow, 'Hospitals, Technology Structure and Goals', in: J. G. March (ed.), *Handbook of Organizations*, Rand McNally, Chicago 1965, p. 910–71.

[4] Cf. R. Castel, 'Le traitement moral', *Topique* **2** (1970) 109–29.

[5] Cf. J. O. Majastre, *L'introduction du changement dans un hôpital psychiatrique public*, Maspero, Paris 1972, p. 211.

[6] For a bibliography concerning the articles appearing during this period, see J. Aymé, Ph. Rappard and H. Torrubia, 'Thérapeutique Institutionnelle', in: *Encyclopédia Médico-Chirurgicale*, 1964.

[7] Cf. J. O. Majastre, *op. cit.*, p. 191.

[8] I. Belknap, *Human Problems of a State Mental Hospital*, McGraw Hill, New York 1956.

[9] E. Goffman, *Asylums – Essays on the Social Situation of Mental Patients and Other Inmates*, Anchor Books, N. Y. 1961.

[10] Like for example Chestnut Lodge analysed by Stanton and Schwartz.

[11] Cf. A. Levy, *Les paradoxes de la liberté dans un hôpital psychiatrique*, Epi, Paris 1969, and J. O. Majastre, *op. cit.*

[12] This can be partly explained by the fact that these are quite recent attempts, and thereby contemporary with the attempt at community psychiatry.

[13] R. N. Rapoport, *Community as Doctor*, Tavistock Publications, London 1959.

[14] W. Caudill, *The psychiatric Hospital as a Small Society*, Harvard Univ. Press 1958, and A. H. Stanton and M. S. Schwartz, *The Mental Hospital*, Basic Books, New York 1954.

[15] Cf. J. O. Majastre, *op. cit.*

[16] See the criticism by C. Perrow, *op. cit.*, and also the distinction established by R. Castel between a *psychosociological approach on the part of the mental hospital* and a *sociology of the psychiatric institution*: in other words the consideration of the total context of the mental hospital and of its social aims (cf. R. Castel, 'L'institution psychiatrique en equstion', *Rev. Franç. de Sociol.* **XII** (1971) 57–92).

[17] Cf. J. Oury, 'Some theoretical problems of institutional psychotherapy', in: *Enface Aliénée*, Union Gen. d'Edit. Coll., Paris (1972) 10–18.

[18] Cf. for example J. Hochmann, *Pour une psychiatrie communautaire*, Ed. du Seuil, Paris 1971.

[19] Cf. for example, M. Woodbury, 'L'équipe thérapeutique', in: *Information Psychiatrique*, 1966.

[20] Cf. P. C. Recamier *et al.*, *Le psychanalyste sans divan*, Payot, Paris 1970.

[21] J. Hochmann, *op. cit.*, p. 191.

[22] Cf. J. Hochmann, *op. cit.*, p. 141.

[23] Cf. J. Hochmann, *op. cit.*, p. 23–24.

[24] R. Castel, *Le Psychanalysme*, Ed. Maspero, Paris 1973, p. 175.

[25] Cf. P. C. Racamier, *op. cit.*

[26] The availability of private subsidies was of help in acquiring staff and equipment.

[27] Cf. J. Hochmann's book, *op. cit.*

[28] Cf. Anna Glogowski, *Déviance et Maladie Mentale*, Mémoire de Maîtrise, Université Paris X, Juin 1973, 52 p., dactyl.

[29] Cf. R. Gentis, *Les murs de l'asile*, Ed. Maspero, Paris 1970.

[30] C. Perrow, *op. cit.*, p. 924.

[31] R. Castel, *op. cit.*, p. 247.

[32] *Op. cit.*

[33] J. O. Majastre, *op. cit.*, p. 247.

III. SOCIOLOGICAL INSIGHTS INTO THE HEALTH SCIENCES

THE SOCIOLOGIST AND THE PROBLEM OF VENEREAL DISEASES

JAN KELUS AND URSZULA SIKORSKA

Institute of Venereology, Warsaw, Poland

In attempting to diagnose the social and behavioural factors operating in a given field of medicine the sociologist must clearly realize that neither his personal nor scientific status gives him an exclusive right to conduct such an activity. Researchers, clinicians and public health authorities in their work of research, treatment and organization constantly encounter problems extending far beyond the traditional sphere of medical interests. Not only do they confront such problems, they also solve them in everyday practice, basing their decisions on some kind of social diagnosis which originates from professional and social experience, commonsense and tradition. According to the well-known mechanisms of functioning of human groups, convictions, attitudes and opinions cease to be property of an individual the moment they are sanctioned by group approval. They integrate the community and furnish its members with a kind of miniature ideology.

When entering into cooperation with representatives of any field of medicine, a sociologist is continually confronted by such established and fixed forms of social diagnosis. From the theoretical point of view they should constitute for him a social fact of extreme importance. If, however, he has any means of conducting empirical research, these established forms should be the starting point and final goal of his activity. In a research project one can always find room to make these diagnoses the object of separate empirical analysis, and the research paper should take the form of a dialogue with them. The sociologist should thus avoid banality and disappointment; for it can happen that his research will lead him either to territory long since discovered or to *terra incognita* of whose existence he will find it hard to convince anyone, sometimes because their very existence, is doubted, or because the names which, in the manner of explorers he will assign to them are not to be found on the social maps hanging in the offices of those financing his expedition.

The matter would seem rather obvious if it wasn't for the fact that the possibilities described above are very rarely applied in research practice. Thus there are many works of practical sociology which, far from containing a dialogue with the established forms of social diagnosis, avoid such a dialogue altogether. This can easily result in a situation where the sociologist takes a triviality dressed up in professional jargon for a truth revealed for the first time.

The aim of the research project described in this paper was an attempt to diagnose significant social and behavioural factors for the treatment and prevention of VD. The research model was based on the suggestions outlined above, i.e. it was assumed that the research was to take the shape of a dialogue with the form of social diagnosis encountered in a given region. This diagnosis is made up of the attitudes and opinions of venereologists, which have been made the subject of a separate study which was integrated with the research project as a whole.

Below we outline the general methods and procedures employed in consecutive phases of the research. It seems to us that in this way we are presenting a model of research which can be examined on a plane extending far beyond the specific problems of VD. Its aim is the description and analysis of a certain group of psycho-social variables which have an important influence on one's behaviour during the course of the illness. One of the most important variables is the definition given this segment of social reality by doctors.

In many other fields of medicine there exists an urgent need for a sociological diagnosis, based on a specific research model of the social and behavioural determinants of health and illness. In this sense our paper constitutes a proposition which should be critically and carefully examined.

PROBLEMS, METHODS AND PROCEDURES

Study I[1]

The choice of variables was based on the assumpiton that they could in theory be divided into two groups: those indicating the probability of contracting VD and those indicating the probability of speedy access to medical help. Because the aim of the research was to provide results of immediate practical use, preference was naturally given to the second group of variables. The probability of contracting VD is unequivocally determined by patterns of sexual behaviour. It is much easier for a venereologist or the author of a health education programme to influence the factors increasing the probability that an individual who has been infected will behave rationally, thus minimalizing the social and individual costs of the illness than it is for him to influence patterns of sexual behaviour. To behave rationally a person must know that he or she is ill and decide to undergo immediate treatment. Hence it should be the primary aim of practical research to establish the degree to which people are informed about VD and the attitudes towards it prevailing in society.

We decided to examine the variables thus defined in a group of subjects who had at some time contracted VD and in a group of subjects who, like the majority of population, had not had this kind of direct experience. In addition we tried to establish whether the two groups differed essentially, i.e. whether we might legitimately attribute to the investigated group of ex-patients any specific sociodemographic or behavioural features. We employed the survey method with the innovation suggested by the specific nature of the problem. This innovation consisted in the mingling with a random sample taken from the population of a certain town of 40,000 inhabitants (hereafter referred to as town N) of a group of ex-patients of the local VD clinic. Throughout the entire period of the investigation the interviewers were not informed that they would contact people other than those composing the random sample. The data were blind coded and the information as to which of the respondents was a former patient was added by the author of the investigation himself at the very end of the coding procedure. This solution not only assured full discretion but also excluded any possible distortions during the process of gathering and interpreting the data. The interviews were conducted in the respondents' homes by a specially trained group of interviewers. The first part of the interview was based on a modified version of a questionnaire used by the Social Psychiatry Unit of the Warsaw Medical Academy to investigate the sense of psychosocial adjustment. It was supplemented by a test known as the Warsaw Scale of Neuroticism invented by Dr. Z. Bizoń. Moreover the questionnaire included, of course, an accurate index of sociodemographic data.

The second part of the questionnaire was entirely devoted to VD. Individual questions or sets of questions dealt mainly with the following, roughly outlined, problems:

1. Knowledge about syphilis and gonorrhoea, i.e. acquaintance with the names of the diseases, their etiology, symptoms, the course they run, their medical consequences and the chances of complete cure;

2. Prevailing attitudes towards VD;

3. Reception of the anti-VD public information programme disseminated by the mass media or by the health education campaign;

4. The degree to which people were informed about the organizational, legal and administrative regulations within the framework of which these diseases are treated and prevented in our country, e.g. the obligation to report contacts, free medical treatment, compulsory serological testing of pregnant women etc.;

5. Attitudes to the above-mentioned questions;

6. The stereotype of a VD-patient.

The random sample consisted of 665 subjects: 368 women and 297 men aged from 20 to 65 were chosen from the voters' lists by means of the standard procedure. The interviewer talked with 567 persons, which amounted to 81% of the whole sample. Eighteen persons refused to be interviewed. The group of former patients was chosen in the following way: 363 residents of town N who had experienced syphilitic or gonorrhoeal infection were selected from the files of the local VD registry. The proportions of men and women were roughly equal. Patients who were still receiving routine medical check ups were excluded. Present addresses could be established only in the case of 215 former patients; the rest had either left town or never been on the files.

Of this group 170 persons were interviewed. When the data-collecting process was completed it was found that the random sample included 10 persons who had also had VD: they were consequently added to the group of ex-patients. In effect we obtained 180 ex-patients (86 men and 94 women) 110 of whom had had gonorrhoea and 70 syphilis.

The data thus obtained were analysed from several points of view. In the random sample of 'healthy' people we tried to establish factors determining the level of knowledge of and the attitudes towards VD, with special reference to age, sex and education, in accordance with standard practice in public opinion polls.

This sample also played the role of an ideal control group. Socio-demographic features as well as the results of tests for neuroticism and social adjustment of ex-patients could in every case be compared with the same parameters for the group of 'healthy' people.

It is the duty of the researcher to notice and draw attention to the drawbacks of the method he is employing. In the case of the research project described we have two critical remarks to make. First, as the attentive reader has already noticed, the group of subjects under investigation cannot unfortunately be treated as a random sample.

On the statistical plane, this restriction made it necessary to apply appropriate procedures: when the group of ex-patients was compared with the control group, the null hypothesis was not formulated as a hypothesis on statistical independence but as a hypothesis that the distribution of the given variable in the population was identical with the empirically assessed distribution of the same variable in the group of VD-patients. Thus, any generalization of the results into the whole population of VD-patients remains a matter of humanistic inference and insight, not being supported by the common abuse of statistics. Second, in trying to avoid certain distortions of the kind to be expected in a situation when a patient is suddenly interveiwed or tested, the moment he comes for medical help, we created a setting which could hardly be called optimal. A respondent trying to conceal the fact of having been ill could declare ignorance or deform the answer in some other way. This was of course taken into consideration in analysing the results.

Study II. The Opinion of Venereologists on the Social and Behavioural Aspects of VD [2]

The opinions which go to make up the existing shape of social diagnosis in the field of interest to us can, of course, be deduced from medical practice and the scientific, health-educational, and organizational activity of venereologists. There arise, however, several difficulties. Many opinions on the matter are not explicitly stated: they require reconstruction and interpretation. One can easily be accused of lack of objectivity when presenting such an interpretation. This is the reason why we decided to obtain some empirical material which would constitute a more direct illustration of venereologists' attitudes towards several essential points connected with the social aspects of VD. We assumed that it might be possible to obtain an insight into the sphere of convictions and opinions which are important not only because they determine the human side of the doctor-patient relationship, but also because to a great extent they mould the social climate attached to this kind of illness.

The investigation was conducted by means of a mailed questionnaire which was sent to 320 medical specialists participating in the All-Polish Conference of the VD Section of the Polish Dermatological Society. We obtained 144 answers, i.e. from 45% of those questioned. Venereologists' opinions on the subjects listed below were of especial interest to us.

1. Social and behavioural characteristics of patients;
2. Reasons for delay in coming to the doctor;
3. Difficulties connected with establishing patients' sexual contacts;
4. An opinion on the actual health-education programme, with particular reference to the question of its deterrent character;
5. An opinion on the criminal and administrative sanctions currently employed and the desirability of their being continued;
6. An opinion on the usefulness of psychosociological research and the expectations arising therefrom.

In addition, a separate set of questions in the questionnaire was preceded by a brief description of the research being conducted (Study I). The group under study was defined, and the doctors were asked if they would care to anticipate some of the results. Thus for example they were invited to express an opinion as to what proportion of respondents would consider syphilis a dangerous illness and what proportion would think it fully curable. They were also asked whether they thought a majority would consider a visit to a VD clinic more shaming than a visit to a mental health clinic. The latter part of the inquiry would appear to have had extremely interesting results. On the basis of it we tried to establish what elements of social diagnosis obtained in Study I differ from the views of representatives of the medical community. In certain situations the difference might obviously be the result of the imperfection of our methods and tools, and we took this into account. Nevertheless, we also noted the fact that frequently the opinions constituting the existing social diagnosis operating in this field are only partially correct or even are totally wrong. Physicians like everyone else and like members of any other professional group are exposed in their individual and social perceptions to the influence of social prejudice and professional deformations and distortions. Cooperation with sociologists, if it is to have any sense at all, should serve to broaden this perspective.

DISCUSSION OF SELECTED RESULTS OF THE INVESTIGATION

In accordance with the assumptions presented at the beginning of this paper any report on an investigation of this kind should take the form of an argument with the social diagnosis currently obtained in the field of venereology. The following remarks are obviously not a report in the technical sense of the word; we intend to publish the complete version in a medical periodical. The necessity of condensation has made inevitable a sharpening of the polemical tone. In our choice of subjects we deliberately emphasized differences, whereas questions on which we find ourselves wholly in agreement with the established view have been omitted in the realization that here we have nothing new to contribute. We assume that some of the obtained results, in view of their general nature, reach far beyond the specific nature of the problem. We hope, however, that like the research model presented above, they may be useful elsewhere.

1. Who is the VD-patient?

The conviction that people contracting VD come in great part from the fringes of society is popular among venereologists. This was confirmed by our questionnaire. Asked who their patients were, the doctors made precisely this observation, defining their patients as

alcoholics	31%	of physicians used this term
demimonde	15%	,,
persons either unemployed or working casually	12%	,,
people frequently changing jobs	8%	,,
prostitutes and their associates	11%	,,
the criminal world	6%	,,
juvenile criminals	13%	,,

In addition, 25% of the respondents described their patients as persons of low intelligence which should be understood rather as persons without education or of poor social background than persons of low IQ.

Attempts to describe patients in any other terms were rarer. In pointing out other social groups or situations where VD contraction is possible, the venereologists spoke mainly of drivers (15%), men traveling on expense accounts (23%) and the inhabitants of workers' hostels (10%). They also describe their patients as 'persons with a strong sexual drive' (9%), persons accepting sexual freedom (10%) and persons leading an irregular sexual life (15%). The above characteristics do not exclude each other and occur in various combinations.

Obviously it is sometimes hard to decide whether a given statement is an objective statement of fact or if it has an evaluative character. In other cases the situation is clear: in 21% of the doctors' opinions we found statements which could only be classified as 'other morally and intellectually disparaging epithets'. In general it can be said that 40% of the respondents' descriptions contain accents of severe moral condemnation.

Comparing the sociodemographic features of the VD-patients with the control group we established that in the case of men the ex-patients differed from their fellows in the random sample in only two respects: they were less frequently raised in the country and less frequently describe themselves as pracing religious believers. The initially observed high percentage of drivers among the ex-patients ceased to be a statistically essential difference when we checked the age factor. The distribution of other variables such as marital status, education, occupation, social standing, income, or job mobility did not vary between the group of patients and the random sample.

Slightly greater differences were registered among the women's group. The ex-patients tended to have relatively lower education, more of them were unskilled workers or lower office personnel and were more frequently divorced.

The percentage of unemployed was the same among ex-patients as in the random sample (for both sexes).

Despite the existence of a whole series of important variables to which our investigation did not extend, the results obtained do not satisfy the assertion that the patients interviewed belonged to the demi-monde. It may be that we were unable to reach representatives of the latter. However the group of patients studied, even if not a true random sample, constituted a statistical majority of persons who in a specific place and at a specific time had contracted VD. We think it likely that in dozens of other small towns there exist many people who have contracted VD and who in sociodemographic terms differ not at all or only insignificantly from their fellow citizens.

The people from the so-called fringes of society are also no doubt on the fringes in the latter group of the group of VD sufferers. This fringe may be considerably larger than it is in the rest of the population (if only because venereal disease is the occupational disease of the prostitute) but it remains only a fringe not a majority.

Let us consider the origin of those generalizations so popular among the medical community and social function they perform. It would appear that, as in all sociological reflections on venereal disease, the key to understanding a whole series of problems is to treat them as arising from – and testifying to – the extent to which our culture suppresses matters connected with sex. On the basis of the Judeo-Christian tradition the sexual life of man has been incorporated into an elaborate complex of sin, guilt and shame. In our society the fact of contracting VD is treated as proof that the individual has violated the social norm restricting sexual contacts to marriage, or in a more liberal interpretation, to some other form of monogamic liaison. The reaction of contempt and aggression to a violation of the norm is so strong that it leads us to think that not only the victims but also the judges are in the face of sex helpless, burdened with guilt and threatened by fear. Consciously or not, many physicians in their opinions and practice identify themselves with this pattern.

The 'social margin' is one of those terms which do not demand precise understanding – in most cases it is used not to describe facts but to give way to emotions.

Sinners are necessary for saints to exist. Similarly, the 'social margin' people are indispensable for us, decent citizens. We need them, among other things, to free ourselves from the responsibility for the fate of every man and for the reality we are creating. It is comfortable not to remember, that even if the social margin exists, it is the effect of the social conditions which are also our creation. And if it does exist it is often worth producing; having thus ensured an object of condemnation we can proceed to satisfy two of our basic needs: to punish and to frighten.

2. Should the Doctor be a Policeman?

In an attempt to establish the opinions of venereologists concerning the use of administrative compulsion and penal sanctions in VD prevention and control our method was as follows:

The doctors were asked to choose one of two given contradictory opinions:

I. "Despite the existence of appropriate legislation in combating VD we make too little use of administrative and penal sanctions."

II. "An increase in the existing use of criminal and administrative sanctions would doubtless do more harm than good."

The first opinion was accepted by 51% and the second by 21% of the respondents. Though the remaining 28% expressed opinions differing from both the above views, without exception they declared themselves in favour of repression.

They asserted that the existing legislation needs to be changed in the direction of stiffer penalties, complained of the dilatoriness of the militia (police) in cooperating with VD clinics, and postulated the introduction of repayment by the patient of the cost of treatment, and fines and corrective labour camps for patients who contract VD frequently.

It is worth noting in passing that the popularity of views of this kind can be seen from the use of terms such as: resistant patient, recidivist, concealment of contacts, etc.

As the answers to other questions in the questionnaire also show, many doctors expected that cooperation with the sociologists would mean that the latter would "make a thorough study of certain groups and milieux associated with the underworld".

A seventy-three-year-old doctor, who was a determined advocate of moderation and tolerance, crossed out this whole page of the questionnaire and wrote in large letters: "A doctor is supposed to cure and not punish – a doctor cannot be a policeman". For this opinion we are deeply grateful to him.

One can point to two sources of the tendencies towards punishment which prevail among venereologists. In psychological terms, this is an expression of authoritarian tendencies. The doctor's profession and his social role contain a fair measure of authoritarian elements. In other fields of medicine authoritarian tendencies manifest themselves of necessity in a veiled manner and undergo various forms of sublimation. In venereology, as a result of cultural conditioning, they can manifest themselves directly. Independently of, or rather parallel with this, tendencies towards punishment flow from the attitudes of intolerance and faith in the efficacy of coercion and repression as a panaceum for all kinds of social ills, which are prevalent in many areas of social life.

Legal rigorism has become in our society a lasting element of our cultural heritage.

In the random sample studied by us, 67% of the respondents asserted that avoiding treatment for venereal disease is punished by imprisonment, when in fact it carries only an administrative penalty. On the other hand a mere 36.7% were convinced that the conscious infection of someone with venereal disease is punishable by imprisonment. The penal code does contain such a provision, but it is a dead letter, which can be seen not only from court statistics but also from the state of legal awareness among the public. Similar percentages of respondents believed, after all, that prostitution (61.5%) and homosexuality (44.6%) are also punished by imprisonment in Poland.

It would appear, however, that in the Polish public's awareness of the law there exists a supposition that for certain offences people are not sent to prison through – as it were – oversight. The vast majority of people who were subsequently asked which of the above acts should in their opinion be punished by imprisonment, simply mentioned them in turn, demanding penalties for prostitution (81.5%), homosexuality (68.7%), infecting someone with venereal disease (80.4%) and evading treatment (87.8%).

What Levi-Strauss described as 'the civilization of penal law' will perhaps outstrip the 'civilization of a sense of law' of many societies.

Our respondents – as decent and honest people – had nothing to suggest beyond imprisonment. They had never, after all, encountered any other suggestions.

The fact must be faced that those venereologists who are in favour of repression and administrative coercion are not alone in their views outside their own milieu either.

3. *Who Treats VD Lightly?*

On the basis of the results of our first investigation, we can state unequivocally that the public is almost universally convinced that syphilis continues to be a very serious illness. Ninety-three per cent of those questioned replied to this effect. A bare 2% were of the opinion that nowadays it is not a serious illness, since if diagnosed at an early enough stage it can be wholly and effectively cured. The remaining 5% had no opinion on the matter. Among patients who had suffered from gonorrhoea the distribution of answers to this question is almost identical with that in the random sample. Thus it is perfectly clear that these individuals do not generalize from their personal experience; the facility of the cure for gonorrhoea and the visible absence of consequences does not lead to a change in ideas on the subject of the more serious of the two venereal diseases. In the group of patients who had suffered from syphilis the proportion of people who did not consider syphilis to be a serious disease only rose to 7%.

Obviously such answers may have a declarative character. This is decisively contradicted however by a further analysis of the results. The statements of those questioned indicate that a genuinely macabre and horrific image of the disease is deeply rooted in society. In reply to the question: "why do you consider syphilis to be a very serious disease?", about one in four answered simply: "It is a terrible disease – the body rots and falls away from the bones". This stereotyped reason – looking as though it had been taken straight from the Biblical descriptions of leprosy – appeared more frequently than any other. The open question form excluded the possibility of distortions arising as a result of suggestive wording.

The universality of these irrational ideas, magnified by fear, is confirmed by the answers to further items in the questionnaire. A considerable proportion of the public doubts that syphylis can be fully cured, and asserts that it is a hereditary disease which, despite treatment, can be passed on to posterity. People are not only convinced that this disease causes serious damage to internal organs, facial disfigurement, disablement and death, but are also inclined to attribute to it such consequences as impotence and sterility.

A casual attitude does indeed occur in relation to gonorrhoea, although it cannot by any means be considered universal. A decidedly easygoing attitude to gonorrhoea we found in 4.1% of the answers from the random sample (almost all men) and in 13.3% of the ex-patients' answers. If we add to this purely factual statements such as "gonorrhoea is not a serious illness, but is easily cured leaving no trace", these percentages rise accordingly to 29.3% and 4.3%.

It must however be emphasized that general ideas on the subject of venereal disease are overwhelmingly dominated by the terryfying stereotype of syphilis; people are perfectly aware of the fact that whether they catch one disease or the other is a matter of pure chance.

Can doctors, who are in daily contact with the treatment of these diseases, have any doubts as to ideas and attitudes prevailing in society? It would appear that they can.

In the second of our investigations we invited the doctors, *inter alia*, to predict what percentage of our random sample would answer that syphilis is not nowadays a very serious disease. The divergences between the doctors' predictions and the distribution of answers actually received are quite unambigous. Only 18% of the doctors estimated the proportion of people who would state that syphilis is not nowadays a serious disease as not greater than 10% – and only their predictions may be considered as being in accordance with the empirical results. One third of the doctors, on the other hand, were inclined to predict that over half of the public does not consider syphilis to be a serious illness.

We obtained further results from the answers to the question, on what principles, in the opinion of the venereologists', should health educational programmes and anti-VD propaganda be based. Fifty-four per cent of the doctors declared themselves in favour of the following opinion:

"In view of the general lighthearted attitude to VD, the publicizing for health educational purposes of the serious, even if at present rarely occurring, consequences of these diseases, is effective and proper". An additional 20% of the doctors formulated their own opinions – although the latter were largely modifications of, rather than counter-proposals to, the above assumption. Decided opponents of propaganda containing intimidating elements found themselves in a minority of about 25%.

The notion that the public treats VD lightly is thus widely held among venereologists. We have shown that this is a false view. It is worth noting at the same time that an exaggerated, fear-filled notion of VD among the public hinders, rather than facilitates, the treatment and prevention of these diseases. Notions of this kind exercise a general influence on such matters as the level of awareness concerning the symptoms of the disease which are of essential significance for eventual self diagnosis. Between the gruesome image of the disease and the fact that, as in the case of syphilis, the symptoms are discrete, non-painful and disappear even without treatment, there is an obvious discrepancy. "Something so terrible cannot have such innocent symptoms", a large proportion of the individuals questioned by us, who would certainly have difficulty in diagnosing the disease themselves in the case of infection, are inclined to think. Health propaganda and education, whether consciously striving to cause or unconsciously causing intimidating effects, generate a level of fear which impedes the assimilation of commonsense and potentially helpful information. Actions of this kind merely help to perpetuate irrational ideas and convictions. If they are intended (as their supporters do not always care to admit openly) to deter people from engaging in certain kinds of sexual behaviour, their efficacy must be doubted.

In our opinion venereal diseases have been neglected by the authorities responsible for public health and for this medical field. Not till the continuously increasing morbidity led us to take the first place in Europe with respect to the number of syphilis cases per head of population* – only then and not a few years earlier – energetic steps were taken to undo the irreparable damage, and the previous views were revised. It is also possible that since the introduction of antibiotics for therapy, many representatives of other fields of medicine ceased to treat VD seriously. The resulting decrease of venereologists' prestige could be the source of possible professional frustrations. On the other hand, the 'medical consciousness' of our society reacted with considerable delay; the common misconceptions about VD are evidently based on the nineteenth century medical pattern. We are suggesting that the attitude of neglect assigned to society can be nothing else but some kind of projection. It is possible that the 'scapegoat' formula is also involved. The results were on some occasion summed up by one of the authors in the following way: a poster stating 'Beware Venereal Diseases' is as ridiculous as a health-educational proposition 'Remember Lung Cancer is No Trifling Matter'.

4. *The Role of Shame: Is It Obvious to All?*

In the medical literature on venerology the various social aspects of the subject are discussed fairly frequently. The fact that few reflections are devoted to the role of shame as a factor hampering people in making up their minds to accept treatment is perhaps attributable to an unwillingness on the part of authors to stress the obvious. After all, even in everyday speech venereal diseases are commonly referred to as shameful diseases. It would appear, however, that that is not the only reason,

In our culture VD is obviously not the only disease where shame may play an essential role in causing the sufferer to avoid or delay the moment of seeking treatment. Desiring somehow to relate this disease to other situations where the patient is branded with a similar stigma we employed the following question: we asked those interviewed which

* The incidence of the early symptomatic syphilis (per 100,000 of population) in the years from 1969 to 1973 in Poland was the highest among the European countries publishing statistical data for this area following the WHO recommendations. The corresponding rates were as follows: 1969 – 51.8; 1973 – 15.9; 1975 – 9.7. (*The Editorial Committee*)

of the three situations mentioned below they would find most embarrassing:

1. To go as a patient to a VD clinic;
2. To go as a patient to an alcoholism clinic;
3. To go as a patient to a mental health clinic.

The largest percentage of respondents in the random sample considered the visit to the VD clinic as being most embarrassing (22.5%). This was immediately followed by the visit to the alcoholism clinic (19.2%), while 7.2% considered the visit to the psychiatric clinic to be the most humiliating. Answers to the effect that "all these situations would be equally embarrassing" were given by 29.7% of the sample, while 12.8% considered that "none of the situations would be embarrassing". The remainder indicated more than one of the given situations.

In passing we should like to point out that the high proportion of answers mentioning the visit to the alcoholism clinic as the most embarrassing situation, came as a surprise to us. Among people with at least secondary education in the 20–39 age group the proportion of such answers was 28.5%, as against 16.9% for the visit to the VD clinic. Strange indeed is the society in which habitual drunkenness is universally tolerated, while alcoholics seeking treatment are condemned to ostracism. It is equally strange that the consciousness of this is greater among young people with higher education.

When we asked the venereologists for their predictions concerning which situation would be considered by the majority of society to be the most embarrassing, we received the following answers:

1. Visit to the mental health clinic – 26.8%;
2. Visit to the VD clinic – 31.9%;
3. Visit to the alcoholism clinic – 21.5%.

Answering the quasi-projective question concerning the causes of delay by VD patients in consulting a doctor, respondents both from the random sample and from the group of former patients mentioned shame far more often than any other possible reasons. Shame was mentioned by the physicians as well, but in first place they mentioned ignorance of or failure to notice the symptoms, or trivialization of the symptoms and failure to take the disease seriously.

In general it would appear that doctors are aware of the role played by shame as a factor impeding rational behaviour in the face of illness, but that their awareness is somewhat less than that of the average man in the street. The feeling of shame associated with VD are fairly assiduously cultivated by means of such devices as the use of such terms as 'sexual hooligans' in popular publications, or films which, besides elements of horror, are shot through with obtrusive moralizing intended to deter viewers from striking up casual acquaintances. Nor need many doctors in their contacts with patients control themselves as much as they would have to were tactlessness to lead by a direct route to bankruptcy. The sinner put to shame has always provided a spiritual feast for the pious.

Understanding of the patient's psychological situation presupposes a capacity for empathy. Condemntaion renders this impossible and makes it pointless anyway.

Doctors often ask patients questions. Many of these questions concern motives – e.g. reasons for delay in coming to the doctor. Such questions obviously must be put, but in putting them it should also be remembered that people are not always aware of the motives for their own behaviour, and are not always able – or do not always consider it desirable – to recount them. Frequently the patient leaves his shame, as it were, outside the door of the doctor's consulting room. Asked his motives for being so late in coming to the doctor he may answer anything or nothing, since he knows that to admit to being ashamed is out of place in this social situation. Such situations are more frequent than is generally supposed.

CONCLUDING REMARKS: DOCTOR AND PATIENT – A RELATIONSHIP OR A BARRIER?

From the extensive empirical material at our disposal we shall permit ourselves to quote one more result in conclusion. It may appear to be taken out of context, but it illustrates perfectly what we want to say. In addition we feel that it is in a sense shocking.

We established, namely, that 25% of ex-patients think that a person who has caught syphylis and is being treated, cannot be sure that he or she will have healthy offspring. This was confirmed by 25% of those who had completed treatment for syphilis.

This result, like the results previously presented, provokes a certain sad reflection. Patient and doctor are mutually involved in a specific social relationship. However they learn little in this way from each other and about each other. Knowing that they live in a world in which a person is seldom listened to in order to be understood, they often say nothing at all. They abandon in advance any attempt to establish human contact, they inspect parts of the body, give injections and hand across the desk the result of the last blood test. Sometimes if they speak it is only to wound. This is ultimately a way of breaking down the barrier, but, like indifference, it leaves a feeling of loneliness.

We know that many doctors in the field of venereology as well do not waste the intellectual and moral chances offered by their profession: the chance of human encounter and the chance to help another human being. Contact with the patient in such cases enriches both parties. Such doctors, instead of condemning, attempt to understand, and in return they are rewarded with satisfaction instead of irritation. In the field which interests us, they understand above all that the patient was driven by a desire which was always an attempt at human contact, even if it were love in its bleakest form.

To those doctors who have understood this, the social sciences have little of substance to communicate.

REFERENCES

[1] The author of this investigation is J. K. Kelus, a sociologist at the Institute of Venereology of the Warsaw Medical Academy. A closer description of the methods applied and some preliminary results can be found in the *British Journal of Venereal Diseases* **49** (1973).

[2] This study was conducted by Urszula Sikorska, on a Research Grant of the Institute of Venereology (unpublished).

DEVELOPMENTS IN THE ROLE OF MEDICINE IN RELATION TO REPRODUCTION*

RAYMOND ILLSLEY

M.R.C. Medical Sociology Unit, Institute of Medical Sociology, Aberdeen, Scotland

1. MEDICAL SPECIALISMS AND ADAPTATION TO CHANGE

In the history of medicine over the last century we have witnessed a proliferation of medical specialisms. Differentiation has occurred in response to many concurrent changes and particularly to advances in medical technology, to changes in the nature and distribution of health and disease, and to differing emphases placed upon specific qualities, behaviour and performance of individuals and populations or the relative importance of an age or sex-group. Advances in medical technology stemming from the health related physical sciences may produce ethical problems in treatment or necessitate organisational changes in the structure of the profession but their introduction can be relatively easily controlled because they are both initiated and mediated through the health professions or through related (and often medically dominated) professions. Changes stemming, however, from general social, economic and political changes in social structure pose questions of a different order, because they may appear to contravene or threaten to override the traditional medical ethics – the image which the profession holds of itself as concerned with the health of individuals, the doctor-patient relationship, and the autonomy of the profession. Clinging with extraordinary dexterity to the notion that medicine is value-free, that the doctor is concerned solely with 'health' and is uninfluenced by social and political ideologies, societal needs can only be accomodated if a social, economic or political goal can be translated into concepts of health. This adaptive process may be profitably viewed from two viewpoints. On the one hand, we may view the process as one by which the medical profession simultaneously adapts to social change whilst retaining its professional identity and ideology. In this sense perhaps it differs very little from other professions such as sociology which conducts a running battle with related applied disciplines such as social policy, social administration and social work or with politically motivated ideologues within its own ranks (c.f. the old controversies "Should sociologists be concerned with applications?" and "Is sociology value-free?"). On the other hand we may view the process from outside medicine and see it as a political process by which controversial political issues are depoliticised and translated into socially acceptable health issues potentially soluble by medical procedures. It is in this sense that Zola [4] talks of the '*medicalising of society*' and sees medicine as an agent of social control. This thesis has been widely explored in recent years, particularly in relation to psychiatry (see Szasz [1], [2], and Wootton [3]). If we take the two ideas together we have the *apparent paradox of a supposedly scientific value-free profession acting as an agent of social control.*

The process of adaptation to change operates with a different emphasis within and between the major branches of medicine – broadly distinguished here as public health, primary medical care, operative medicine, internal medicine and the so-called fundamental medical sciences. If we examine the internal organisation of medicine either in terms of segments of the medical curriculum, or the names of medical departments in a teaching hospital, or the titles of their professors, it is evident that differentiation has proceeded along different lines – and at times very confusing lines – within each major branch. Departments and sub-specialities have arisen which have differentiated themselves by differing or by a combination of differing criteria. The historical process by which this has occurred requires further study, and here I give only illustrative examples. One *distinguishing* criterion is clearly technical skills or procedures such, for example, as surgery itself, anesthetics, radiology. Another criterion stems from parts of the body or from specific malfunctions located in particular systems, e.g. E.N.T. or oto-rhino-laryngology, orthopaedics, opthalmics, dentistry, cardiology, gynaecology, etc.; specific location also, of course, implies related skills and technology. Symptomatology partially distinguishes such categories as psychiatry, dermatology and much of internal medicine. Others clearly focus around care and treatment – general practice, rehabilitation, pharmacology. Among the most interesting are those which specialise in a particular age or sex-group – paediatrics, geriatrics or obstetrics, where the skills may be highly diffuse and where the profession frequently acts largely as a co-ordinator of other specialist contributions. The classifications or criteria cited above as illustrations are not mutually exclusive; that is to say particular sub-specialisms may be classified according to two or more criteria or may themselves contain further sub-specialisms which straddle boundary lines, e.g. psychiatry, neurology, neurosurgery, neuropsychiatry, etc.

The major branches of medicine have evolved specialisms and sub-specialisms in response to differing pressures. If one studied the emergence of specialisms out of the general area of surgery it would probably reflect fairly adequately advances in the fundamental sciences and medical technology. Others, however, and this applies particularly to public health, internal medicine and medical care, have been more powerfully influenced by changes in the nature and distribution of illness or by the changing emphasis placed by society upon an age or sex group, or specific forms of behaviour, or levels of performance. In this sense the history of psychiatry would be distinguished not so much by responses to technology or by the proliferation of sub-specialisms as by changing attitudes towards deviant behaviour and by the successive (or overlapping) application of alternative ideologies. Its retention of a virtually identical label over the decades therefore hides fundamental changes in the nature of the discipline. In this sense it has some analogies with the field of public health which has successively responded to the changing nature of illness and the structure of health services, retaining its identity but continuously changing its name as it moved through phases of concern with infectious disease, wider epidemiological interests, the prevention of illness (other than infectious disease) towards its current preoccupation with the organisation of health services. Since institutional titles change slowly Departments in different countries and universities concerned with virtually identical problems may variously be known as public health, epidemiology, social hygiene, social medicine, preventive medicine, community health or medicine or even (at W.H.O.) the strengthening of health services.

I am here mainly concerned with specialisms which, retaining the same apparent image and title, have nevertheless responded heavily to changing ideologies or been the buttresses of a particular social and political ideology and I have chosen obstetrics and gynaecology as the case example.

2. OBSTETRICS AND GYNAECOLOGY: AN EXAMPLE OF RETARDED ADAPTATION

In terms of traditional definitions and roles obstetrics and gynaecology are separate specialisms although in practice most obstetricians are also gynaecologists and the two subjects are taught and carried out within the same department or service. Whilst both relate to the functioning of the female reproductive system, obstetrics has referred to the 'normal' process of pregnancy and childbirth, whereas gynaecology has been concerned with malfunctioning of the system outside pregnancy, or even outside the childbearing period. The borderline, however, is by no means clearly drawn, especially in recent years and for the purpose of this analysis may for the most part, be considered separately. At some points the roles are complementary – the gynaecologist who helped the infertile woman to conceive also supervised the resulting pregnancy. On the other hand the gynaecologist who decided whether or not the pregnancy should be terminated had, as his special obstetric responsibility, the task of ensuring that each conception proceeded without interruption to term.

In most countries obstetrics developed out of the previous combined responsibilities of the general practitioner and the midwife. The impetus and the opportunity for the development of the profession emerged from the high death rates for mother and child in childbirth and the advances in technology which rendered childbirth both safer by reducing infection and less painful. Reduction of risk increasingly seemed to imply hospitalisation where skilled obstetric management and treatment and emergency facilities were immediately available. Counterbalancing risk reduction, however, was the removal of the childbirth from the familial and cultural environment of the mother into the medical/scientific milieu of the hospital. Depersonalisation might be mitigated by various procedures but the most common situation in advanced industrialised societies embodies many, and at times, all the following characteristics:

a) Regular ante-natal care from early pregnancy onwards in clinics staffed by a variety of regular specialists and occasional consultants.

b) Delivery in hospital contexts followed by a brief recuperative period.

c) Management of pregnancy, childbirth and puerperium by teams of specialists including obstetrician, anaesthetist, endocrinologist, dietitian, paediatrician, specialists in particular conditions (cardiology, diabetes) and a succession of ante-natal nurses, midwives and post-natal nursing staff each exercising their particular skills and translating the risk-laden but familiar process into a depersonalised clinical and safe exercise.

This is not a back-to-nature cry but a statement of the managerial back-ground which may throw light on issues of professional ideology. Essentially, from the medical viewpoint pregnancy and childbirth became converted into physiological and endocrinological processes and into the monitoring of these processes to identify and intervene medically and surgically in the event of abnormalities or complications. Each event, each process was made amenable to a body of scientific laws and derived procedures. Hospitalisation meant that each pregnancy was seen as a separate clinical event, supervised by teams which had changed in their individual composition, although the role-positions remained. Continuity was maintained by detailed records systems. The product of conception was the responsibility of a different specialist. In most cases, and until recently counselling and prescription concerning contraception did not exist as part of the system but might be provided by still further, separately administered clinics or voluntary agencies. The adoption of these procedures meant that the obstetrician could seal himself behind his medical/scientific walls and eschew responsibility for social, political, moral decisions.

The detachment of the pregnancy and labour from preceding or succeeding events or from the surrounding socio-cultural environment was reinforced in other ways.

a) Until relatively recently, not only were pregnancies seen as separate events rather than as part of a patterned reproductive history, they were seen as influenced by the events, experiences, and context of pregnancy itself. Thus if complications occurred their origin was sought in the physiological processes of that particular pregnancy or the potentially harmful experiences of the pregnancy period – bad housing, infection, pregnancy nutrition, physical work or psychological stress. The perspective which views the events and outcome of pregnancy and labour as the final resultant of an accumulation of injuries, deprivations etc. sustained over the previous 25 years of childhood and adolescence, is of relatively recent origin – at least in so far as obstetric teaching and practice are concerned.

b) Not universally, but typically, the obstetrician was concerned with the individual woman and her pregnancy on a kind of shop-keeper-customer basis (even if no financial transactions were involved). The reproductive health and efficiency of populations, as opposed to individuals, might be the concern of the demographer, the epidemiologist or the public health doctor, but not of the hospital-located obstetrician or gynaecologist. Thus public policy might affect the conditions under which the obstetrician worked, but policy itself, being essentially political and value-laden was not initiated by the obstetrician except in so far as it could be justified on health grounds. This generalisation applies with differing emphasis in different national systems, the public health aspect having been incorporated into the maternity services of some countries for several decades whereas in others the shop-keeper-customer relationship still predominates.

Does the scientific medicalisation of pregnancy and childbirth mean that the scientific ideology of traditional obstetrics was value-free, emptied of social and political content? Recent developments in the practice of abortion strongly suggest the opposite, that, in fact, obstetricians by confining themselves within a limited scientific framework, have been upholding the established political and social morality and indeed acting as moral policemen by withholding their scientific expertise where its application would supposedly threaten the institutions of marriage and family, the traditional relationship between the sexes, and at times might run counter to official goals for population expansion. Thus the accepted scientific ideology has acted as a barrier to change. This argument is expanded in the following section.

3. ABORTION ON HEALTH OR SOCIAL GROUNDS

Abortion, legal or illegal, has been practised in many societies over many centuries. Legislation against abortion, however, was widely enacted in advancing industrial societies in the 19th Century, the first major reversal to this legislation occurring, although with some hesitation and rescindment, in the USSR in the inter-war period. Legalisation was later introduced into other East European countries following the Second World War but again reversals or restriction of criteria have occurred from time justified either on grounds of health or of population decline. In the remainder of the advanced industrial world debate about the legalisation of abortion has been more heavily concentrated and centred particularly upon the 1960s.

In fact there have been at least two debates, conducted by different protagonists, motivated by different pressures and conducted in widely differing rhetorics. The first debate is perhaps merely the culmination in the 1960s of a long-drawn-out movement which itself began in the middle of late 19th century with gradually increasing control over infant and child mortality, the pressure of surviving children on the families of the middle classes, the motivation of these classes, either by restraint, by vicarious pleasure with prostitutes, or by crude methods of birth control, to limit or to space their conceptions. Complex inter-woven tendencies were involved which are merely listed here: the introduction of more advanced industrial technology and the consequent need for a more highly-educated population more able to innovate, to link means and ends using first principles rather than accepted dogma; more widespread education and the parallel secularisation of society; reduced need for labour as capital intensive industries developed; the introduction of women into both education and the labour force and other influences towards equality of the sexes; more recently changes in sexual morality and sexual behaviour and the direct and indirect impact of improved contraceptive methods. The debate stemming from these developments and issues was primarily social and economic and conducted in terms of a political religious and ethical rhetoric. The viability of fundamental institutions (marriage and family) was frequently raised, as was sexual morality, the role of women and more broadly the right of individuals or couples to determine their lives through family planning of all varieties on the basis of criteria important to them rather than imposed upon them externally. The churches conducted a connected debate in religious and metaphysical terms.

Obstetricians and gynaecologists, considering the centrality of the topic to their professional field, took only a sporadic, and rarely an initiatory, role in this debate. Contraception received only the scantiest, if any, attention in the medical student's education. Until the development of the oral contraceptive, facilities were the commodities of barbers, slot-machines and pharmacists. The professional associations of obstetricians and gynaecologists were equivocal on the moral issues and frequently condemnatory. Individual doctors, for the most part, left practice to a handful of specialists or of voluntary agencies and in conselling were prone to use their personal social and moral values as the source of advice. In refraining from the debate they were upholding the scientific objectivity of their professional ethic, but at the same time were implicitly supporting established values and institutions.

The abortion debate (as opposed to family planning generally) was more embarrassing because gynaecologists were the only qualified technicians who might perform abortions with maximum safety. Their refusal to perform, or to campaign in their favour, was therefore tantamount to a total prohibition of safe abortion. By refusing, they, in effect, acted as moral policemen, the ultimate implementors of anti-abortion legislation. Nor, of course, was abortion always illegal, so that, in countries without anti-abortion legislation, they were interpreting the public welfare and upholding, not the law, but their professional rules and ideology. Debate within the profession, however, could not be forever avoided. To be professionally acceptable, however, it had to be carried out in terms of health and medicine. A review of research papers produced in Western industrialised societies over several decades reveals a shifting emphasis. Early work centres around issues of life and death. The probable death of the mother if pregnancy continued was frequently the first criterion adopted as a valid ground for abortion. But death could not always be guaranteed and therefore probabilities and hypothetical outcomes were introduced. Suicide was a much researched outcome – but action had to be taken on the basis of threatened suicide or attempted-but-failed suicide, and again limited ability to predict left judgement in the hands of the gynaecologist (or consultant psychiatrist). The linking of rubella to foetal malformation, and later, other means of predicting congenital defects provided other medical grounds (without necessarily solving the ethical dilemma). Early contenders for becoming acceptable criteria were existing psychosis in the mother or the probability of post-partum psychosis. Psychosis may be one of the most certain of psychiatric diagnoses but that still leaves a wide margin of error. Even larger degrees of error and judgement must be involved in predicting whether continued pregnancy is more likely than termination to regenerate pre-existing psychosis, to exacerbate existing psychosis or produce post-partum (or post abortal) psychosis. The introduction of psychiatric criteria into the debate inevitably widened the area of research and discussion, and opened opportunities through which abortion might be approved on medical criteria which could not be opened through the use of somatic complications. This was particularly the case with pregnancies to young unmarried girls, particularly those in the middle classes. Past obstetric complications could not be used because they were rarely predictable; fewest complications in any case occurred among young healthy girls and therefore somatic criteria would rarely be applicable. Suicide or psychosis were too rarely occurring to be frequently used as criteria and ultimately the medical debate opened up to deal with neurosis, personality defects, psychological vulnerability etc. Being diagnostic or explanatory categories used and accepted in general psychiatric medicine they could be held to constitute medical/scientific grounds and yet open up the pathway to abortion on social grounds. Somewhat similar considerations apply to abortion on the grounds of the potential impact of unwanted pregnancy and motherhood on the child or on existing children.

A vast research literature now exists into the relationship between pregnancy, abortion and psychiatric illness and abnormality. Very few firm results have been obtained, partly for methodological reasons, partly because psychiatric terminology, classifications and diagnoses are usually a poor basis for hard epidemiological research and partly because the questions asked were largely irrelevant to the problem, being based on the assumption that abortion is a unitary phenomenon rather than a simple technical operation with a multitude of culturally imposed meanings.

During the period of liberalisation leading to abortion law reform psychiatrists were increasingly drawn into the decision-making process, essentially to provide medical/scientific validation for decisions taken on humanitarian grounds. Psychiatry was thus the Trojan Horse through which abortion was introduced into medical systems which could not adapt themselves to cultural change. The unreality of the psychiatric criteria has subsequently been demonstrated in societies such as Great Britain and the United States, where, following more liberal legislation, the psychiatrists are much less likely to be consulted about the decision, and where they themselves are beginning to question their professional relevance in decision-making.

4. DISCUSSION

In the earlier section of this paper I discussed specialisation in medicine and the proliferation of sub-specialisms whose title and roles signified advances in technology, changes in the nature of illness, or the changed importance attached to particular age and sex groups or particular types and levels of performance etc. I took obstetrics and gynaecology as a case example of those medical specialisms which despite unchanged nomenclature nevertheless showed internal ideological and role changes as a response to changing social structure. My thesis has been that, apart from its technical content, obstetrics and gynaecology fulfilled another function – that of social control, of preserving established institutions and normative sexual behaviour. Resistance to change was achieved by the adoption of medical/scientific criteria which, seemingly neutral, nevertheless supported the status quo. When conflict between professional ideology and contemporary culture became irreconcilable, acceptable scientific criteria were needed to effect the change in professional practice. The service was performed via psychiatry which, through its loose terminology and diagnoses and its closer relationship to social behaviour, was able to supply the validation required.

It is unlikely that we have seen the final developments in this process of adaptation. Recent evidence (e.g. the massive new involvement of WHO in matters of family planning and population change) suggests that the abortion controversy signalled one phase, perhaps a crucial stage, in the de-medicalisation of maternity services. Alternatively we might say that, having medicalised sexual and reproductive behaviour and begun to absorb social and psychological perspectives, obstetrics and gynaecology is adapting to changes in social structure and to linked ideologies. The rate of adaptation varies sharply between medical systems and in some the change is as yet barely discernible.

This analysis has ignored many relevant issues (those, for example, relating to population and national power) being focussed upon the mode of transformation. The simultaneous occurrence of similar movements in other disciplines (note the emergence of such terms as social paediatrics, social psychiatry and community medicine) indicates that, despite its idiosyncratic features, the adaptation in obstetrics and gynaecology is merely a special case of a more general tendency.

BIBLIOGRAPHY

[1] T. S. Szasz, *The Myth of Mental Illness: Foundations of a Theory of Personal Conduct*, Hoeber–Harper, New York 1961.

[2] T. S. Szasz, *The Manufacture of Madness*, Routledge and Kegan Paul, London 1971.

[3] B. Wootton, *Social Science and Social Pathology*, Allen and Unwin, London 1959.

[4] I. K. Zola, 'Medicine as an institution of social control', *Sociological Review* **20** (1972) 487–502.

REFERENCE

* Direct reprint requests to: Raymond Illsley, M.R.C. Medical Sociology Unit, Institute of Medical Sociology, Aberdeen, Scotland.

THE USE OF THE CONCEPT OF SOCIALIZATION IN THE STUDY OF REHABILITATION

ANTONINA OSTROWSKA

Institute of Philosophy and Sociology, Polish Academy of Sciences, Warsaw, Poland

Interpretation of social phenomena in sociological categories requires a sociological theory. Such a theory makes it possible to formulate problems in the appropriate scientific language, and facilitates construction and verification of hypotheses. According to many authors a sociological theory has three essential functions [1]:

i. it is instrumental in the codification of the existing knowledge;
ii. it serves as a guideline for research by determining the boundaries of our knowledge;
iii. it serves as a starting point for research, it helps to eliminate errors and acts as a control on observation and interpretation.

These three functions of the sociological theory indicate that it may have some bearing on the study of rehabilitation. Moreover, when applied to this field it seems to have one more, particularly important, function:

iv. it provides recommendations for social engineering.

A sociological theory can be translated into an aggregation of practical recommendations of a social engineering character that have a direct impact on social practice. These relations are shown in the diagram:

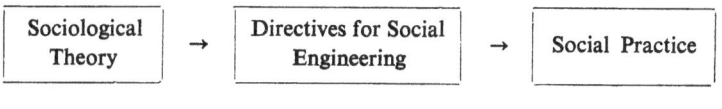

Sociological Theory	→	Directives for Social Engineering	→	Social Practice

In this article I shall try to show what sociological theory implies for rehabilitation process.

The question of rehabilitation may be approached from several angles. It is commonly assumed that rehabilitation affects all spheres of life, and is – or should be – studied from many points of view: medical, physical, psychiatric, sociopsychological, vocational, etc. And yet, these numerous and independent approaches have not so far been unified into one theory, which would be able to combine several fragmentary points of view and mediate between them, so as to offer a uniform conception of the rehabilitation process. I wish to suggest such an interpretation of the rehabilitation process in terms of a sociological theory that could be a step in this direction.

The choice of a sociological theory and its justification are dependent on the sociological analysis of possible approaches to social rehabilitation. It is thus necessary first to define what rehabilitation is – and what it is not – and to establish what processes and behaviors can be so described.

Many authors divide rehabilitation into three basic aspects: medical, psychological and social. The social aspect, with which I shall be mainly concerned here, aims at bringing the subject back into his social situation where he is expected to reasume his former tasks or adapt himself to new ones, and where he is also expected to take up the new roles which are open to him in his medically new situation. This definition of rehabilitation evidently contains elements of learning and of adaptation.

Four stages of the rehabilitation process can be distinguished [2]:

(1) relinquishment of the previous roles;

(2) identification with the new roles;

(3) self-improvement in the new roles;

(4) integration of the new roles within the totality of roles performed.

This approach, stressing the learning of new roles, adaptation and socialization, is not an isolated view. In the sociomedical literature there are many conceptions that relate rehabilitation to the process of learning and to adaptation to new roles, but not always have been expressed in the terminology adopted in this paper.

A related conceptual framework has been for example proposed by Edward Suchman [3]. He postulates the following scheme for the analysis of the rehabilitation process:

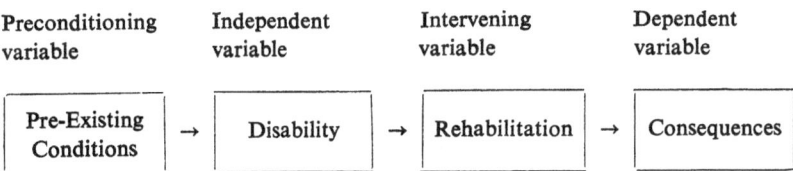

Preconditioning variable		Independent variable		Intervening variable		Dependent variable
Pre-Existing Conditions	→	Disability	→	Rehabilitation	→	Consequences

In other words, Suchman points to the development of certain consequences of disability depending on various primary and secondary conditions. This general scheme can be made more specific. Among the conditions preceeding disability—in which we are interested since they have certain implications for the ensuing course of the rehabilitation process and its final consequences—there are preexisting medical conditions (seen as the subject's medical characterization) and also conditions of a psychological and social character.

The same can be said of rehabilitation, or the intervening variable in the scheme. Comparatively speaking, this concept raises the fewest difficulties, since it has often been operationalized for purposes of research and study. Similarly, the consequences, or the dependent variable, may also be separately examined within all spheres of conditions preceding disability and involved in the rehabilitation process, i.e. medical, socio-psychological, etc. But in the case of disability it is not enough to say that it has medical, psychological and social aspects. The problem is more complicated, and if we are trying to solve it, it is not only because it is important in itself, but also because its solution may become useful in the conceptualization of the rehabilitation process. There are different types of rehabilitation corresponding to different kinds of disability. Numerous rehabilitative techniques have to be administered in different proportions to differing types of disability. In certain circumstances medical treatment dominates, in the other minor medical assistance is accompanied by appreciable effort in social rehabilitation.

The last point brings us to the crucial question: how should we differentiate disability? Obviously more than one criterion can be used. Medicine can differentiate impairment according to medical variables, distinguishing for example types of sickness, treatments applied, etc.

No such classification, however, has so far been invented although it seems to be a general view that it is indispensable for further studies. I cannot attempt to give such a classification here. It should rather be produced by physicians and specialists in various other fields. Here, I wish only to stress how great is the need for a classification, and that it is not only physicians who are aware of it. The social consequences of paraplegia differ for instance from those of the amputated limb or schizophrenia. Very often a sociologist cannot solve the problems which interest him because he does not have a dependable medical classification of disabilities. In these circumstances several sociologists studying the process of rehabilitation – make up their own classifications of the disabled individuals on the basis of demographic and social characteristics of patients dating back to their history from the period prior to injury, and on the basis of the social consequence of disability. Examples of this are the works of Saad Nagi [4] and Safilos Rotschild [5].

Apart from the difficulties involved in making an exhaustive classification of disabilities, it seems that for the purposes of sociological analysis two dimensions are essential:

(1) reversability of disability;

(2) stigmatization, or the stigma produced by the negative public attitude towards certain forms of impairment.

Both the disabled individual and those about him view his impairment as non-stigmatizing if it is temporary and can be removed completely or to a considerable degree by proper medical treatment. But even the existing negative attitude can be considerably abated by the course and range of the rehabilitation process applied.

In our culture all manifest incapacity is stigmatized and viewed negatively by the public: witness such commonly heard names and phrases as: 'freak' or 'blind as a bat'. This disfavor is not without influence on the type of social rehabilitation chosen. The public attitude toward incapacity must be taken into consideration by social rehabilitation teams. Those are not, of course, all the variables to be considered – there still remain the social characteristics of the disabled individual and numerous variables connected with his own assessment of his incapacity – but it seems that the two social characteristics mentioned above are of primary importance.

These two dimensions may intersect:

	Reversible	Irreversible
Stigmatizing	Cleft palate	Paraplegia
Non-stigmatizing	Broken leg	Coronary heart disease

They reflect the degree of social revulsion vis-à-vis incapacity: from the mildest – non-stigmatizing and reversible, to the strongest – stigmatizing and irreversible. This classification of patients implies that rehabilitation teams should modify their procedures according to the patient. This is furthermore connected with varying social consequences.

Research into the rehabilitation of the handicapped cannot be isolated from an analysis of the disability that has been the cause of their incapacity. This kind of analysis reveals what can be substituted for the roles formerly performed by the patient, which of these roles he can reasume without rehabilitation, and which he must learn anew. A simple analysis of his disability cannot settle the problem entirely, of course. Other social characteristics of patient undergoing rehabilitation have to be considered also (the pre-existing conditions). Their range has been discussed by many researchers (particularly those concentrating on the handicapped family environment) and their conceptualization seems to be easier.

*   *
*

The foregoing consideration of rehabilitation shows that a more general theory of socialization and adaptation would be adequate. It would provide a platform on which social rehabilitation could be clearly seen as a species of socialization and adaptation on the part of the handicapped person to new roles (or to the reassumption of his former roles under changed conditions). The literature dealing with socialization shows, however, that there are some difficulties in using this concept. The term itself and the studies that use it refer more often to children than to adults, and do not deal with older age groups which may also be initiated into communities, confronted with the need of adopting new values and patterns of behavior, and expected to learn new roles. The question of adults socialization is more frequently found in the sociology of politics (transmission of political ideas and values); whereas in psychology, anthropology, sociology of education, etc., the term seems to allude exclusively to children and young people. It is only natural in these circumstances that socialization literature consists mainly of studies that have little bearing on the process of adults' rehabilitation.

Any attempt of drawing a more detailed picture of rehabilitation within the broader and more general framework of the socialization process must make use of the differentiation introduced by J. O. Brim [5] between legitimate and illegitimate socialization. The former pertains to situations in which it is believed that an individual has not yet mastered a really socialized role (he may for example be a student who acquires the capability to assume his prospective roles in the course of studying at university). Illegitimate socialization applies to situations in which there is a public belief that an individual should have learned certain roles earlier (for example those of a parent or a spouse). When the need for resocialization is regarded as legitimate some formal institutions or public mechanisms are invoked to provide for that role. If it is considered illegitimate there are generally no such institutions.

The resocialization process constitutes a parallel case. Resocialization may also be legitimate or illegitimate, depending on whether the existing norms of behaviour have been previously socialized or not. A criminal is expected to have known legitimate norms earlier—his resocialization is hence illegitimate. Legitimate resocialization applies to situations in which an individual had been legitimately socialized but due to certain changes in his health and fitness found himself impelled to change the form of his socialization. An example of such resocialization may be the rehabilitation process of a disabled person. A handicapped individual had socialized certain roles and then found out that he had to change or modify them.

Such a distinction based on the concept of socialization is important since it shows how to locate the rehabilitation process within the socialization theory.

Some interesting suggestions for the analysis of the rehabilitation process may also be found in the works of political sociologists, particularly in their analysis of socializing institutions. There is a certain analogy between their observations and mine. According to H. Laswell the process of political socialization can be reduced to five questions concerning general interpersonal relations: "a) who, b) learns what, c) from whom, d) under what circumstances, e) with what effects?" These are sufficiently general questions to encompass analyses of all kinds of socialization, including the rehabilitation process. They can be answered by determining:

(a) the characteristics of the individual undergoing the process of socialization or rehabilitation;
(b) the nature of the message being socialized;
(c) the characteristics of the socializing (rehabilitating) environment, persons and institutions, and whether the process is executed in an organized and controlled manner;
(d) the circumstances surrounding socialization (rehabilitation): the social context and traits of the environment in which the rehabilitated subject is to be found, types of social interaction, social situations, etc.;
(e) the measurement of the effects of socialization, or the degree of success in rehabilitation.

This model can be utilized for description of rehabilitation process itself and also for classification and synthesis of innumerable studies already existing in this field.

Certain difficulties cropped up when we attempted to find an answer to the last question in the scheme presented above, i.e. when we tried to determine the degree of success in rehabilitation. Although it is fairly easy to establish the degree of success in medical or purely physical rehabilitation – by applying medical tests, or so-called daily activity scales – the measuring of social adaptation is still problematic. Similar problems are usually encountered whenever a social scientist attempts to measure the effects of socialization. The existing scales of socialization are criticized for their apparent inability to differentiate individuals who have been successfully socialized from those who have only succeeded in becoming conformists.

It is also interesting to see into types of motivation that initiate the process of socialization. On the one hand we can find cases where socialization has been embarked upon because it was expected or required by others. On the other hand, we can find cases of socialization which has been started by the individuals concerned unaided. It has traditionally been assumed that the requirements of the group or the milieu which the individual aspires to join are more important. The second type of socialization which is undertaken by the individual without inspiration from his group has not been so thoroughly studied. This type of socialization covers all forms of activities which are performed in order to change the roles which are found unsatisfactory by the individual in view of his expectations concerning his own personality, behaviour, life style, etc. Very often this type of socialization coincides in mature persons with notable changes of personality. It seems that this form of socialization is particularly important for rehabilitated persons. Sometimes, when a person's physical impairment is viewed negatively by his group, usually because it is connected with visible disfigurement, the victim is not expected to assume his former roles, and moreover is persuaded from doing so, and his reasumption of previously severed contacts with 'healthy' people is deliberately discouraged. In such a situation a complete return to society may be brought about by the solitary efforts of an individual to complete his adaptation.

So far I have been concerned with the possibility of utilizing the theory of socialization for a systematic classification of problems in the field of rehabilitation. But the socialization theory may also serve a more practical purpose in connection with rehabilitation. I will try to show now how verified contentions may be adopted to rehabilitative practice. Let us take the example of socialization limitations.

Limitations to socialization are encountered mostly in dealing with older age groups. From the point of view of the rehabilitated individual two barriers impede the process of his rehabilitation:

(1) biological;

(2) attachment, familiarity with previously socialized roles.

The success of resocialization depends to a great degree on a successful surmounting of these barriers.

Biological barriers, like age, physical fitness, etc., definitely affect the success of rehabilitation and must always be taken into account.

Among factors that hinder the socialization of adults there is one that needs to be clearly emphasized. The resocialization of a disabled person is more difficult than other socialization processes because it is not initiated by the anticipatory socialization. Nobody tries to prepare himself for his future roles, modified by his decreased fitness, with the possible exception of people, with congenital defects. Very often the transition from the normal roles which a person could perform before his injury to the set of very limited roles open to him after it is a very traumatic experience resulting in a dramatic loss of vitality, a desire to have no contacts with people, and inability to undertake prolonged attempts at adapting to the new social and medical conditions.

As regards repeated socializations, it has been established that the behavior deeply ingrained in previous socializations is proportionately more resistant to change. An attempt to modify it is often connected with a disturbance of the entire system of values, modes of behavior, conceptions of life patterns and roles.

But there are also other factors that impede the process of socialization. It has been established for example that "the more an individual feels himself rejected the more likely he is to become dependent and unable to identify with new roles". Certain obstacles may be inherent in the socialization process itself. It has also been proved that when it is carried out in a repressive or overprotective manner, or if it is inconsistent and produces conflicts, it will have little impact on the subject apart from stimulating his aggressive tendencies.

Besides, there may also be barriers unrelated to the subject undergoing rehabilitation. They may be erected by the character of the rehabilitation institutions and their functioning. The more congruent the action of the socializing agencies, the more smoothly and rapidly the process of socialization develops. If on the contrary there are numerous conflicts among these agencies, the process is slowed down and its results are more uncertain. But there are also factors that can minimize the limitations to socialization, namely the motivation of the persons being socialized, the prestige of the socializing individuals and institutions and, finally, the totality of the subject's social conditions.

All these various approaches, tendencies and rules and many others, not mentioned here can be directly applied to the rehabilitation process. They provide explicit advise on how to control the rehabilitation process, how to organize rehabilitation teems, etc. Besides, it seems that these factors should be taken into account in all studies and research programs on rehabilitation currently under way. The recent study conducted in Poland on patients who had recovered from myocardial infarction has shown how fruitful can be a study on limitations and motivation for rehabilitation to elucidate this process [7].

* *
*

The aim of this paper was to demonstrate how social rehabilitation can be analyzed in terms of socialization theory and what its place is in that theory. It was also indicated that rehabilitation may be analyzed with reference to the models created in socialization theory.

Naturally, the propositions advanced here do not exhaust the problem. They rather suggest what lines of research seem to be fruitful and how the results obtained should be utilized. Moreover, in this brief review, I have shown how the available data on rehabilitation can be systematized. The type of presentation proposed should help to fill a gap in the literature devoted to the rehabilitation of handicapped persons.

BIBLIOGRAPHY

[1] T. Parsons and E. A. Shils, *Toward a General Theory of Action*, Harvard University Press, Cambridge Mass. 1959.

[2] J. B. E. Cogswell, 'Rehabilitation of the Paraplegie', paper presented at Vth World Sociological Congress, Evian 1966.

[3] E. Suchman, *A Model for Research and Evaluation on Rehabilitation Sociology and Rehabilitation*, ASA, 1965.

[4] Saad Z. Nagi, *Readings in Disability – Policies and Programs, an Analysis of Organizations, Clients, and Decision-Making – Mershon Center*, The Ohio State University, Columbus Ohio 1973.

[5] Constantina Safilios-Rothschild, *The Sociology and Social Psychology of Disability and Rehabilitation*, Randon House 1970.

[6] O. G. Brim Jr., Adult Socialization, International Encyclopedie of the Social Sciences, Vol. 14, New York 1964.

[7] J. Bejnarowicz, A. Ostrowska and M. Sokołowska, 'Social Rehabilitation', in: *Investigation into the Effect of Medical Rehabilitation and of Therapeutic Procedure on Vocational Rehabilitation of Patients with Recent Myocardial Infarction, Final Report*, Warszawa 1969.

SOCIAL STRUCTURE AND HEALTH: METHODOLOGICAL AND SUBSTANTIAL PROBLEMS WITHOUT SOLUTIONS

MANFRED PFLANZ

Institut für Epidemiologie und Sozialmedizin, Medizinische Hochschule Hannover, Hannover, Federal Republic of Germany

I. AN INVESTIGATION IN POLAND 125 YEARS AGO

About 125 years ago on February 20, 1848, one of the most important and most admirable studies in the history of social epidemiology was begun. Although much work has been done in the field of the relationships between social factors and health the study we are talking about here remains unique in its hypothesis, its realization and its conclusions.

How did this study come to pass and what are its results and conclusions? In January of 1848 reports in the Prussian newspapers concerning a catastrophic disease newly broken out in Upper Silesia became increasingly urgent and frequent. At this time Upper Silesia was under Prussian rule. The government department responsible had not yet received any reports from local public health authorities either about the nature of the disease or about such a disease problem having been noted at all. Only after being pushed by public opinion the government department sent Dr. Barez to Upper Silesia with instructions to make himself acquainted with the situation. The Minister of the Interior, however, refused him authorization for any effective intervention. So the only thing he could do was to try and adopt a scientific approach to the problem of the epidemic. Thus the 26-year-old Privatdozent from the University of Berlin Dr. Rudolf Virchow was ordered to accompany Dr. Barez on his trip to Upper Silesia. Virchow, soon to become the most outstanding and brilliant anthropologist and pathologist of his time, began work on February 20, 1848, covering in less than three weeks the areas of Rybnik, Pszczyna, Żory and Mikołów. In the paper he published immediately after the completion of his inquiry Virchow [1] reported on the number of diseased persons, the number of deaths and the results of the *post mortem* examinations. He it was who realized that the disease in question was not typhoid fever, as first supposed, but typhus.

More important than his pathological findings, however, was the fact that Virchow carefully analysed the social and political circumstances under which the epidemic had developed. He made himself acquainted with housing conditions, nutrition and also with agricultural production. In the oppression of the population by the state, its officials, the hierarchy of the feudal system and finally by the church, he found the main reasons for poverty and starvation and consequently for this epidemic. His demands were: Complete and undiminished democracy, freedom, education, prosperity, and national reorganization for Upper Silesia. If there exists a model study in the field of social structure and health it is this report by Virchow on the typhus epidemic in Upper Silesia. The combination of precise observation and historical and political knowledge, generalized conclusions and detailed, realistic political demands is unique.

In this auditorium I can forgo a closer explication of Virchow's survey since there is unlikely to be any medical sociologist who does not know this study. What cannot be omitted, however, is the very deplorable fact that in the past 125 years we have learned so little more about these problems. The reaction of the Prussian government 125 years ago, disgraceful as it was, should not lead us to the assumption that a similarly shocking neglect could never happen nowadays and in our countries. It is my opinion that any European state in a similar situation might react today in a similar way, that is by showing inadequacy combined with an attempt at concealment, being more concerned about saving face than saving human lives.

At the same time we have to admit that medical sociology and social epidemiology were, really, filling volumes with empirical, theoretical or simply speculative studies but did not help a bit to gain more freedom, to diminish social injustice or to solve any other social problem in which the roots of today's epidemic diseases must be seen.

II. THE ABSENCE OF DEFINITIONS

In dealing with Virchow's analysis of the typhus epidemic it soon becomes obvious that he not only made a contribution to the special problem of 'social factors and typhus' but was also dealing with the more general question of 'social structure and health'. When looking for a precise definition of 'social structure' in literature we meet a chaotic mass of different definitions. Kroeber[2] says in his *Anthropology*:

" 'Structure' appears to be just a yielding to a word that has a perfectly good meaning but suddenly becomes fashionably attractive for a decade or so – like 'streamlining' – and during its vogue tends to be applied indiscriminately because of the pleasurable connotations of its sound. Of course a typical personality can be viewed as having a structure. But so can a physiology, any organism, all societies and all cultures, crystals, machines – in fact everything which is not wholly amorphous has a structure. So what 'structure' adds to the meaning of our phrase seems to be nothing, except to provoke a degree of pleasant puzzlement."

I would like to add in parenthesis that Kroeber could not have any idea of the incredible abuse later to be made of the word 'system' – a word as fashionable and insignificant as the word 'structure'. Thus in many publications nowadays either of these words can easily be replaced by the other without changing the meaning of the sentence. This is done so to make the paper as fashionable as possible and to conceal the lack of precise concepts. Stanley Udy jr.[3] expresses himself in nearly as sceptical a fashion as Kroeber, when he says:

"The concept 'social structure' is, paradoxically, so fundamental to social science as to render its uncontested definition virtually impossible. Basic concepts in particular seem likely to suffer from this difficulty, since their primordial character demands that they provide an effective link between the field of inquiry and the particular approach, or even the personal philosophy of the individual scholar. Various controversies, both apparent and real, are thus especially likely to surround the use of such concepts. In the case of 'social structure', some of these difficulties are purely terminological and are, hence, more easily resolved than may appear possible on the surface. Others derive more fundamentally from disagreement over the basic philosophical assumptions appropriate to social research. And still others reflect substantive theoretical problems, which seem likely to persist even when there is agreement over terminology and basic philosophy."

These preliminary remarks, however, did not prevent Udy from giving a definition completely devoid of any meaning at all:

"We shall define 'social structure' very broadly as the totality of patterns of collective human phenomena that cannot be explained solely on the basis of human heredity and/or the non-human environment."

These remarks might authorize me to forgo a definition within this framework. Instead of a definition I shall later give some examples of the fact that health is especially dependent on those features of social life which some authors believe to be the essential aspects of social structure.

The definition of health is not any better. There is a lot to be said about the definitions of 'health' – they are bombastic, trivial, tautological, meaningless. Only one thing cannot be said about them: that there exists any 'pleasant puzzlement."

Every medical sociologist can be sure to get all the applause he cares for, if only he emphasizes that we should now turn away from the consideration of diseases and bestow our attention upon health and health problems. But nearly always when this term 'health' is used in connection with concrete facts it is a matter of illness or disease. 'Health insurance' is in fact sickness insurance, and public health does not promote health in general but is meant to treat or to prevent diseases.

Recently there have been attempts to establish a continuum from health to disease on a scale measuring the degree of impediment to everyday life. The medical sociologist has to sympathize with these endeavours because this operationalization of the term 'health' is mainly done by using social criteria.

Nevertheless the fact must not be neglected that those scales presuppose social criteria, the validity and meaning of which have first of all to be proved. They are based on role-performances and achievement expectations not yet proved to be as generally valid as theorists of health measuring seem to take for granted. So it might not have happened by chance that these movements towards a generally valid measure of health were started by mathematicians and economists. Practising physicians are clearly displaying reserve about any attempt to make health ascertainable or even measurable.

Facing these different points of departure chosen by sociologists, mathematicians and physicians it does not seem very likely that within the next few years we shall arrive at a definition and operationalization of the term 'health' which will satisfy both theoretical and practical requirements.

Therefore in the following there shall be no more talk about health, but only about various groups of diseases and ailments. If neither social structure nor health are clearly defined, there does not seem to be any point in trying to bring the relation of these two concepts into a theoretical framework however helpful this would be. The real difficulties of our subject are, however, to be seen both in inadequate methodology and in a specific political and ideological perspective.

III. METHODOLOGICAL PROBLEMS

The methodological problem can be described in the following way: The development of psychometrics has had a considerable influence on sociology. Nearly all methods used in empirical social research are based on observation or inquiry of individuals. Attitudes, opinions, values, interpersonal relationships, motivations and behavior patterns are still the essentials in empirical social research. They refer primarily to individuals and are to be correlated with sociological categories – if at all – only in so far as sociological theory can be used for the interpretation of the results – often enough like a *deus ex machina.* It will be emphasized that this methodological field is highly developed. Reliability, validity, item analysis, scaling, factor scores are only a few of the magic words every student of sociology is taught today, which characterize those techniques he will have to apply later on. That these techniques are by no means always used where they should be, and often enough are used as an end in themselves, is a separate chapter.

A second task is to determine and classify social structures. Generally, two kinds of variables can be used here: Aggregate data, and global data. Aggregate data are originally obtained from individuals but afterwards aggregated into higher statistical units. The average income of the employed population or the percentage of individuals with less than 8 years of education are just two examples of aggregate data.

Global data are not gained from individuals, though of course the kind of global data which is significant in sociology concerns human beings as well, that is to say human beings in a community. Some global data are easily obtained, as for example the political or economic system of a nation or the main financial ressources of the health services. Some of those global data can only be measured on nominal scales or they cannot be measured at all because they have only a qualitative character. Much global data can be obtained only with difficulty. Anomie, disorganization, industrial society are terms we permanently use but even today there do not exist any generally acknowledged rules how to operationalize those terms to the extent necessary for the establishment of corresponding global data.

In trying to put the concepts of social structure and health into a meaningful relationship for empirical research the problem of measurement is not even the most important one. The difficulties begin already with the unanswered question of which data and variables we shall use. In general we apply such data as official statistics supply us with. In many countries there exist highly developed statistics containing an immense amount of aggregate and global data of high quality. These are the data we work on, but as we find ourselves almost in a pioneer state we hardly ever ask ourselves whether these are the data and variables we really need and whether they are of any significance for our problem. Looking at the few existing studies – some of which we shall be talking about in more detail – one cannot avoid the suspicion that we do not at all have at our disposal those data which are necessary to find any significant correlations between social structure and health.

The next problem consists in combining the variables into a specific variable structure which might be an indicator as well as a model or even an image of the social structure. Up to now there have been two methods of approach. Either you can choose a completely intuitive proceeding which is based on subjective evidence, emphasized with the more vehemence the less evident they are to other people. The other possible approach starts from the mathematical methods of factor analysis, especially cluster analysis, or the regression model. Here it should be asked whether these really are procedures adequate to the hypothesis or whether they are third rate procedures forced upon the researcher because there do not exist any first class or at least second class procedures. Again it has to be stated that even these inadequate methods are not fully made use of. Even if an intuitive or mathematical compilation is not – as so often happens – completely forgone, the assumptions under which alone the application of these methods is permitted are hardly ever pertinent.

And nobody has seriously applied himself to the question of what units those aggregate or global data are utimately to be correlated with. M. Haas,[4] for example, in his paper called 'The Study of Biopolitics' works with the mortality data from 72 countries using these countries as points of departure in the analysis without regard to their different sizes. Similar ridiculous experiments have been in the field of urban ecology. Some of the statistical units are too big, others too small. There does not even exist any reasonable definition of what a society with social structure actually is. I don't underestimate the intense discussion of these questions by the structuralist school of anthropology. The answers they found, however, were hardly suitable for empirical analysis of the relationships between social structure and health.

Nations are units extremely important for the ecological analysis. Bertram M. Gross[5] has shown in an admirable compilation what little agreement exists in classifying social structures into nations. Even less agreement can be obtained regarding the measuring of social structures by social indicators. Nor is there anything justifying the hope for a speedy achievement of corresponding indicators for nations. Gross comes to the conclusion that:

"Progress in the collection of social indicators will be slow and uneven... The maturation of social accounting concepts will take many decades."

It follows as an additional difficulty for our special topic that health in itself is an essential indicator for social systems and social structures. Equally at a loss we seek reference units in historical studies, trying to achieve a longitudinal approach as the epidemiologist calls it. I do not want to hurt my historically oriented colleagues' feelings, but it seems to me that sometimes beautiful and impressive words help to conceal the lack of constructive criteria which might allow us to develop empirically ascertainable hypotheses as to the correlation between social structure and health in historical perspective.

It would be a mistake to assume the methods for the ascertainment of health or – to be more precise – of the major diseases to be merely an epidemiological problem and as such easily solved. As far as the surveys are based on official or semi-official statistics there exist two sources of errors depending on structural issues, thus preventing an objective evaluation of the epidemiological situation:

1. deliberate concealment, and
2. ignorance.

In seeking countries cooking their statistics of suicide we do not have to go as far as India, we might find them quite nearby. In other countries the statistics on communicable diseases are manipulated, especially serious cases like cholera or smallpox. Ignorance and inadequacy in working out official health statistics is not distributed at random but as a function of structural issues. An explanation is not necessary here. But even the results of epidemiological primary surveys are biased by structural features. The attitude towards disease and performance, the assessment of need and the feasibility of treatment are essential elements of the social structure modifying any epidemiological result.

IV. IDEOLOGICAL AND POLITICAL PROBLEMS

It might be possible to overcome some of the methodological problems within a reasonable time. But medical-sociological thinking about diseases does not happen in a vacuum, and we can only practise methodological purism or *Wertfreiheit* (science free from value-commitments) by shutting our eyes to our society. We are surrounded by official ideologies from state, party or parties and other forces which have gained power in some universities in the so-called capitalistic industrial societies. We are not only surrounded by those ideologies but many medical sociologists are part of these ideologies, their promotors and high priests. There is probably hardly any medical sociologist living who has not succumbed to the temptation of talking about the relationship between social structure and illness. Though there exists one difference strictly dividing them into two separate groups. The first consider the structure of their own society as promoting diseases, and the others only accuse the structures of other societal systems of being agents of illness.

The entire rhetoric in this field – some more examples shall be quoted later on – is without any practical consequences. Whatever the official statements of health policy might be, how much or how little the medical sociologists try to interfere in this field, it is everywhere the individual, the single citizen, the patient, who is held responsible for his health. There is no state in the developed regions, nor any political grouping, willing to change its own structures for the sake of the population's health – which does not prevent them from giving advice to and making claims on other states, ideologies or groups. – Everywhere one appeals to some kind of 'health ethics' on the part of the citizen, he is held responsible for any health risking behaviour. As has been already mentioned, science concentrates on motivations, values beliefs and attitudes to find out why people do not act like official medicine demands, instead of concentrating on the examination of those structural barriers which perhaps make the prevention of disease impossible.[6]

We shall deliberately omit here the problem of whether it would after all be desirable from the social point of view to undertake any structural changes in order to prevent diseases, knowing that success would be doubtful and that dangerous secondary side effects cannot be completely ruled out. The only point I want to emphasize here is that while everywhere great discussions are going on about the influence of social structure on disease, nowhere are practical conclusions being drawn with regard to research and the health system – conclusions some people might even be afraid of. Of course no state, no political party can afford to announce clearly, that deliberately avoidable diseases are put up with because there are other values and goals deemed to be of greater importance. It is not my intention to proclaim health to be the highest achievable value to which everything else is to be subjected. It only has to be admitted that all the talk about great successes regarding productivity, military efforts, life expectancy, physician-population ratio, tax yield and so on is only meant to conceal the fact that health is not of primary importance.

To sum up what has been said above: Our scant knowledge of the relation between social structure and health cannot merely be explained by difficulties in definitions and methodology; at least as many difficulties are to be seen in concealed, vested ideological interests which impede a more intense scientific or practical pursuit of this problem.

V. PRIMITIVE SOCIETIES AND DISEASE

Structuralist conceptions are to be seen behind the popular idea that in primitive, illiterate, simply structured societies those diseases do not exist which are usually summed up by the merely ideological term of 'civilization-diseases', which is to say specifically, psychiatric and psychosomatic diseases. Unfortunately we only know very little about the diseases occurring in illiterate or primitive populations. Difficulties of access, conditions prohibitive to diagnosis, small populations, low life expectancy, and, in particular difficulties in linguistic communication concerning health, are some of the problems impeding an adequate epidemiological-sociological survey. By virtue of the uncomplicated and agreeable examination method involved, blood pressure has often been the topic of such surveys. In many primitive populations the level of blood pressure was found to be low in general, the average blood pressure in older people not being higher than in younger ones. Hypertension with its complications was found to be non-existent. But such facts are not only to be found in primitive populations. Exactly the same was true for many population groups in Central and Eastern Europe during the last years of the war and the years immediately following it. Native studies in foreign countries have showed that these characteristics are also to be found in population groups which cannot be called primitive. Two examples of such groups are: 1. Iranian miners living near the city of Esfahan, and 2. The Ewe, living in Ghana, adherents of the native natural religion. Neither groups could not be described as primitive, but their state of nutrition was rather poor, as in the population groups in Central Europe during and immediately after the war. If surveys carried out among primitive populations can teach us something about the correlations between social structure and health then we have either so far failed to understand these lessons or, on the other hand, we might not yet have hit upon the right line of questioning. The few and contradictory data we have obtained hitherto certainly do not allow us to draw any essential inferences about the subject of social structure and health.

VI. MACROSOCIOLOGICAL STRESS MODELS

The method of correlating aggregated data with frequencies of diseases has already been mentioned in this paper. Unfortunately there does not yet exist any sufficiently sophisticated and elaborate concept for this problem. This means that the two studies to be quoted here also suffer from deficiencies.

M. Haas [7] began with the hypothesis "that levels of foreign and domestic violence are a function of societal conditions and processes that become manifest in the form of deaths due to psychogenic causes, such as suicides and heart diseases". To test this hypothesis, data for all significant causes of death – 46 in all – were collected for 72 political units along with death rates due to foreign and domestic violence. However, the hypothesis could not be confirmed. Foreign and domestic violence did converge as part of an over-all medical underdevelopment cluster. Psychogenic causes of death, which emerge within the developed cluster, are unrelated to political casualties in the mid-twentieth century.

Without any doubt the hypothesis was justified and made sense; the particular results, however, are irritating. There are correlations to be found between causes of death which one could never find within one country. The reliability and validity of dependent and independent variables are to be doubted and after all political units showing enormous differences in size and importance were used for the statistical analysis.

Similar mistakes mark the study by Dodge and Martin [8] which is based on the assumption that the incidence and prevalence of chronic diseases vary with the measure of socially induced stress. On the other hand the degree of socially induced stress in a special population varies correspondingly with the stability and permanence of social relationships and the degree of status integration. As in such ecological analysis the single states of the U.S.A. are taken as statistical reference units and only official statistics, especially census data, were available, this hypothesis could not be convincingly operationalized. High rates of divorced or widowed people as such are taken as essential indicators of low status integration, these again correlate negatively with mortality in arteriosclerotical disease, malignant diseases, liver cirrhosis, and diabetes.

The methodological problems in such studies have already been mentioned. An especially weak point in Dodge's and Martin's survey is that the authors were not sufficiently aware of this deficiency. Indeed remarkable, however, is the inadequacy of the methods to the designed stressmodel. In the chain of events leading from socio-structural factors to the individual disease, the authors believe that different social structures and organizations expose different people to different socio-psychological experiences. These differences in living through and coping with socio-psychological experiences create varying degrees of stress for the single individual in the population.

Using their methods, however, no verification is possible. The authors correlate aggregate data with aggregate data without dealing with the psychological aspect of their model which is how social events are to be experienced to become effective as a stress. I reviewed this survey so detailed because it is plainly the prototype of a research approach often chosen to elaborate the topic social structure and health. It nearly always leads to ecological fallacies, especially if ecological data are interpreted on an individual level. For in these surveys the indicators used have also to include some criteria of the social structure which is possible both in global and in aggregate data. In interpreting the results every effort has to be made not to succumb to the temptation to deduce pathogenetic chains for individuals.

VII. CONCLUSIONS

Rudolf Virchow made a survey in 1848 of a standard not previously achieved by anybody. He linked empirical observations to socio-structural data and, drawing conclusions from this, made proposals nobody at first cared about. Later on, many other researchers after Virchow understood poverty and its causes to be an essential factor in the genesis of diseases. The success achieved in health policy by diminishing poverty proved these researchers to be right. Wherever poverty, lack of education and absence of freedom were largely eliminated, many diseases connected with them disappeared without any preventive medical measure.[9] Even if no social structural hypotheses were explicitly laid down, all the observations and actions on the connections between poverty and disease were based upon them.

In this paper several kinds of approach have been shown, and all upon close examination have turned out to be wrong. A retreat to a primitive social structure would probably produce no real positive effect on health.

We assume social structures and health to be connected but quite obviously up to now we must have been using the wrong methods, as we do not have any valid proof for this assumption. The results of our studies did not help in finding any possibility of exerting a positive influence on diseases without increasing the social costs too much. Our question is: Which aspects or variables of the present social structure are responsible for the increase of those diseases which are most frequent in industrialized countries today, such as cardio-vascular diseases, or cancer of specific localization? Trying to solve this problem takes several different steps.

1. Physicians have to be convinced that solving this problem will take more than merely medical means. 2. We are in dire need of thoroughly new theoretical approaches, but the search for an all-embracing theory should be stopped. 3. Methodology has to be widely improved. 4. After reiterated tests by replicative studies political conclusions must be drawn from the results. What we are in need of is medical sociologists with a high level of independence, who are able to recommend preventive measures – measures which are useful socially with regard to health as well, and which are acceptable to society.

REFERENCES

[1] R. Virchow, *Mittheilungen über die in Oberschlesien herrschende Typhus-Epidemie*, Berlin 1848.

[2] A. L. Kroeber, *Anthropology*, New York 1948, 2nd ed., p. 325.

[3] S. H. Udy, jr. 'Social Structure: Social Structural Analysis', in: *International Encyclopedia of the Social Sciences*, Vol. 14, New York 1968, p. 489–494.

[4] M. Haas, 'Toward the Study of Biopolitics: A Cross-sectional Analysis of Mortality Rates', *Behav. Sci.* **14** (1969) 257–280.

[5] B. M. Gross, 'The State of the Nation: Social Systems Accounting', in: R. A. Bauer, *Social Indicators*, MIT Press, Cambridge, Mass. 1966, p. 156–271.

[6] Chr. von Ferber, *Gesundheit und Gesellschaft. Haben wir eine Gesundheitspolitik?.* Stuttgart 1971.

[7] M. Haas, *op. cit.*

[8] D. L. Dodge and W. T. Martin, *Social Stress and Chronic Illness. Mortality Patterns in Industrial Society*, Univ. of Notre Dame Press, Notre Dame, London 1970.

[9] T. McKeown, *Medicine in Modern Society*, George Allen and Unwin Ltd., London 1965.

TOWARDS SOCIOMEDICAL HEALTH INDICATORS*

JACK ELINSON

Division of Sociomedical Sciences, Columbia University School of Public Health, New York, N.Y., U.S.A.

The stagnation of total mortality rates over relatively long periods of time in economically developed countries has reduced the value of mortality rates as indicators of the health status of populations in these countries. The insensitivity of mortality rates is quite noticeable in the United States where there is little to suggest that the increase in health services over recent years has resulted in improvements in the level of health. Even the infant mortality rate, long regarded as the most sensitive index of the level of health, is no longer a particularly useful indicator, despite the fact that the infant mortality rate of the United States suffers in comparison to that of many industrial nations [13]. The principal residual value of infant death rates is to reveal contrasts in health status within limited geographic areas as in large cities, as exemplified by a recent analysis in New York City [27]. Mortality rates are also useful for the assessment of specific diseases, but the present behavior of mortality rates have made moot the value of statistics of deaths from all causes as a measure of health in countries like the United States. The usefulness of biomedical indicators for population – based measures of health status is declining.

Nearly two decades ago (1957) the World Health Organization [32] recommended that mortality data in various forms – life expectancy at birth, the infant mortality rate, the crude death rate and the proportionate mortality rate for ages fifty years and over – be used as indicators of level of living for international comparison. The great virtue of mortality data is the availability of a long and generally comparable series of statistics. There is, as yet, not other body of routine statistics that provide diagnostic data for a country as a whole. Indeed, a principal reason for the W.H.O. recommendation is that mortality data are available for many countries.

The inadequacies of mortality data have been summarized by Moriyama [33] as follows:

– In countries where the need for statistical information is greatest the data are non-existent or of poor quality.

– While high lethality conditions, e.g., lung cancer are well represented, nonfatal conditions, e.g., arthritis, do not have the same probability of appearing in the statistics.

– The relationship of mortality and morbidity has not been clear.

– As chronic non-infective disease has increased, the interpretation of mortality statistics has become more difficult, particularly in cases of multiple, potentially fatal, chronic conditions.

It is paradoxical but what has been the most successful international effort in developing uniform statistics with respect to mortality, the World Health Organization's publications of '*International Classification of Diseases, and Causes of Death*' [21], now in its eight revision, has inhibited, if not stultified, the development of non-lethal measures of the health status of populations.

The inadequacy of and dissatisfaction with mortality rates as a measure of health level have led to demands for morbidity rates and "even other measures of social well being" [29]. It is useful to distinguish between biomedical and sociomedical measures of morbidity. Biomedical measures of morbidity include [17]:

(1) Tissue alterations, viewed as such and judged by pathologists to be causes of death – e.g., 'atherosclerosis', 'carcinoma'.

(2) Records produced by physiologic measuring equipment – e.g., the electrocardiogram; and the interpretations by specialists – e.g., cardiologists – of such records as the 'right bundle branch block'.

(3) Judgements rendered by clinicians in the form of a 'diagnosis' after considering 'all the evidence' – e.g., 'coronary artery disease'.

It is usually not possible to conduct pathological analyses of human tissues on populations who are not in medical facilities, e.g., in clinics, hospitals, or morgues, so that it is ordinarily not possible to extrapolate from such selected groups to general populations. Many physiologic measures and clinically diagnostic judgements can, however, be applied to population samples, sufficiently large, such that generalizations with respect to health levels of the total populations from which the samples are drawn can be made with statistical confidence. The U.S. National Health Examination Survey [35] provides an example of this procedure on a national basis; and there are a number of examples of the application of biomedical measures to smaller, community populations [26].

Intermediate between biomedical measures and sociomedical measures are measures of functional physical capacity necessary to carry out what have been called 'activities of daily living': bathing, dressing, toileting, feeding, walking. Such measures, which are usefully applied to evaluating the effectiveness of medical intervention in cases of disabling chronic disease [24], could conceivably also be addressed to general populations. The periodic reports of the U.S. National Health Interview Survey on 'limitation of activity' [34] by reason of illness constitute perhaps the best single example of an application of this notion of functional physical capacity on a national and continuing basis.

The principal advantages of the concept of 'limitation of activity' are that persons can be characterized in degree, not merely as to presence or absence (as with death of disease); and that the number of useful dimensions can be kept to a few for purposes of national data and need not be proliferated in the fine detail which might be needed for individual assessment and care. Furthermore, it is possible to collect such data reasonably reliably from large populations by means of household sample interview surveys.

An alleged disadvantage [45] of the U.S. National Health Interview Survey procedure is its reliance on self-report in a household interview. It is clear that such reports of functional disability do not necessarily reflect physical disablement. The significance of tests of physical movements in assessing physical impairment has recently been investigated in Great Britain [23]. The relationship between physical impairment and dependency has also been extensively explored in that country [20]. These studies empirically demonstrate the conceptual distinction between physical impairment and social dependency. While these two variables are related, they are two indicative dimensions and one cannot be used to predict the other.

Attempts to break out of the conceptual straitjacket of biomedical indicators of health are beginning to be made. A direct stimulus for this new effort is dissatisfaction with the limitations of death rates for describing the health status of populations. An indirect stimulus, but nevertheless a pervasive one, is what has been identified as the 'social indicator movement' [41]. Social indicators refer to indicators of societal well-being generally; sociomedical health indicators constitute a subset of social indicators.

Sociomedical health measures imply an assessment of a valetudinarian individual's condition in relation to others. Measures of social disability are perhaps the best example. The inability to perform in a social role as worker or student, or as spouse or parent, as a consequence of illness or disease is a sociomedical measure of the level of health. The U.S. National Health Interview Survey approaches this concept in its definition of disability as inability to carry out 'usual activities' [34], leaving the burden of defining 'usual activities' to the respondent – worker, student, retiree or housewife. The use of social disability as a measure of health level of a national population has been extensively elaborated by Daniel Sullivan [42, 43] of the U.S. National Center for Health Statistics. Social disability has been suggested as the least common denominator not only for physical illness, but for mental and psychological illness as well [16, 19]. Of course, social role performance is often dependent upon many other variables besides health. Some investigators are attempting to go beyond pure measures of functional capacity and activities of daily living, but still avoid the complexity of social role performance.

Among sociomedical health indicators, in addition to social disability measures, for which operational definitions are being attempted are: typologies of presenting symptoms; behavioral expressions of sickness; appraisals of the quality of life, so-called positive mental health, and, indeed, of happiness; and professional and lay assessments of unmet needs for health care.

A leading epidemiologist [12] has claimed that "...a large proportion of ambulatory patients (perhaps as high as 60 percent) never receive an orthodox diagnosis". He further states that "...there is increasing awareness that for many patients the labels developed in textbooks of medicine just do not fit the clusters of complaints seen in ambulatory care situations", and that "...a new classificatory system needs to be developed... (which) would be based upon the clusters of presenting symptoms and complaints and ideally should include the patient's perception of these". The international Classification of Diseases is oriented toward inhospital morbidity data and is overly specific for ambulatory cases [30]. Among efforts to create a typology of symptoms, for example, are those described by Argentinian sociomedical scientists who used two dimensions only: seriousness of symptoms and prognosis, with three degrees of each dimension, such that all conditions with which patients present themselves for health care may be classified in a nine-fold typology [39]. A practical application to which this typology has been put was to estimate the probable needs or demands for care for a defined population. Furthermore, by adding a third dimension of probable need/demand for health care a tridimensional typology of disease was created.

One of the more ambitious efforts to develop sociomedical measures which may be more sensitive to health care intervention is the 'Sickness Impact Profile' [5]. This is a comprehensive and systematic attempt to translate or depict all illness in behavioral terms. 'Sickness Impact Profile' is an attempt to develop a measure based on behavioral expressions of sickness to evaluate the effects of ambulatory programs, by focusing not on disease, a professionally defined entity, but on sickness (a state which is perceived by the sick person and often by nearly anyone else because it is manifested behaviorally in observable aspects of behavioral functioning). In this profile, 14 categories of behavioral items were developed:

Social interaction (other than family);
locomotion;
sleeping and resting;
eating;
work around the house;
work outside the house (occupation);
travel and confinement (mobility);
body movement;
speech and communication;
hobbies and recreation;
mental activity (mentation);
family relations ('persons with whom I live');
feeling-state items;
dressing and toileting.

We have also the efforts to design indicators of positive mental health and quality of life. Traditionally, mentally ill individuals who are in treatment have been categorized with respect to: psychoses, psychosomatic disorders, mental retardation and deviant behaviour. The measures used as indicators of mental illness have been: biochemical assessments, genetic characteristics, behavioral syndromes, psycho-physiologic items, utilization of mental illness facilities (i.e., psychiatrists, mental hospitals) and role-functional capacities [8]. There has been much debate with respect to the degree to which it is possible to classify a person as mentally ill without reference to the behavioural norms of his community. Nevertheless these are all negative measures of mental health.

In opposition to the clinical psychiatric notion that the absence of mental illness is coincident with mental health [3], the sociologist Marie Jahoda [22] issued a call in 1958 for research on concepts of positive mental health and provided a classification of mental health concepts which included such terms as: attitudes toward the self, including a sense of identity; self-actualization; resistance to stress; autonomy; empathy; environmental mastery, including adequacy in interpersonal relationships, adequacy in love, work and play, and problem solving. The challenge of operationally defining 'positive mental health' and applying measures of it to general populations was taken up by Bradburn [6, 7]; and application to large populations in different cultures has proven feasible [31]. Such efforts to do 'happiness research' have customarily been denigrated in the past, but more recently such august bodies as the U.S. National Research Council have sponsored large scale serious efforts [10] to measure the quality of life.

In a report being delivered this same week at the annual meeting of the American Sociological Association in New York City results from several national surveys on measures of perceived life quality are being presented [2]. About thirty different measures of a person's sense of overall life quality are described. Included in the quality of life measures are affective perceptions of family life, money, fun, housing, recreation, housework, health, schools, neighborhood, weather, friends, job, getting along with people, and so on.

Objection may be raised that such measures of positive mental health and perceived quality of life are too subjective. At the other end of a continuum we find perhaps the most objective measures in the field of dental health. Dental disorders are usually chronic, but are not usually dysfunctional. In this field the same measure frequently has the virtue of being not only a measure of a condition, but also a measure of treatment provided. For example, the decayed-missing-filled index is used as an additive measure of caries; and is not only a measure of disease condition but is also a measure of met and unmet needs, or of treatment provided. Currently measures of oral health status are being applied internationally in a W.H.O. study in Australia, New Zealand, Bulgaria, Federal Republic of Germany, Japan and Norway. The study will attempt to provide objective data on the relation of various structural features of health systems to national needs [15].

The indicator pie may also be sliced by introducing special sets of indicators which are age-group relevant. Just as it is common biostatistical practice to age-standardize populations when making comparisons in mortality or to refer to age-specific death rates for diseases, the notion of indicators for living populations differentiated as to age-group seems reasonable. For example indicators of health status and functioning have been developed for older people with chronic disease [25]. Similarly, appropriate methods of assessing adolescent health status are being explored [9].

Perhaps one of the most important ways of looking at the purposes of sociomedical health measures is to indicate the extent to which medical knowledge is being applied in a given society or to a specified population. This approach directs attention away from the biological aspects of disease in a population and toward the discharge of social responsibility for the organization and delivery of health care. Thus it is possible for the prevalence of disease to vary independently from the provision of care. It can be argued that the provision of care when needed is more easily recognized as a social responsibility in populations that have achieved the prevention of preventable diseases and that have arrived at the stage where the prevalence of disease is largely of the currently unpreventable variety. Whether needed care is being provided becomes then the measure not so much of the health of a population, but rather the assessment of social capacity to care for the sick. Thus it is possible to state what proportion in a given population are receiving needed care; and populations can be compared as to degree of neglect. Needed care of course is a reflection of the state of medical knowledge at any given point in time. Paradoxically as medical knowledge advances, recognized needs for care may concomitantly become greater. Nevertheless whether knowledge is being applied can be determined for individuals and for collections of individuals or large populations by means of sampling [11, 44].

Some economists object to the concept of 'needs for care' on the ground that 'needs' are either undefinable or infinite, or both. What will be regarded as needs is a function of both objective conditions and social values.

The usage made here of the term 'Sociomedical Health Indicators' is consciously value-laden. Values are imposed by a total society or any of its segments. Some investigators may prefer another use of the term 'indicators' as a quantitative expression of any social variable without value connotations. Such value-less usage has its place in sociological analysis or description, but is *not* intended here.

In the field of health the question of values is so implicit that it almost never arises. The term 'health' itself has value connotations; as do 'disease', 'disability', and even 'discomfort'. An approach which appears to escape the onus of valuation is based on a proposed application of psychometrics [14]. In this concept, health is regarded as relative to a group context rather than as an absolute condition. [1] The value-loadings of various indicators are not known quantitatively; undoubtedly they vary within and between societies. This is a subject for future empirical research [37, 38].

We are in agreement with the notion that as soon as one addresses oneself to social indicators, one is talking about a redistribution of power [4]. Interest groups are served by the indicators that are put forth. Indicators, in the sense that we use the term, are clearly policy-oriented.

A clear example (in the United States) of the socio-political consequences of a health status index may be seen from a brief historical review of infant mortality statistics [40]. Infant mortality data justified the founding of the U.S. Children's Bureau (1912), focused the attention of physicians on prenatal care, and led to a concentration of maternity care in hospitals. Although many other health problems could have been candidates for concentrated activities, at the turn of the century care of infants was given priority because infant mortality was so high.

Infant mortality statistics have served not only as an index of a nation's health status, but more importantly as a mobilizing agent for research and for expansion of legislative and other activities.

Current sociopolitical pressures (in the U.S.) revolve more about economic issues (concern with the delivery of health services), and about organizational issues (concern with making health services more responsive to health care needs), and only secondarily with the issue of raising the level of health of the population. Current concerns in the U.S. are about the role of hospitals in health maintenance activities, e.g., in more effective use of manpower, changes in technical services and in types of personnel and in more effective organization of medical records. Current goals are to lower or contain costs of health care and to distribute health care more equitably. One of the more interesting sociopolitical issues is a concern with methods of assuring the quality of health care. 'Professional Service Review Organizations' have been proposed as one such method. It is argued that criteria developed by the medical profession are likely to add to the costs of medical care and to protect the provider rather than the consumer of medical care. The focus of such measures is on process rather than outcome of medical care since it is easier to measure and change process than to affect outcome.

Despite what seems obvious policy implications of health indicators a recent inquiry [18] among hospital administrators, public health planners and legislators revealed a marked unconcern in such measures. Hospital administrators appear to be quite uninterested in health status indicators: the organizational goals of hospitals are to provide hospital services efficiently without regard to their effect on the health status of the community. At best, hospital administrators might be concerned with 'case treated' indicators rather than with the health status of populations, geographically defined. Some health planners are looking for a single overall national health index, analogous to the Consumer Price Index. Legislators, and other policy makers, on the other hand, show more interest in the evaluation of specific health programs than in indices of the health of the general population. Who, then, cares about health indicators? Global thinkers; top policy makers, occasionally; monopolistic trade unions such as the American Medical Association, who when a national health indicator goes up or down feels a reflection on their self-image; and social reformers who would like to influence health policy.

The role of social scientists in the development of indicators is reflected in the recent establishment of a Center for Coordination of Research on Social Indicators, the Social Science Research Council, and funded by the National Science Foundation [36]. The U.S. Government has established a Clearinghouse for Health Indices as a responsibility of the National Center for Health Statistics [28]. The United Nations System of Demographic Manpower and Social Statistics is asking member nations to participate in the collection of data over nine subsystems, among which are health, population, income, education, crime, social mobility, etc.

We believe it is important to recognize that the development and application of sociomedical health indicators, and social indicators generally, since they represent operationally defined and measurable expressions of social goals must inevitably exert some influence on social policy and social action. To measure is to point the way to policy. It is also worthy of note that especially as the level of education of the general population rises, popular conceptions of health more and more will join with the professional and be reflected in sociomedical measures as well as biomedical. A prominent health policy maker [46] in the United States has proposed a theory that the medical care system is anxiety-motivated, and that he is therefore not interested in measuring the health of population groups in terms of mortality or disability, but in terms of satisfaction. As philosophers have pointed out:" ...one thing (a person) knows better than anyone else in where the shoe pinches his own foot".

BIBLIOGRAPHY

[1] C. A. Akpom, S. Katz and P. M. Densen, 'Methods of Classifying Disability and Severity of Illness in Ambulatory Care Patients', *Medical Care* **11**, No. 2. Supplement (1973) 125–131.

[2] F. M. Andrews and S. B. Withey, 'Developing Measures of Perceived Life Quality: Results from Several National Surveys', for presentation to the Annual Convention of the American Sociological Association, New York City, August 1973 (mimeographed).

[3] W. E. Barton, 'Viewpoint of a Clinician', in: M. Jahoda (ed.), *Current Concepts of Positive Mental Health*, Basic Books, New York 1958.

[4] R. Bauer, (ed.), *Social Indicators*, MIT Press, Cambridge 1966.
[5] M. Bergner, presentation before Seminar on Sociomedical Health Indicators, Columbia University, April 13, 1973, on the Sickness Impact Profile being developed at the University of Washington, Department of Health Services, in cooperation with the Group Health Cooperative of Puget Sound.
[6] N. M. Bradburn and D. Caplovitz, *Reports on Happiness: A Pilot Study of Behavior Related to Mental Health*, Aldine, Chicago 1965.
[7] N. Bradburn, *The Structure of Psychological Well-Being*, Aldine, Chicago 1969.
[8] M. Braren, presentation before Seminar on Sociomedical Health Indicators, Columbia University, May 11, 1973.
[9] A. F. Brunswick and E. Josephson, 'Adolescent Health in Harlem', *American Journal of Public Health*, Supplement, October 1972.
[10] A. Campbell, 'Aspiration, Satisfaction, and Fulfillment', in: A. Campbell and P. Converse (eds.), *The Human Meaning of Social Change*, Russell Sage Foundation, New York 1972.
[11] W. Carr, presentation before Seminar on Sociomedical Health Indicators, Columbia University, March 9, 1973, on the Meharry Studies of Unmet Needs for Health Care and Services (Nashville), Samuel Wolfe, Principal Investigator.
[12] J. C. Cassell, 'Information for Epidemiologic and Health Services Research', *Medical Care* **11**, No. 2, Supplement (1973) 76–80.
[13] H. C. Chase, 'The Position of the United States in International Comparisons of Health Status', *American Journal of Public Health* **62** (1972) 581–589.
[14] Martin Chen, presentation before Seminar on Sociomedical Health Indicators, Columbia University, March 23, 1973.
[15] L. K. Cohen, presentation before Seminar on Sociomedical Health Indicators, Columbia University, March 16, 1973.
[16] J. Elinson, 'Base Lines for Assessing Change', in: L. C. Kolb, V. W. Bernard and B. P. Dohrenwend (eds.), *Urban Challenges to Psychiatry*, Little, Brown, Boston 1969.
[17] J. Elinson, 'Methods of Sociomedical Research', in: H. E. Freeman, S. Levine and L. G. Reeder (eds.), *Handbook of Medical Sociology*, Prentice-Hall, Englewood Cliffs, N. J. 1972.
[18] S. B. Goldsmith, presentation before Seminar on Sociomedical Health Indicators, Columbia University, February 2, 1973.
[19] E. M. Gruenberg, 'The Social Breakdown Syndrome – Some Origins', *American Journal of Psychiatry* **123** (1967), 1481–1489.
[20] A. Harris, *Handicapped and Impaired in Great Britain*, Her Majesty's Stationary Office, London 1971.
[21] *International Classification of Diseases*, Adapted for use in the United States, Eighth Revision, U.S. Department of Health, Education and Welfare, Public Health Service Publication No. 1693, Washington.
[22] M. Jahoda, *Current Concepts of Positive Mental Health*, Basic Books, New York, 1958.

[23] M. Jeffreys, J. B. Millard, M. Hyman *et. al.*, 'A Set of Tests for Measuring Motor Impairment in Prevalence Studies', *Journal of Chronic Diseases* **22** (1969) 303–319.

[24] S. Katz, A. B. Ford, T. D. Downs and M. Adams, 'Chronic-Disease Classification in Evaluation of Medical Care Programs', *Medical Care* **7** (1969) 139.

[25] S. Katz, A. B. Ford, R. W. Moskowitz, B. A. Jackson and M. A. Jaffe, 'Studies of Illness in the Aged: The Index of ADL, a Standardized Measure of Biological and Psychosocial Function', *Journal of the American Medical Association* **185** (1963) 914–919.

[26] I. I. Kessler and M. L. Levin (eds.), *The Community as an Epidemiologic Laboratory, A Casebook of Community Studies*, The Johns Hopkins Press, Baltimore 1970.

[27] D. M. Kessner, J. Singer, C. E. Kalk *et al.*, *Infant Death: An Analysis by Matternal Risk and Health Care*, National Academy of Sciences Printing and Publishing Office, Washington 1973.

[28] D. Krueger, presentation before Seminar on Sociomedical Health Indicators, Columbia University, March 2, 1973.

[29] M. Lerner and O. W. Anderson, *Health Progress in the United States, 1900–1960*, University of Chicago Press, Chicago 1963.

[30] A. H. MacFarlane and G. R. Norman, 'Methods for Classifying Symptoms, Complaints, and Conditions', *Medical Care* **11**, No. 2, Supplement (1973) 101–108.

[31] N. Matlin, 'The Demography of Happiness', Puerto Rico, Master Sample Survey of Health and Welfare, Series 2, No. 3, Department of Health, Commonwealth of Puerto Rico, San Juan, December, 1966.

[32] 'Measurement of Levels of Health', Technical Reports Series **137**, World Health Organization, Geneva 1957.

[33] I. M. Moriyama, 'Problems in the Measurement of Health Status', in: E. B. Sheldon and W. E. Moore (eds.), *Indicators of Social Change: Concepts and Measurements*, Russell Sage Foundation, New York 1968.

[34] National Center for Health Statistics, 'Health Survey Procedures: Concepts, Questionnaire Development and Definitions in the Health Interview Survey', Publication No. 1000, Series 10, No. 25, Public Health Service, Washington, May, 1964.

[35] National Center for Health Statistics, 'Plan and Initial Program of the Health Examination Survey', Publication No. 1000, Series I, No. 4, Public Health Service, Washington, July, 1965.

[36] R. Parke and N. Zill, presentation before Seminar on Sociomedical Health Indicators, Columbia University, May 4, 1973. See *Social Indicators Newsletter* **1**, No. 1 (1973).

[37] D. Patrick, *Measuring Social Preference for Function Levels of Health Status*, doctoral dissertation in sociomedical sciences, Columbia University, 1972.

[38] D. L. Patrick, J. W. Bush and M. M. Chen, 'Toward an Operational Definition of Health', *Journal of Health and Social Behaviour* **14** (1973) 6–23.

[39] J. Segovia and H. Goglio, 'La Variable Enfermedad en el Estudio de la Demanda de Servicios Medicos', *Medicina Administrativa* **2**, No. 4 (Buenos Aires 1968).
[40] S. Shapiro, presentation before Seminar on Sociomedical Health Indicators, Columbia University, February 9, 1973, on Sociopolitical Pressures for a Health Status Index.
[41] E. B. Sheldon and H. E. Freeman, 'Notes on Social Indicators: Promises and Potential', *Policy Sciences* **I** (1970).
[42] D. F. Sullivan, 'Conceptual Problems in Developing an Index of Health', National Center for Health Statistics, *Vital and Health Statistics*, Series 2, No. **17**, Public Health Service, Washington, May, 1966.
[43] D. F. Sullivan, 'Disability Components for an Index of Health', National Center for Health Statistics, *Vital and Health Statistics*, Series 2, No. **42**, Public Health Service, Washington, July, 1971.
[44] R. E. Trussell and J. Elinson, *Chronic Illness in a Rural Area: The Hunterdon Study*, Harvard University Press, Cambridge 1959.
[45] U. S. National Health Survey, 'Health Interview Responses Compared with Medical Records', Public Health Service Publication No. 584-05, Public Health Service, Washington 1961.
[46] Vernon Wilson, Health Services and Mental Health Administration, from statement made at a Washington conference attended by health policy makers.

REFERENCES

[1] In this approach health dimensions are identified, e.g., blood pressure, and then individuals are rank ordered with respect to each dimension according to their deviation from a norm. The norm need *not* be a statistical norm, e.g., arithmetic mean, but any predetermined quantitative range. This range may be determined subjectively by physicians' judgement or objectively by finding the relation between measured dimensions of health and mortality for specific groups – much in the way that tables of ideal body weight were developed as they related to mortality. Once the 'ideal norm' for each health dimension has been located, one can: (a) find individual deviations from the norm, positive or negative (adding a constant to all distances to get rid of the negative scores); (b) appropriately weight those deviations which represent a greater threat to health than others, if this occurs; and (c) compute new deviation scores, based on a distance scale. The measures then become commensurate for various dimensions, which can then be weighted or not as desired, according to the risk represented by deviations along each dimension. It is then possible to sum the variances of a number of single measures, whether related or independent (if the measures are correlated, then that factor must be included in judging the total variability), having converted them into standard scores, and so to arrive at a composite index of positive health.

A SOCIAL SCIENCE BASIS FOR CONCEPTUALIZING FAMILY HEALTH*

HANS O. MAUKSCH**

University of Missouri, Columbia, Missouri, U.S.A.

The increasing prevalence of emerging programs in family health care and the growing popularity of family medicine as an area of commitment for physicians in the United States invites a careful look at the nature of this new area of specialization and at the assumptions which are implied by this development. A brief look at the background of family medicine and a juxtaposition of the medical model and a construct of the family will suggest that the acceptance of the family as a target for health evaluation and health care requires serious reassessment of traditional practices.

The development of modern medicine is linked to the advances in the biological sciences achieved largely during this century. Fundamentally, the biological sciences have enabled the physician to acquire an impressive understanding of intra-organismic processes and structures. These laboratory advances have been associated with the fascination with smaller and smaller units of analysis. They have helped medicine to move from the organism to the organ, from the organ to the cell, and from the cell to molecular properties. Thus scientific medicine has achieved success and acquired new capabilities at near exponential proportions. The understanding of illness processes and the capacity of countering them has given rise to a huge body of knowledge. This has caused an increasingly fine division of expertise and fostered the proliferation of intra-professional specialty groups. Recently, significant movements have occurred, essentially representing a counterforce to the direction which medical science has taken during the last fifty years. Some of these developments are linked to a recognition of the complexity inherent in the translation of medical science into effective delivery of patient care [42]. Other voices have called attention to accessibility and availability of care, while others have raised the issue that health fundamentally rests within processes of the community and of society [28]. All of these trends represent a change from preoccupation with disease and a move towards an inclusion of health as proper concern of medicine and of the health professions [12].

Although some of the voices calling for change have come from outside the health field, it is important for the development of this paper to emphasize that significant pressure for new directions in medicine has come from within the profession [44]. Some of these developments focus on new approaches to the care of patients. The notions of 'primary care', 'comprehensive care', or 'continuing care' all represent modifications in the application of medical science and the inclusion of patient oriented factors into the practice of medicine. Two of these developments have taken the path of suggesting new areas of specialization and thus have laid the ground work for distinct domains of expertise, of knowledge, and of practice. The emergence of Community Medicine and of Family Medicine are significant in that their field of specialization is neither an organ system or a disease syndrome but rather in both instances, a designation of social categories.

Obviously, other categories of medicine have existed which were not oriented to disease categories. Public Health, Preventive Medicine and Epidemiology have been on the scene for a long time. Social Medicine has been primarily a European speciality with varying meanings attached to the label. Nevertheless, the aforementioned developments represent a more forceful bid for expanding the concept of medicine.

The emergence of family medicine is symptomatic of a complex sense of discomfort within the health professions and by the public at large regarding the depersonalization and episodal discontinuity associated with the scientific advances of clinical medicine. As suggested above, family medicine is associated with an almost cyclical rediscovery of the human, social, and cultural aspects of health and illness and also with a growing sense of concern about the gap between medical capabilities and the ultimate effectiveness of medical intervention.

In some quarters, family medicine has served as a synonym for 'primary care' and, frequently, for general practice. In the eyes of a large segment of the medical profession the activities of the general practitioner are thought to be synonimous with family practice. Another trend, particularly in Internal Medicine and in Pediatrics, has claimed the term Family Practice as mantle for those who emphasize patient care and health maintenance and who seek a respectable alternative to the research laboratory. Then there are those who indeed seek a new concept and who are groping towards an innovative mode of using the family as a focal point for health care. Thus, Family Medicine as a label on the current medical scene combines those who are genuine innovators, those who seek to counteract the laboratory emphasis of the academic medical center, those who respond to the whims of fashion, and those who want to give new status to General Practice with the aid of a new name.

This paper is stimulated by the emergence of family medicine. It seeks to link the emphasis on family-oriented health care with a conceptually innovative framework capable of fostering scientific inquiry, a body of unique expertise, a new mode of delivering health services. This paper seeks to suggest an approach to a rigorous basis for family medicine. The point of departure for such a basis must be an examination of the family itself.

A vast amount of work on the family has been accumulated in sociology and in anthropology. Concern with the family can also be found traditionally in the literature of psychology [2] and psychiatry [17, 34, 49]. This paper, obviously, will be based heavily on the concepts of sociology even though an attempt will be made to argue for an approach which is not confined to any of the traditional disciplines. On the contrary, one major contention of this paper is that an adequate model of the family cannot be confined to the consequences of social processes, but must include consideration of the biological implications of the continuing coexistence of several organisms with different organismic properties.

It is interesting to note that even in the examination of sociological scholarship the criticism has been made that a majority of the contributions to this literature deal primarily with the individuals in the family rather than with the family itself [46]. The traditional approaches in the sociological literature define the family as a network of interacting personalities and roles, as structural arrangements of positions, as status networks or as institutions representing the performance of cultural tasks [41, 24, 23, 6]. While all of these approaches are valid and contribute to certain important perspectives, an examination of the properties of the family itself is less frequently seen. The influence of systems theory has probably stimulated most of the attempts to achieve systematic understanding of the family itself [8].

The development of a family model requires a definition of the family. The traditional concept of the procreational unit, including mother, father, and one or more offsprings may still be numerically the prototype of the family. Yet, an inquiry into a primary human unit cannot confine itself to this definition but must look for more generic properties [45]. Although this paper will continue to use the term 'family', the questions to be raised must be tested against the most basic conditions of human grouping. One of these is obviously the coexistence of more than one human being involving continuous, presumably permanent sharing of living facilities [4]. A perception of reciprocal obligations, a sense of commonness and sharing of certain obligations toward each other and towards others are suggested as other criteria. One of the key questions to be raised in a definition of the unit to which our model applies is the nature of the sense of unity and of the network of obligations. While it is clear that a husband and a wife are *a priori* subsumed under this model, there may not be normative consensus whether two members of the same sex linked through homosexual attachment and living together, would fit. How about two friends who, without the involvement of sexual relationships, share a home for a long period of time? Moving from co-generational to cross-generational examples we can travel from the traditional home with two parents and any number of children to the single parent with young children, to the home consisting of an adult living with one of the parents. There are other cross-generational possibilities.

The term family is a culturally sanctioned label suggesting normative as well as possible scientific properties. A point of scientific departure might be to raise the question about the conditions under which the coexistence of individuals and the development of interpersonal and psychologically and culturally meaningful relationships give rise to processes and consequences which cannot be adequately explained within the framework of the participaitng individuals. From the point of view of health and health care this approach permits the raising of fundamental questions about the response of the organism to its involvement with other organisms. While the network of interaction of role, personality, and status are the major concepts used in the social linking of the members of a human unit, there are few concepts which express the linkage of physical coexistence of biological organisms. In order to explicate this point of view certain assumptions have to be made about the components of the social unit which we have called 'the family.' These assumptions will be sellped out in the following paragraphs.

This basic human unit consists of two major components: the unit members and the 'linking processes'. The unit members are schematically suggested to have several simultaneous identities. Every member of a family unit is an individual, subject to investigation and understanding within the framework of individual analysis: biologically, psychologically, or socially. Every member of a family unit is a participant in various relevant social systems and social categories and participates in the definitions and behaviors appropriate to those social categories. The perspectives of individual characteristics and of social categories are richly represented in the literature of the appropriate disciplines. Thirdly, however, a family member functions as a component of the family unit itself, infusing into the family system the biological, psychological, social and cultural properties of his other two identities. What is suggested here may be obvious on the surface only. There may be several individuals with identical patterns of blood pressure, circadian rhythms, intelligence quotients, assertiveness, body weight and other individual properties. These indentical individuals cease to be identical when evaluated as members of their respective families with w'dely differing companions. The individual data emerge as interactive forces with the properties of these other members and thus differ in, in fact, meaning and behavior. In the unit perspective these properties take on system meanings, modified by the properties of the other members [29, 22, 55, 21]. Similarly, social and cultural characteristics such as values, skills and role performances which may adequately describe a person in his various social settings do not necessarily predict the intra-family processes in which this person functions as a unit member.

It is suggested that individual properties take on different analytic and predictive characteristics when examined within the unit perspective and when seen as infusion into the system rather than as primarily individual definitions. Although these three perspectives on the individual are abstractions they are conceptually meaningful and are essential to a proper conceptualization of the family. This suggested pluralistic view of the unit members also obviates the frequently asked question whether the family is an open or a closed system. Through the pluralistic view of the individual we can simultaneously accommodate a view of the family unit as being defined by boundaries as well as seeing it in continuing interaction with social processes.

A second major assumption about the individual needs to be spelled out. In order to achieve a fully adequate framework for studying the family unit, distinctions between the biological and the social processes need to be obviated. The literature abounds with protestations of the unity of the human organism [9, 14, 25]. Research in this area has been primarily in the field of psychosomatic medicine and, therefore, has been largely illness oriented [43]. Yet, an observation of the day-to-day realities in professional as well as in public situations belies this unity and testifies to the fact that the duality of mind and body is still the core of our usual behavior [3]. In order to provide an adequate framework for coexisting members of a family unit, it is essential that the following assumption be made and tested: within the individual member there is a unity of life processes and social, psychological, physiological, and biochemical processes are interrelated, interdependent and frequently merely different facets of the same phenomenon. Changes in adrenal functions, body weight, fluid balance, fatigue reduction, or vascular functions may have as corollaries changes in moods, attitudes, behaviors and relationships.

The area in which we have come closest to a unitary concept of human behavior is sexuality. But even here the comprehensiveness of the literature is spotty. Although there are data on the social, psychological and biological unity of sexual intercourse, the sensations of love, affections, and attraction has not yet been adequately examined for their biological basis. The threshold of sexual arousal is known to be subject to symbolic, behavioral interpersonal, physical, and physiological stimuli [35, 17, 36]. Yet except for some animal research [39], this obvious example of the unity of the organism has rarely been approached from a framework which cuts across the convenience of traditional academic disciplines.

The unit member is seen, therefore, as a component of the family unit who infuses into the family process idiosyncratic and societal factors. The unit member also is characterized by the integrity of the organism which denies the separation of social and biological processes although they are frequently manifested separately and are subject to either discrete or unified analysis.

This sets the stage for describing the linking processes as being all those emissions and infusions which occur among the unit members. This definition includes, obviously, the traditionally noted network of social relationships ranging from adaptations between personalities to implementations of socially defined divisions of labor. It includes modes of relating and the emergence of meaning in verbal and in other forms of communications [19]. It also includes heretofore not adequately researched intra-organismic adaptations. Are there differences in the response of human organism to sharing a bed in close physical proximity during sleep? How do such differences, if they occur, affect the biological function of sleep, the relationship of the individuals and the nature of health of the participants? How do the interactions of biological rhythms of unit members affect these members, their relationships and their health maintaining processes [33]?

Postulating these linking processes without specifying substantive categories permits us to raise certain generic questions about the very process which we identify as the family unit. Whether these linking processes are biological or social, whether they involve the interchange of the husband-wife role dyad, or the adaptation of differing fatigue cycles, certain common questions can be asked. Do the linking processes emitted from the unit members match and fit, do they compete and conflict? Are they imposed by some members on others or is there learning, adaptation, or compromise? Is there a degree of modification of individual or societal properties required for a unit member to sustain any of the linking processes? Linking processes may be stress creating or stress reducing; they may be pleasurable or they may be characterized by discomfort. Of the total range of linking processes one can postulate that there are some which enhance the family unit while others represent a negative linking property. Some linking processes may be positively functional by creating linkage through agreement, consensus and adaptive fit. Positive linkage may, however, be identified with conflict; conflict being possibly a bonding mechanism [51, 18].

The linking mechanism may be primarily in the social sphere or may be fundamentally biological. However, one of the avenues of research which needs to be explored is the likelihood that linking may cut across the traditional analytic categories. Clinically, and anecdotally there is ample material to suggest further inquiry. Changes in relationships related to changes in health status have been amply documented [27, 40, 10]. Personality changes may not be associated only with one's own biological condition but may occur, at least selectively, in response to changes within the biological makeup of another unit member.

It is worth noting that this essay suggests a framework for investigation and for the development of a model which would organize a body of knowledge. However, this effort is so rudimentary that the very assumptions used here to suggest the direction of research should be first subject to test and to validation. It not only seeks to avoid an *a priori* definition of the family but it also seeks to avoid the inclusion of normative judgments. In its simplest terms, it says that when individuals coexist under certain conditions certain processes will occur on various levels which may either enhance or diminish the unity and identity of this family unit. Just as this model avoids the question of good and bad, it seeks to avoid an existing set of assumptions about health and illness. The health of the unit and the health of the individual are assumed to be interdependent [37]. However, these two foci of health may not be synonymous. Whether a smoothly functioning family unit is truly healthy or whether the involved subjugation of one family member to unit cohesion is, indeed, pathology must be a question to be investigated scientifically as well as philosophically. Whether a father's ulcer, a son's trip on drugs, a daughter's obesity, or a mother's neurosis may be indeed separate phenomena or represent different manifestations of the same problem in the family unit is also open to question [53].

Having made an attempt to develop a concept which encompasses the family as an entity distinct from its component individuals we can now proceed to examine the ramifications which this construct has for health. First of all, there is the implication that in a unit forming network any dysfunction which affects any component of that unit may and frequently will in some ways affect the entire unit. This can be observed as changes in the component members or as alterations of the processes which link the unit members within the system. Carrying this thought somewhat further, we can distinguish between the health of the 'family' as a functioning unit and the health of the components who, as sociobiological organisms have individual health statuses and are subject to individual illness risks. Within this framework the absence of health may be illness in the traditional organismic sense [37]. It also may involve pathology of the linkages, although observable as disease manifestations in the individual members. Health threats may also involve a breakdown of the linkages such as seen in family disorganization, loss of affection, interpersonal conflict, status differentiation or other forms of dissonance or discord.

If one conceptualizes illness as representing a form of 'breaking down', one can establish a comparative analytic framework which permits the establishment of criteria to evaluate these factors which may cause, facilitate, hinder, or prevent the breaking down process, be it microbial invasion, diseases of stress, marital discord, incompatability of roles, headaches, or starvation. It may seem far fetched but even resistance to infection can be examined within the total network of family patterns, habits, and maintenance and meaning of individual health just as we look at the family for factors affecting drug addiction, criminal behavior, emotional crises, or breakdown of intra-family communications [38]. The involvement of social factors in infectious disease is clearly implied in Lerner and Anderson [31]. We know that the same threatening forces, whether microorganisms, social temptations, stress or hunger do not necessarily have the same effect on every organism. Yet, we have thus far, by and large, sought the causes for resistance or vulnerability within the individual rather than within the social network. This is particularly true of somatic disease. In the so-called social problems, psychiatrists, psychologists, and social scientists have called attention to family influences. From the point of view of family health care, however, it is important to establish this frame of reference as basic and as a supplement or alternative to predominantly single-organism focus.

This approach provides the opportunity of developing a data base and a set of perspectives which would permit an expanded evaluation and, hopefully, more effective intervention in the natural career of health processes which characterize the role of health and illness in family life. Thus, the family as it is established includes the development of health values, health habits, and health risk perceptions as an integral part of the emerging family network through the characteristics of the family founding individuals. This includes the biological and emotional strengths and vulnerabilities as well as the cultural and subcultural norms, values, and habits which they bring into the system. The main argument of this essay is that the resulting pattern is not merely additive of individual characteristics or a mirror of the larger culture, but that, in a profound and scientifically researchable sense, the unit itself represents a health relevant commodity which is unique and distinct from its contributing cultural, social, and biological components.

Every family has its own 'health estate' [52]. This health estate is the syncretic product of all of the forces which the family members contribute within the context of their culture, their awareness of health relevant knowledge, and their unique individual ways of introducing these factors into the emerging family. The family health estate incorporates those objective conditions which can be assessed by observation or examination of the individuals' blood pressure, vital capacity, and various laboratory data. It includes the levels of physical conditioning, dietary and sanitary habits, and even the health consequences of such factors as the adequacy of the fit of the shoes that are worn. But it also includes the levels of conscious emphasis on these factors or behaviors, their importance and priority within the hierarchy of family health values. It includes the consideration whether the contents of the family health estate are consensual family property or whether all of it or some of it are issues of stress or intra-family discord. The family health estate involves behaviors, knowledges, attitudes and values, but it also involves role and task allocations within the family system. Do all share equally in the health agendas or do 'mothers' carry the burden? Do physicians and nurses reinforce segmental family health tasks by focusing on mother and omitting father? Family health care which approaches family health maintenance or illness care with stereotypical expectations of 'who does what' or 'what are priorities' may indeed fail in the long run although the patient's chart may show short run success [32].

The family health estate is an integral part of all of family life. The concept of a 'symbolic family estate' was developed by Farber. While Farber's work applies to knowledge of extended kin networks, the basic premises are applicable to health and illness related behavior [15]. This is an obvious assertion which should not be necessary. However, although the literature shows the correlation between the onset of certain individual diseases and crises in life style, these insights have not become internalized components of family health assessment. In an epistemological sense, the expansion of the notion of health from purely biological specimen to an integrated macro-organic framework changes the traditional self-contained boundaries of the concept of physical illness to an open system which demands that health and illness be viewed or, at least, be examined as part of a larger set of processes of which illness is but one ingredient.

This applies to the stages of health: (1) health attainment, (2) health maintenance, (3) disease prevention, (4) illness susceptibility, (5) illness management, (6) recuperation and reintegration, (7) illness consequences and (8) modification of the family health estate. These eight stages are not exhaustive. They subsume, for instance, health maximization, which is the much neglected effort to discover and pursue increased levels of health for family members and for the family itself. Also, permanent disability, chronic disease, and the amputation of a family component through death are subsumed under the above suggested eight stages.

Admittedly, there could be many questions and issues where the family framework will add nothing to the knowledge gained by the study of the individual organisms. It is suggested, however, that the absence of relevance be established rather than assumed. This applies to the question of accident proneness, to the etiology of ulcers, and to heart disease. It applies to migraine headaches and to the conditions under which infections and diseases are the response to microorganismic invasions. It also applies to the more obviously family based etiologies of obesity, dental neglect, food habits, and emotional disorders.

One area in which the concept of the family health estate may be particularly useful is in the evaluation of child rearing and in the establishment of a health framework and health goals in the process of growth and development. The family context of washing hands, of brushing teeth, the family meaning of the dinner table, of desserts, of getting injections, of sports, all represent modes by which a child learns health as a state and health as a process [26]. Health can be a conscious priority, it can be an aesthetic byproduct, it can be a prerequisite for the valued outdoor life. It can be simply an economic necessity or conversely it can be dysfunctional. Health is something that may be taken for granted or something that has to be maintained through conscious effort.

The diet which enhances sex appeal may resemble in calories the diet which seeks to maximize disease resistance and longevity, but the similarity ends there. Because every single health behavior is shared by family members as an integral part of the whole family world of meaning, the nutritionist or the physician had better be aware of the context of the diet rather than merely of its content. Effective assistance and care is as linked to meaning as it may be to substance. Thus, the concept of the family health estate serves as an organizing principle for knowledge not attainable by inquiring into the properties of the individual family member. It also serves as a conceptual bridge to the network of agendas which the family has to balance as its priorities and as effort demanding concerns.

In addition to judging the effectiveness of the illness oriented therapeutic prescriptions, the consequences of medical intervention on the entire family system must be evaluated. The physician who places a husband on a low calorie or a low sodium diet is affecting the family system. He may only view this diet as a modification of intra-organismic nutritional processes within that individual. If, in a traditional family, shopping, cooking, and serving is done by the wife, and if, thus, she becomes the operational guardian of the physician's intent, the delicate balance of the intra-family network of dominance, power, initiative, and claims has been altered. The physician has become a potential accomplice in shifting power to the wife or in facilitating the channeling of other labile intra-family issues into the negotiation between the wife as the implementor of the physician's prescription and the husband as the recipient of these meals. Food may have been successfully modified medically, but may range in its message to the recipient from conveying hostily to subjugation, from loss of love to castration.

Other examples of such phenomena can occasionally be found in the literature and they occur in the anecdotes of practitioners [2, 16]. To discharge a patient after recovery from a myocardial infarct without assessing the modifications in family structure and family process is like repairing the leg of a table without concern whether the table upon the reattachment of the leg will, in fact, be evenly balanced and sturdy [50]. The return into the family network of a family member who has been removed due to illness changes the person's participation in the family health estate and frequently requires serious professional assistance.

It does not matter whether those issues ought to be the concern of the physician, the nurse, the social worker, or any other member in the gallaxy of health functionaries. What does matter is that the family as a target of health care and as a conceptual autonomous unit requires professional perspectives which go far beyond the commonly observed approaches to problems and complaints.

As mentioned earlier, the family health estate is involved in a network of other task systems of the family. Thus, when a physician has a choice between two medications to be given to an eleven year old child, his deliberation should include not merely the pharmacological comparisons between these two drugs, but also other, appropriately evaluated factors. If one medication requires that it be taken every two hours and if the other one lends itself to a six hour interval, consideration should be given to its affecting the competition between the family health tasks and the stresses on the independence-seeking aspects of the socializing process; they will be strained less if a child is summoned less frequently.

An excellent example of the issues argued in this paper can be found in the study of those who are in the process of losing a family member through death. The working with the family and with the dying person requires not only an understanding of the processes by which human beings tend to grope with and cope with death and dying, but it also requires an assessment of the total family's perception of the consequences of death to what they perceive to be their family estate [13, 5]. The departing family member may deprive those who remain behind by taking the symbolic essence of their family into death, or this symbolic family concept is experienced to be a legacy which must be assumed by those who remain. This makes a great deal of difference in the aid and assistance given to those who die or to those who remain.

The number of examples that can be offered to illustrate the relevance of the family concept to the planning and implementing of care and cure are legion and range all the way from compliance with medication requirements [54] to the reintegration into the family of those who are handicapped [30]. The most challenging, although least studied area in which the family concept could be a significant addition to health care is in the tasks of health maintenance and health maximization. Except for very few and frequently quite esoteric investigations, very few questions have been raised about the health consequences of the arrangements which characterize the every day life of any family unit. There has been practically no research in the potentially significant question of the stress consequences of physical proximity between continuously associated organisms who more or less differ in biological rhythms, physical and psychological properties, and other idiosyncratic characteristics. Even the simple question of the conjugal bed has apparently not been subject to research except for the dramatic sexual moments. The much less dramatic relationship between the organism's tasks to be accomplished during sleep and the physical proximity of another organism deserves some attention [48]. At least on the anecdotal level, there is room for the hypothesis that not all people who sleep togethei rest equally well doing so. How much stress is incurred by the marital juncture of two people whose biological rhythms are seriously at odds; they impose consciously or unknowingly stresses on themselves in order to accommodate each other and in order to facilitate those other linkages required by the maintenance of a family unit. Does learning occur, supportive of health needs or are there cost bearing adjustments?

The approach proposed in this paper provides ways of expanding the range of proper targets for different types of health care services. It provides a basis upon which a group of physicians and other health professionals can build a claim for uniqueness of approach and for developing family health care as a domain of special expertise. This discussion offers an avenue of investigation and a vast new range of research problems within which a specialty can develop its own pursuits and accretion of knowledge.

Several comments about the implications of this suggestive direction need to be spelled out. For one, the significance of the social, cultural, and psychological segments which are part of the anatomy and physiology of the family unit require that the knowledge, practice, and research basis of family health care must incorporate the social sciences as major intellectual resource areas. However, let this point be misunderstood, this does not imply diminished concern with the biological spheres. On the contrary, the implications of this paper clearly require an innovative and integrative synthesis of the diverse disciplines needed to develop the investigative capabilities for answering the questions about the nature of linkages in human groups and about their relationships to the health and illness of the unit and of its component members.

The implications of this paper point to health and to illness as process and as the product of continuously interacting forces within the unit, among its members, and within each component participant. Therefore, this paper also calls for a departure from the 'cause and effect' model of illness. Illness, as a variant to health status must be sought within the framework of pluralistic interactions. Above all, however, the arguments offered in this paper argue that a total understanding of illness care within a family framework must consider traditional disease manifestations as one of several possible responses to stress or to disruption. Research into the process of illness must then include as a hypothesis the possibility of alternate manifestations, which may not lie within the medical sphere.

Ultimately, the position taken in these pages is based on the assertion that the most fundamental area of needed research is a broadly interdisciplinary approach to research in the maintenance, enhancement, and preconditioners of health itself. Family oriented research in the social sciences has, understandably, been much more prolific than the biological sciences which have been either disease oriented or have looked at the basic molecular processes in which they have achieved such notable success.

In a sense, the cognitive style with which the family health estate has to be conceptualized, understood, and influenced stems from the approach of sociology and from some of the other social sciences. The point of view developed here offers not only an additional and new approach to the health care system; it also is, hopefully, an invitation to additional approaches in family research. Because of the practical utilization of sociological theory in this field, reciprocity of the development of new theoretical questions is likely to be enhanced. Sophisticated and thoughtful application of heretofore not utilized theoretical constructs may not only significantly benefit the fields of practice, but also may spur on the development of basic research and theory.

The implications of this paper go beyond the acquisition of knowledge and the development of a specialty in family health care. Family practice was, at the beginning of this paper, identified as an attempt to develop a field of specialization in medicine which is neither disease nor organ oriented. The implications of the argument presented in this paper carry over into the entire process by which we educate and socialize health professionals, particularly physicians. The skills of assessing, evaluating and assisting the needs of the family health unit requires not only new areas of substantive knowledge but also the acceptance of complexity, ambiguity, and imprecision. It requires a change in the total approach to health care, including a different set of emphases in history taking, a different definition of relevance and significance and, above all, a change in the fundamental role of the health care practitioner within a family health network. To the traditional model of repair and restoration must be added the model of accommodation, fac ilitation, and enablement.

At best this paper is a preamble and a search for synthesis in response to the frustration about the gaps between disciplines and professions. It is an attempt to suggest where the road should be bu ilt rather than the actual construction of the highway.

BIBLIOGRAPHY

[1] Paul Adams, 'Family Characteristics of Obsessive Children', *American Journal of Psychiatry* **128** (1972) 98–100.

[2] American Public Health Association, *A Model for Planning Pa tient Education*, Baltimore, American Public Health Association, Public He alth Education Section, 1970.

[3] Kurt W., Back 'Epidemiology Versus Cartesian Dualism', *Social Science and Medicine* **5** (1971) 461–468.

[4] Donald W. Ball, 'The 'Family' as a Sociological Problem: Conceptualization of the Taken-for Granted as Prologue to Social Problems Analysis', *Social Problems* **19** (1972) 295–307.

[5] C. M. Binger, A. R. Ablin, R. C. Feverstein, J. H. Kushner, S. Zoger, and C. Mikkelsen, 'Childhood Leukemia: Emotional Impact on Patient and Family', *New England Journal of Medicine* **280** (1969) 414.

[6] Carlfred B. Broderick, 'Beyond the Five Conceptual Frameworks: A Decade of Development in Family Theory', *Journal of Marriage and the Family* **33** (1971) 139–59.

[7] G. W. Brown, J. L. T. Birley and J. K. Wing, 'Influence of Family Life on the Course of Schizophrenic Disorders: A Replication', *British Journal of Psychiatry* **121** (1972) 241–58.

[8] Walter Buckley, *Sociology and Modern Systems Theory*, Prentice-Hall, Englewood Cliffs, New Jersey 1967.

[9] John A. Clausen, 'The Organism and Socialization', *Journal of Health and Social Behavior* **8** (1967) 243–252.

[10] S. Cobb, S. Kasl, J. R. P. French and G. Norstebo, 'The Intrafamilial Transmission of Rheumatoid Arthritis, VII, Why do Wives with Rheumatoid Arthritis Have Husbands with Peptic Ulcers?', *Journal of Chronic Diseases* **22** (1969) 279–293.

[11] S. Deutscher, F. H. Epstein and M. O. Kjelsberg, 'Familial Aggregation of Factors Associated with Coronary Heart Disease', *Circulation* **33** (1966) 911–923.

[12] Rene Dubos, *Mirage of Health*, Anchor Books, Garden City, New Yrok 1959.

[13] W. M. Easson, 'The Family of the Dying Child', *Pediatric Clinics of North America* **19** (1972) 1157–65.

[14] Bruce K. Eckland, 'Genetics and Sociology: A Reconsideration', *American Sociological Review* **32** (1967) 173–94.

[15] Bernard Farber, *Kinship and Class: A Midwestern Study*, Boise Books, New York 1971.

[16] Vida Francis, Barbara M. Korsch and Maria J. Morris, 'Gaps in Doctor Patient Communication', *New England Journal of Medicine* **280** (1969) 535–540.

[17] K. Freund, 'A Laboratory Method for Diagnosing Predominance of Homo- or Heteroerotic Interest in the Male', *Behavioral Research Therapy* **1** (1963) 85

[18] Edward Gross, 'Work, Organization and Stress', *Social Stress* (Sol Levine, and Norman A. Scotch, eds.), Aldine, Chicago 1970, pp. 54–110.

[19] Edward T. Hall, *The Silent Language*, Doubleday, Garden City, New Jersey 1959.

[20] Gerald Handel (ed.), *The Psychosocial Interior of the Family: A Sourcebook for the Study of Whole Families*, Aldine, New York 1967.

[21] E. Harburg, S. Kasl, J. Tabor and S. Cobb, 'The Intrafamilial Transmission of Rheumatoid Arthritis, IV, Recalled Parent-Child Relations by Rheumatoid Arthritics and Controls', *Journal of Chronic Diseases* **22** (1969) 223–238.

[22] C. G. Hayes, H. A. Tyroler, J. C. Cassel and C. Hill, 'Family Aggregation of Blood Pressure in Evans County, Georgia', *Archives of Internal Medicine* **128** (1971) 965–75.

[23] R. Hill and J. Aldous, *International Bibliography of Research in Marriage and Family*, University of Minnesota Press, Minneapolis, Minnesota 1967.

[24] R. Hill and D. R. Hansen, 'The Identification of Conceptual Frameworks Utilized in Family Study', *Journal of Marriage and the Family* **22** (1960) 299–311.

[25] L. E. Hinkle, Jr., 'Studies of Human Ecology in Relation to Health and Behavior', *Bioscience* **15** (1965) 517–20.

[26] David Holland, 'Familization, Socialization and the Universe of Meaning: An Extension of the Interactional Approach to the Study of the Family', *Journal of Marriage and the Family* (1970) 415–427.

[27] Thomas H. Holmes and Richard H. Rahe, 'The Social Readjustment Rating Scale', *Journal of Psychosomatic Research* **11** (1967) 213–218.

[28] D. Hooper, Roger Gill, Peter Powesland and Bernard Ineichen, 'The Health of Young Families in New Housing', *Journal of Psychosomatic Research* **16** (1972) 367–74.

[29] B. C. Johnson, F. H. Epstein and M. O. Kjeisberg, 'Distributions and Familial Studies of Blood Pressure and Serum Cholesterol Levels in a Total Community – Tecumseh, Michigan', *Journal of Chronic Diseases* **18** (1965) 147–60.

[30] Barbara Korsch and H. L. Barnett, 'The Physician, the Family and the Child with Nephrosis', *Journal of Pediatrics* **58** (1961) 707–715.

[31] Monroe Lerner and Odin W. Anderson, *Health Progress in the United States: 1900–1960*, University of Chicago, Chicago 1963.

[32] Theodor J. Litman, 'Health Care and the Family: A Three Generation Analysis', *Medical Care* **9** (1971) 67–81.

[33] Gay Gaer Luce, *Biological Rhythms in Human and Animal Physiology*, Dover Publications, Inc., New York 1971.

[34] Olga R. Lurie, 'The Emotional Health of Children in the Family Setting', *Community Mental Health Journal* **6** (1970) 229–235.

[35] N. McConaphy, 'Penile Volume Change to Moving Pictures of Male and Female Nudes in Heterosexual and Homosexual Males', *Behavioral Research Therapy* **5** (1967) 43.

[36] W. H. Masters and Virginia E. Johnson, *Human Sexual Response*, Little, Brown and Company, Boston 1966.

[37] David Mechanic, 'The Concept of Illness Behavior', *Journal of Chronic Diseases* **15** (1962) 189–194.

[38] Alfred Messer, 'Mechanisms of Family Homeostasis', *Comprehensive Psychiatry* **12** (1971) 380–88.

[39] R. P. Michael, G. S. Saayman, and D. Zumpe, 'The Suppression of Mounting Behavior and Ejaculation in Male Rhesus Monkeys (Macacamulatta) by Administration of Progesterone to Their Female Partners', *Journal of Endocrinology* **271** (1968) 421–431.

[40] Jerome K. Myers, Jacob J. Lindenthal, Max P. Pepper, and David R. Ostrander, 'Life Events and Mental Status: A Longitudinal Study', *Journal of Health and Social Behavior* **13** (1972) 398–406.

[41] Ivan F. Nye and Felix M. Berardo (eds.), *Emerging Conceptual Frameworks in Family Analysis*, The Macmillan Company, New York 1966.

[42] B. Picken and G. Ireland, 'Family Patterns of Medical Care Utilization', *Journal of Chronic Diseases* **22** (1969) 181–191.

[43] 'Quizzing the Expert: Linking Stress and Personality to Physical Disease', *Hospital Physician* **8** (1972) 26–31.

[44] Robert E. Rakel, Howard F. Conn and Johnson W. Thomas (eds.), *Family Practice*, W. B. Saunders Company, Philadelphia 1973.

[45] Roy H. Rodgers, 'Toward a Theory of Family Development', *Journal of Marriage and the Family* **26** (1964) 262–70.

[46] Betty J. Ruana, James D. Bruce and Margaret M. McDermott', 'Pilgrim's Progress II: Recent Trends and Prospects in Family Research', *Journal of Marriage and the Family* **31** (1969) 688–98.

[47] Frederick Sargent II and Demitri B. Shimkin, 'Biology, Society and Culture in Human Ecology', *Bioscience* **15** (1965) 512–516.

[48] Barry Schwartz, 'Notes on the Sociology of Sleep', *The Sociological Quarterly* **11** (1970) 485–499.

[49] M. Siegelman, 'Family Background of Alcoholics: Some Research Considerations', *Annals of the New York Academy of Sciences* **197** (1972) 226–29.

[50] M. Skelton and J. Dominian ,'Psychological Stress in Wives of Patients with Myocardial Infarction', *British Medical Journal* **5858** (1973) 101–03.

[51] Jetse Sprey, 'The Family as a System in Conflict', *Journal of Marriage and the Family* (1969) 699–706.

[52] Sidney M. Stahl, 'Illness Among the Aged: A Study of the Determinants of the Perception of Levels of Health in an Indigent, Urban Population', Unpublished Doctoral Dissertation, University of Illionis, Urbana, Illinois, 1971.

[53] S. Leonard Syme, 'Clinical Biases in Social Epidemiology', Paper presented to the American Sociological Association Meetings, Miami, Florida, 1966.

[54] Daisy M. Tagliacozzo and Kenji Ima, 'Knowledge of Illness as a Predictor of Patient Behavior', *Journal of Chronic Diseases* **22** (1970) 765–75.

[55] W. Winklestein, S. Kantor, M. Ibrahim and D. L. Sackett, 'Familial Aggregation of Blood Pressure', *Journal of the American Medical Association* **195** (1966) 160–62.

REFERENCES

* This is an original version of the paper published in *Social Science and Medicine* **8** (2), September 1974.

** The author wishes to express sincere appreciation to David Stagner and to Roger Francis for research assistance and to Sidney Stahl, David Stagner and to Ingeborg Mauksch, for critical reading of the manuscript.

VALUES IN THE MEDICAL PROFESSION *

ECATERINA SPRINGER

Institute of Philosophy, Rumanian Academy of Social and Political Sciences, Bucharest, Rumania

It is perhaps no exaggeration to say that the medical profession is a strange one, whose status differs from that of other modern professions. This contention is based on an assessment of the features which make it peculiar.

Any socially recognized profession (as medicine most undoubtedly is) necessarily regulates its performance according to various modes of social control. It is practiced according to a set of standards which are generally exact and handled explicitly enough to allow for a clear assessment. Medicine is outside the reach of such objective control. This is due primarily to the difficulty of determining suitable criteria. In common sense terms, however, there is one obvious criterion: the patient's return to health. Unfortunately, this criterion is analytically imprecise and therefore inadequate. Moreover, inconsistency apart, one would find very few branches of medicine whose results were measurable in this manner.

But society, unable to control medical activity by normal means, exerts instead a strong social pressure on medicine. This pressure has many aspects: social organization of medical care, prescriptions for physicians' role behavior, and manpower, pressure to discover general measures to cope with a wide range of diseases. [1]

We are concerned here with two different things: the failure to control medical performance, and the attempt to exert strong pressure on medical activity. These are not contradictory, just different. A physician is supposed (and to a certain degree under specific circumstances obliged) to do all that his professional tasks demand and skills permit in order to cope with major social demands, but the outcome of his actions depends not only on what he is doing, but also on a very complex set of independent factors.

The medical profession is characteristically esoteric in the field of medical acts and judgements and fairly exoteric regarding the object of these acts: the sick person.

Thus, the basic relationship in medicine, that between physician and patient, is singular. In this relationship, two persons of the same kind find themselves face to face, but the relationship is one of subordination and even, it may be said, of submission, because the patient's will is subordinated to that of the physician. But, oddly enough, this submission is freely given.

Providing appropriate medical care presupposes an intimate knowledge of the patient as a whole human being. In dealing with his patient, the physician generally finds himself in the position of intruding into the private life of the patient. He is supposed to approach the whole man, not a particular illness.

Doctors commit themselves to observe perfect secrecy regarding their patients.

Furthermore, a physician often deals with matters of life and death, and often he or she has to cope with this in the face of considerable uncertainty.[2] There are as many uncertain elements in medical care as there are certain ones.

But the physician is faced not only with social and professional requirements. He is expected to perform a specific role which is often likely to exceed his duties.

Finally, the medical profession involves much greater responsibility for the physician than that usually placed on an individual who practises a profession. It is a threefold responsibility: professional, social and personal. Profesionally, the physician is called upon to overcome an adversary which is often poorly understood – disease; socially, he is called upon to restore a man to society intact; and personally, he is involved in his profession to a greater extent than other professional men because of his power over pain and evil.

Obviously, all these are ideal features; however they are especially relevant to the medical profession. To a greater or lesser extent, problems like responsibility, uncertainty, social pressure and so on are real and deserve our attention.

The specific conditions of providing medical care suggest other aspects of the medical profession. According to social and community contexts, the practice of medicine acquires some peculiar features: it varies in terms of the formal organization of the profession, its hierarchical structure, the pressure of time and the flow of patients, the high cost of medical care, the scarcity of physicians and medical facilities, the network of medical institutions, the organization of medical training, etc.

All these factors exert many, sometimes contradictory, pressures on physicians. The compulsion is expressed not only in the norms of professional conduct, but also in values. Each of the above features is linked to particular sets of values.

There is a wide range of values related to the medical profession. Most of them are social and professional.

By values related to medical profession I mean those standards of desirability which play an important part in medical activity. Some of them are characteristic of other professions too, but in medicine they are more evident. Others are specific to the medical profession. Among the former we may note a high degree of responsibility, a strongly developed sense of duty, a greater honesty. Among the latter there are: devotion to others, the commitment to help those in need, the great value assigned to human life.

The professional values encountered in this field are more pressing than elsewhere because the physician, by virtue of what he can do and what he is doing, is involved in the whole existence of his patient.

It may be assumed that because values in the medical profession depend on the social conditions regulating professional practice, they can vary according to special changes occurring at the societal level. The impact of social changes upon medical activity involves to some degree a value change as a final result.

In contemporary socialist Rumania there are two such major changes in the medical profession: 1. the implementation of a system of free medical care; and 2. the provision of free medical training. These macrostructural changes have multiple consequences.

Because medical care is supported by the state, there are many possibilities of medical policy effecting a special pattern and network in the provision of medical care.

The fact that medical care has become free for the patient, has implications for all strata of society. Currently, access to medical care is one of the basic rights enjoyed by the whole population. Everyone who is ill has the opportunity to seek and receive competent medical care.

This change has necessitated others. It has involved different kind of relationship between physician and patient. Being free from financial constraints in seeking help, the patient, whatever his income, can receive the medical care he needs. There are no more economic barriers to receiving medical care and advice. As a consequence, the former link between illness and poverty has become obsolete.

The existence of free medical care eliminates the competition among physicians in search of clients. The doctor's practice, treatment, prescription, and observance of medical standards are no longer dependent on a client relationship. Medicine and medical practice are now under the charge of society, which facilitates efficient intervention in organizing and controlling medical institutions. Moreover, it is now society which guarantees the status of the physician. Freed of the competition of private practice, being a salaried person with a guaranteed income and position in the societal hierarchy, the physician is no longer concerned with improving his social position in order to earn his living.

Free medical training means that young men of all social classes can have access to the medical profession; formerly medical training was available only to those coming from a wealthy background because of the great financial burden assumed by the family of the young man during his training and the beginning of his career. Thus the number of those who want to enter the medical profession and can realistically expect to do so has rapidly increased.

There are now conditions for a careful selection of those entering medical school. This provides a significant opportunity for social planning concerning the number of physicians and the various branches of medicine according to the needs of a continually developing medical network. Because concern for health is constantly increasing, the need for medical care is very great, especially in rural areas.

These are the general conditions and changes that have occurred at the social level.

There is also another circumstance to be taken into account: a physician practises his profession in a particular social organization providing medical care and in a particular community.

Generally speaking, the physician's status represents for much of the population a high standard of living and a high degree of professionalism. Moreover, he may sometimes be viewed as a model for the community. First the medical profession, second the social organization of medical care, and third community pressure, are all factors affecting in one way or another the specific values related to the medical profession and held by a given medical body.

The physician's status itself involves a value judgement: physicians are supposed to be dedicated men, who place their patients' welfare above their own; they are supposed to be valuable members of society. But it is possible to find differences or discrepancies between assigned values and those currently held by physicians.

Given the characteristic features of the medical profession and given the societal changes that have occurred in medical activity it is worth undertaking a study of the value aspect of the medical profession, taking into account the values currently held by physicians.

In order to investigate the whole body of physicians in a community, a medium-sized community was selected, the town of Lugoj, in the Timis district.

It may be assumed that community size is a significant factor in relation to some aspects of medical activity.

What is especially relevant when the community is of small or medium size? In a big city, the physician is known only in the narrow circle of his clients. Obviously, in a smaller community he is known and recognized in a much wider circle than that consisting of his present or potential patients. The physician himself is more often than not in a position to have a social and personal acquaintance with a large range of members of the community. In such cases he can escape only seldom from the many influences stemming from the community. His social, professional, and personal behavior is controlled because he is a very visible figure in the community. Undoubtedly, this produces another kind of pressure. In such a community the doctor is the target of a wide set of demands and expectations coming not only from his patients, but from many others, because he is viewed both in his professional and in his social role.

The physician is often a general advisor on problems not related to health alone. He is at hand when required and he may intervene rapidly when his help is needed. On the other hand, he often plays an active role in the prevention of many diseases and so he contributes to improving the general health of the community.

In Lugoj at the time of survey hospital personnel with higher education consisted of about 80 physicians working in the two hospitals and out-patient clinic.

The data were obtained by circulating a questionnaire to all the physicians in the community. 73% of these were returned, providing an adequate sample on the basis of which assertions could be made about the entire physicians' community of the town.

Presumably, values related to the medical profession are likely to be more pertinent in some areas than in others. Here we are concerned with findings relating to the following lines: career choice, professional values held by the medical staff, relationships between physicians and patients, and differences in value system according to age and sex.

The changes in medical care and practice have led to the emergence of new criteria for career choice. These apply to the sample because most of the physicians under study graduated after the changes had occurred.

The main stress was put on the problem of motivation. How are physicians motivated to choose their profession?

The major motive indicated by the subjects was the attraction their felt towards this profession. 87.7% of them gave this motive for their choice of career.

For some of them this meant the high social status of the profession. A few of them reported that their choice also reflected the wishes of their families' – or that this was the sole motivation – and three stated that their choice was random.

Nobody reported that their choice was dictated by the profitable character of the medical profession. Though I have not enough data to support an explanation, the reasons may be one or both of the following: 1) career choice generally takes place at an age when the individual holds mainly romantic values, 2) the medical profession in the present Rumanian social context is really not a very profitable one, or at least it is no more profitable than any other profession requiring higher education. Thus, the quest for money does not account for the choice of career.

The attractiveness of the profession is a universal reason. It consists of several elements: the desire to give help, the desire to be useful to society, compassion for those who are ill, the hope of doing good, the need to develop one's skills in order to help others. [3] One may note that these elements are highly consistent with those involved in the physician's status.

Together these components may be characterized by a single value, namely 'altruism'. The choice of the medical profession involves a cluster of values centered around an altruistic core.

There is general agreement among physicians concerning the value which made them choose their profession. Certainly, this value is one of the best expressions of the specific features of the medical profession and of the new social conditions in which medicine is practised.

'Altruism' is also the basic social value specific to the medical profession. It expresses one's willingness to devote oneself to others.

The professional values held by those involved in treating the sick may be analysed by studying the relationships between physicians and nurses in their professional activity.

Formally, the relationships between doctors and nurses are hierarchical. The former have higher status, higher income, higher professional skills and greater knowledge than the latter. In this hierarchical structure the nurses are supposed to carry out the physicians' professional commands and to help in dealing with the patient. Professionally, these relationships consist also in a division of tasks between doctors and nurses.

The concrete relationships may vary considerably. Asked what professional features they expect of the nurses in their team, the physicians mentioned a number of features. Most of them (26) placed honesty first; 15 valued the nurses' professional skills; 14 wanted the nurses to contribute more to the process of treatment; 8 assessed conscientiousness; 8 required them to be disciplined and 6 demanded kindness.

Some of these features are evaluated as high social values in the value system of society. In respect of their content, they are not independent, but it is supposed that as a group they characterize a type of personality.

It must be stressed that, in this field, the theoretical distinction between values and norms no longer holds. Most of these features are values as well as norms.

'Honesty' is a general value, accounting for the whole behavior of an individual. It is viewed in the societal value system as the individual's basic feature.

The claim for professional skills makes it necessary for nurses to try continually to keep up with advances in the professional field. By asking the nurse to be active in the relationship with the patient, the physicians emphasize the nurses' obligation to perform and even to go beyond the tasks assigned to them by the physicians. 'Conscientiousness' is a value concerning mainly the attempts to do one's job as best one can.

The discipline required of nurses is worth commenting on at length. Every physician has to cope with great pressures of time and work. But this pressure must not be allowed to threaten observance of the necessary standards of medical care. In order to avoid any such negative influence, the nurse must perform a very important task by scrupulously carrying out the doctor's prescriptions and treatment. Very often, the effectiveness of the medical care as a whole depends on the nurses' role performance (especially in the hospitals). The tremendous importance ascribed to this norm does not appear here very clearly. But I assume that this feature must be recognized in the two values previously mentioned: honesty and conscientiousness.

Finally, kindness refers to the manner of handling the patient. This requirement expresses the nurses' duty to reassure the patient and put him at his ease as much as possible.

It was discovered that the central value in the relationship between physicians and nurses is 'competence'. It is by far the most highly evaluated and has the richest content.

In other words, it may be asserted that the set of exceptations expressed by the physicians in relation to their nurses means that they want them to have a broad professional and social orientation, that is physicians expect their nurses to be 'cosmopolitans', [4] to use Merton's terminology.

To go a step further, all the physicians are aware of the importance of continuing their studies. Nowadays, a doctor is supposed to keep up with scientific developments in medicine in order to be able to perform adequately in his profession. This is a value and a duty as well.

Every physician in the survey asserted his concern with improving his professional knowledge. But their answers enable us to divide them into three ranked groups. On the bottom are ranged those who stressed reading professional materials only. Next are those who add to reading professional debates with their colleagues. Finally there are those who themselves carry out scientific research, experiments, innovations. For all physicians, however, reading remains the principal means for keeping up their professional knowledge.

The relationships occurring between physicians and patients are by far the most important in the medical profession. The survey design focussed on the physicians' expectations concerning the behavior of their patients.

The most frequent expectation is trust (28 doctors), followed by respect (24). Moreover, the patients are required to maintain discipline (12 doctors) and 6 physicians expect their patients to be frank.

Trust is a professional as well as a social claim. It is the inner condition making medical practice possible. Although the evidence is not clear-cut, it may be said that trust is required not only in relation to the physician, but also to the whole profession to which he belongs. This claim is more frequently expressed by those physicians practising in a branch of medicine where immediate and long lasting success is possible.

What about the expectation of respect? It is a clear reaction to the community's impact on medical practice.

The relationship between physicians and the public is here more often an informal, very close one. It frequently happens that doctors are treated too familiarly. By demanding respect, physicians resist excessive familiarity. It is, of course, a status claim. But it is also related to some professional features which may be damaged by this familiarity: for example, the patient's willingness to conform to the physician's instructions may be impaired.

There is another claim which clarifies all these: discipline, by which the patient is required to conduct himself strictly according to the doctor's orders so he may recover his health.

Candor, like trust, is an expectation: the doctor is in a position to render help only if he is properly informed about his patient's disease.

There are a few physicians who add some rather surprising demands: they don't want their patients to expect them to do wonders; or to consider them sorcerers. That is an expression of humility manifesting high professional awareness.

The evidence shows that 'cooperation' is the value which best depicts the physicians' expectations of their patients.

But do physicians feel these expectations are fulfilled by their patients? Their answers display a kind of disappointment: only 18 of them think their patients are conforming to their claims. Most of them are uncertain, 5 say they don't know and two give no answer. Although the answers show a significant correlation with the respondent's age, they seem to be, as such, a strong expression of that feature of the medical profession mentioned above: uncertainty, the major hazard of the medical profession. Each difficult case and each failure may disrupt the fragile relationship between physician and patient.

Age and sex differences are not very sharp, so one cannot speak about variations caused by differences in generation or sex.

By age, the physicians were divided into three categories: the first consisting of those aged 25–35, the second of those aged 35–45, and the third of those over 45. Age plays some role regarding professional characteristics, expectations regarding the patient, and self-confidence. Related to the respondent's sex, these differences are still weaker.

The consensus displayed by the sample concerning the values that account for career choice makes irrelevant any possible difference related to age. One can only say that career choice that is random or motivated by family expectations is more frequent in men than in women.

The variable of improving professional knowledge displays some differences: the young doctors fall in the middle of the scale, the physicians in the second age group at the middle and top, and those in the third age group at the bottom and top. There is a single woman at the top of the scale in this field.

The young physicians more often than the other two age groups expect trust and less often demand respect in their relationships with their patients. The other age groups are very similar. In this respect, there is no difference between men and women.

Assessments of the patients' conformity to the physicians expectations varies according to age: all doctors in the highest age group report a high conformity, those in the second age group a rather good conformity and only 25% of the young doctors report a high conformity. It seems that men have greater authority than women, but the difference is not great.

With increased age, there is an improvement in the physicians' assessment of their own personal activity: the older the physician, the greater his reported professional success.

This survey found out that there is a cluster of values characterizing the medical profession. These values (altruism, competence, cooperation) are more than professional values. They all have great social significance.

Where and when are these values learned? Primarily, of course, at school and during the physicians' training. But their assimilation and sometimes their creation is mainly social and occurs in the professional career of the physician. There is also a good deal of social learning by various means involved here. It may be said that these values reflect to a high degree the social conditions of medical practice in Rumania.

REFERENCES

* This paper is based upon an article previously published in the journal 'Tribuna'.

For the present version the author expresses her gratitude to Professor Michael Cernea for his suggestions and helpful criticism and to Katherine Verdery for help in editnig the text.

[1] For a general approach to the problem see O. Berlogea, O. Neamtu and V. Krasnaseschi, 'Sociologia sanatatii' (Health Sociology) in: *Sociologie generala*, M. Constantinescu (ed.), Ed. st., Buc. 1970.

[2] David Mechanic, 'Medical Sociology – A Selective View', The Free Press, New York, 1968, pp. 91–95.

[3] Cf. Patricia L. Kendall, 'Medical Sociology in The United States', *Sc. Sci. Inform.* **2** (1963) 32.

[4] Robert K. Merton, 'The Role of the Nurse: Locals and Cosmopolitans', *NSNS News Letter*, Fall 1962.

IV. THE HEALTH SYSTEM

THE HEALTH SYSTEM AND THE SOCIAL SYSTEM*

MARK G. FIELD

Department of Sociology, Boston University, Boston, Mass. U.S.A.

The major intent of this paper is to present a synthetic view of the health system as an integral component of the social system for which it performs a series of critical functions and from which, in turn, it receives a number of problematic supports or resources. As such an attempt is made to place the health system in its proper perspective, i.e. not at the exclusive center of sociological interest but alongside a group of complementary and differentiated sub-systems, each one performing its own tasks and necessarily competing for the scarce resources necessary for the performance of these tasks. My conceptual scheme is 'structural-functional' and derives, in its greater part, from the insights elaborated by Talcott Parsons and his view of society as an equilibrium-maintaining system, and made up of meaningfully interrelated sub-systems in such a way that change in one sub-system is potentially bound to affect other sub-systems and the system as a whole.

The basic departure point for an examination of the health system (which I will define below) is the functional problem it attempts to cope with. This problem is the incapacitation or the inability of the individual to perform expected social roles because of illness, trauma or premature mortality. It is thus possible to conceive of 'health' as a strategic resource of the social system, because of its bearing on the ability of individuals to act, and the health system as a defense mechanism aimed at the preservation, the repairing, the conservation and the enhancement of that resource. Thus in addition to the highly *personal* aspects of illness, trauma and early death (suffering, anxiety, lack of self-actualization, dependency and demise), there is a *societal* component in their potential and actual impact on institutionalized role performance. The illness of a chief of state or of industrial workers have repercussions that often extend well beyond personal discomfort.

The response to ill health and its consequences can be defined as both cultural and sociological. *Cultural*, that is, in the development of definitions and attitudes toward illness and schemes or techniques to deal with it. And sociological, in the emergence of health institutions and an increasingly occupationally differentiated body of individuals (health personnel) who are entitled, expected, and mandated to deal, on a specialized basis, with illness.

Broadly speaking, I would like to emphasize, at the cultural level, four responses to illness that are analytically different: religious, magical, pastoral/supportive, and technical/medical. These four responses can be arrayed in a two-by-two table, along the dimensions of pre-modern and modern, and of meaning and means:

	Pre-modern	Modern
Meaning	1. Religious (symbolic meaning)	2. Pastoral/supportive (expressive meaning)
Means	3. Magical (ritualistic means)	4. Technical/medical (instrumental means)

1. The *religious* response to illness and death may be described as one that encourages their acceptance as the result of some higher force(s) or power over which man has little or no control, and whose designs are often mysterious. The religious response thus attempts to provide 'symbolic meaning'. For example, in the case of premature death that otherwise makes 'no sense', the stock phrase is, "The Lord giveth and the Lord taketh away, blessed be the name of the Lord".

2. The *magical* response is an attempt to actively deal with illness seen as the result of the actions of gods, divinities, or other occult forces that must be palliated, neutralized, or in some fashion affected so that they, in turn, will affect the course of illness. It is an attempt to secure favorable outcomes, and is epitomized, in the modern world, by the familiar phrase: "If you want to help the patient recover, pray for him as you have never prayed before". This response thus provides 'ritualistic

means' to deal with illness. The administration of certain drugs, whose effect is doubtful or nil but hopefully harmless, may also be likened to a kind of magic associated with the need to 'do something'.

3. The *pastoral/supportive* response may be described as the provision of psychological help and support, of 'tender loving care' to the anxious and often emotionally regressed patient, particularly in the light of the association of illness and injury with possible permanent disability, dependency, suffering, and death. The psycho-emotional support and reassurance must include a strong fiduciary element, and reassurance to the patient that the health personnel 'care' for him in the dual etymological sense of 'love' and 'treatment'. In an evolutionary sense, its prototype is probably the mother-child relationship. This response thus provides 'expressive meaning'.

4. The *technical/medical* response is the provision of services aimed at dealing with illness and trauma in scientific-objective and verifiable terms, both in the conceptualization of etiology and the application of remedial measures. It is usually conceived as an active intervention, as doing something to and for the patient, epitomized by the stock phrase that "the physicians are doing all they can to save the patient's life (or limb or health)". This response provides 'instrumental means'.

The above list is probably not exhaustive but it may be assumed that some mix or profile of such responses is present in the 'medical' response from primitive society to the present, and could be subjected to comparative analysis. Given the aleatory aspects of health and illness, and the uncertainty of outcomes, one can doubt that the magical/religious aspects are slated for extinction, even in the most scientific medical system. And by the same token, primitive or prescientific medicine includes empirical elements resulting from an observation of causality grounded in reality, and not simply magico-religious elements. But I also suggest that with time and the development of science, the medical response has tended to differentiate itself into two major complementary streams, the magico-religious on one hand, and the pastoral-technical on the other hand. Each of these has tended to become the focus of different occupational and professional roles. This then leads to an examination of the process of the emergence of differentiated roles and of individuals dealing with the illness problem of society.

It may be correct to assume if one adopts an evolutionary-historical perspective on the development of societal responses to illness that, in very simple, primitive type societies, there were no differentiated cultural elements nor roles concerned with health and illness. Indeed this concern was everybody's, and was taken care of within the context of the family/kinship/community. But with the rise of folklore and of techniques centrally focused on health and illness, there emerged a body or corpus of individuals who, on a part time basis, and later on a full-time basis were concerned in a specialized manner, with the provision of custody, treatment and the care of the sick. Probably in the early phases of that development the same occupational role included priest, magician, pastor, and doctor altogether. In the contemporary society, and particularly in the last hundred years, under the impact of increased available knowledge and techniques, the priest-magician role has tended to formally differentiate itself from that of the pastor-physician. It is around the latter function that modern medical roles have clustered. Certain tensions to which I shall refer later, have developed in the mix of these two last functions, and it is not inconceivable that in the future we shall witness a further differentiation between two specific 'medical' roles: one centered on the pastoral/supportive aspects of treatment, and the other more centrally focused around the application of technological/medical means.

Health personnel and health facilities operate within the context of a 'health system'. Conceptually, the health system of any society is that totality of formal commitments, resources and activities that the society 'invests' or sets aside for the health concern in contrast to other concerns, whether this be the polity, industrial and agricultural production, general education, national defense, communications, and so on. Semantically the term 'system' may lead to some confusion in this instance, particularly in view of the fact that it is usually not a tightly organized and managed web of activities and facilities working in concert with each other. One might use the words 'sector' which is too static, or 'program' which in most instances it is not, and I will therefore stick to 'system' and contend it is possible to cast a conceptual net around it for analytical purposes.

There will always be a certain amount of indeterminacy as to the exact boundaries of the health system, but such boundaries are necessary if one wants to deal operationally and comparatively with that system. In one sense, a society is also a system and everything is connected with everything else. By definition then, physicians and allied health personnel are part of the health system, as are hospitals, clinics, and pharmaceutical plants. But are housing, or agriculture or general education or transportation, or the general economic level (all of which certainly have a *bearing* on health) part of the health system? To say yes would be absurd and would make analysis practically impossible. But is, for example, the American pharmacist who dispenses drugs and sells all sorts of notions part of that system? I might answer 'yes' insofar as he executes doctors' orders and fills prescriptions. When he sells toothpaste or candy or cigarettes, the answer would be 'no'. The mother who calls in a physician, and nurses a sick child would not be a member of that system, nor would the construction worker who builds a hospital. However, the ambulance driver, the hospital carpenter or dietician, the medical secretary would be. I shall return to this thorny question of 'health personnel'.

There remains yet another conceptual difficulty. How does one define the health system at the macro-sociological level when there are a variety of cultural definitions of health and medical practices (for example, the co-existence in some countries of so-called modern medicine along with traditional medicine or medicines, as in India, Southeast Asia, China etc.)? And when there is a multiplicity of institutional arrangements for the provision of health-related services (for example, in the United States the private practice of medicine, public medicine, the Veterans Administration, the Kaiser-Permanents or the Health Insurance Plans)? My answer is, that for the time being, I would define the health system of any society as the *aggregate* of its health practices and systems. Later on, a society by society analysis could be mounted of the systems, their co-existence, or competition, or their struggle for recognition and legitimation.

The essential task of the health system is to cope with the threats and consequences of illness, trauma, and premature mortality. These 'incapacitating' aspects may be called the *Functional Problems* which the health system seeks to mitigate or neutralize. They are sometimes referred to as the five D's, though the list might be extended:

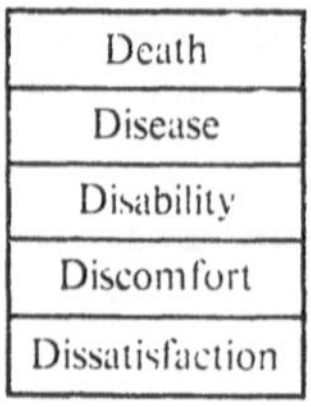

To cope with these, the health system must provide a series of services which, briefly listed, consist of the following six *Modalities*:

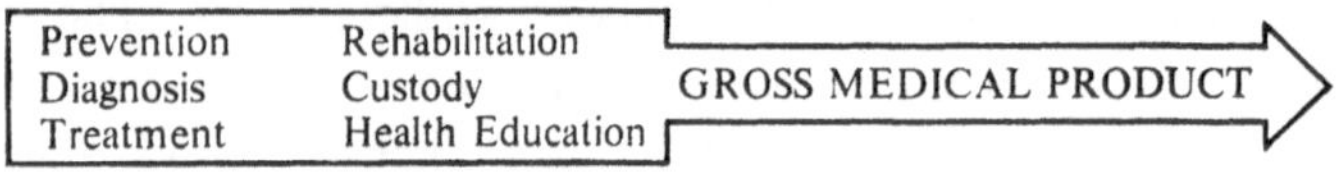
Prevention
Diagnosis
Treatment
Rehabilitation
Custody
Health Education
GROSS MEDICAL PRODUCT

The totality of these services for any chosen time period can be termed the Gross Medical Product (GMP) of the society, and consists of transactions that go from the health system to society's health problems. A physician who sees a patient in consultation, a nurse who dresses a wound, a hospital admission and stay, or a ride in an ambulance to the emergency room, all contribute to fashioning the GMP. The health system, furthermore, can be said to consist of one external and two internal components. The external component are the multiplicity of services that constitute the GMP just mentioned: these activities are what the system is all about, this is what society expects and demands from its health system, i.e. outputs aimed directly at the health problems. The internal components, education and research, provide outputs that remain essentially within the health system (though in the final analysis they are indispensable in making it possible for the health system to perform its tasks). The education component provides 'socialization' in the health professions whether this be in medical schools, nursing schools, schools for X-ray technicians or dieticians. The education component in addition provides for the selection, recruitment and replacement of health personnel because of attrition caused by retirement, invalidity, emigration and death. General schools (elementary and secondary) whose graduates might go into a variety of fields, cannot thus, be considered a part of the health system, though again they have a bearing on it. The research component yields the knowledge and techniques essential for health professionals to perform their tasks. It is basically an elaboration, in the health areas, of the state of knowledge, science and technology in the world at large (for example, the application of laser beams in surgery, radio isotopes in diagnostics, or computers in data analysis or record processing). The health system and its functions can be diagrammed as follows:

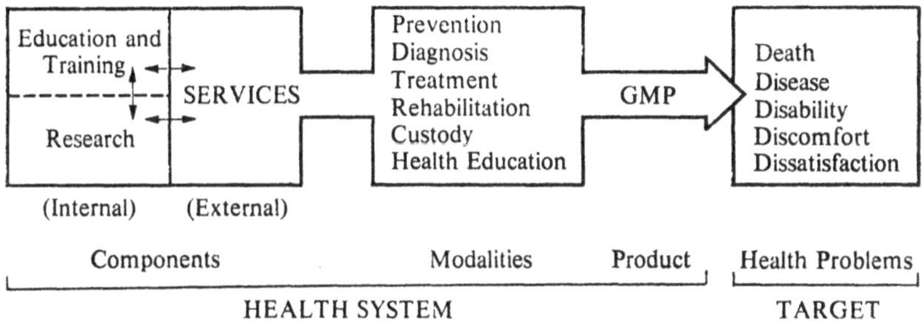

As a differentiated 'service' sub-system of society, the health system cannot generate its own resources and thus requires a complex of structural supports from its society. Without these it simply could not operate. I have delineated at least four such categories of societal supports:

1. The health system (and its practitioners) must enjoy legitimacy, including a specific mandate (a social contract, so to speak) and trust. The services which the health system provides must be seen as both proper and desirable. To a very considerable extent, the 'proper' or 'legitimate' response to illness is affected by the value system of society. That value system in turn influences the 'mix' of medical responses mentioned earlier. Thus the medical response of an active, 'mastery-of-nature' modern society will be quite different from that of a society that emphasizes acceptance of the world and passivity. In societies where different medical traditions exist or co-exist, there is a struggle for recognition, legitimacy, supremacy, and monopoly on the part of the different practitioners (modern medicine versus chiropractice versus Christian Science in the U.S.; Western and Ayruvedic medicine in India; traditional Chinese and Western medicine in Mainland China).

2. In order to provide services, the health system needs a cultural resource in the form of knowledge and techniques, i.e., the art and science of medicine. In contemporary society, this element is constantly being modified by research, practice and experience and is, as seen earlier, affected by the general state of scientific knowledge in the world. At the same time, and increasingly so, organizational and administrative knowledge becomes an important 'cultural' resource for the health system. It should be pointed out that this resource is, basically, non-finite, since it can be used over and over again without decreasing it. For example, once a technique has been developed it becomes part of the cultural fund of the health system. On the other hand, availability of knowledge techniques and technology have enormous implications for the utilization of other finite resources, particularly manpower and economic outlays.

3. The health system requires a contingent of personnel who operate within that system. This corpus includes all those whose work formally takes place within the health system or are directly contributory to that system. As hinted earlier, not only physicians and nurses, but technicians, aids, helpers, and those in auxiliary and ancillary occupations that are directly supportive of health personnel. It is thus empirically possible, for any society, to differentiate between those members of the labor force who are in the health system from all others; and within the former category, to distinguish between the different types of occupations and specialties; and among these, those who are active (and in what capacity), inactive, or in training.

4. The health system must receive from the larger society economic resources (in the form of capital and equipment) and compensation (in the form of transfer payments for services performed). The former (capital and equipment) makes it possible for the system to obtain the 'tools' it needs (or means of medical production, whether these be hospitals, drugs, instruments, and so on). The latter (transfer payments) makes it possible to acquire the services of personnel since even the most dedicated persons working full time in health, cannot attend to their own needs, such as food, housing, clothing, etc. It is theoretically possible, by aggregating all these resources (or expenses), to compute what percentage of the Gross National Product goes to health, and then to further redefine that percentage in terms of the different services or

subsectors of the health system (hospitals versus physicians' salaries, etc.).

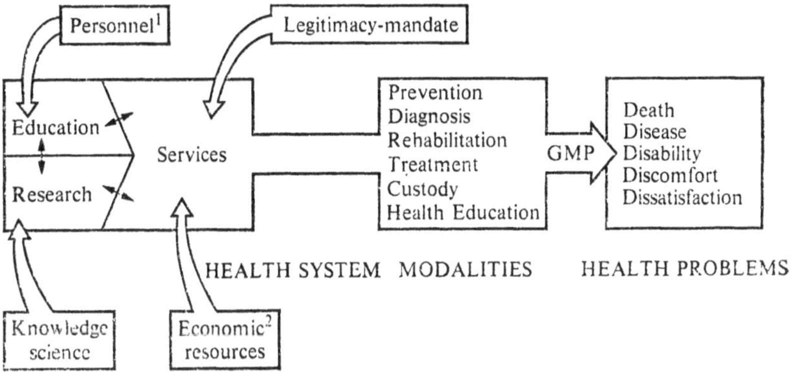

[1] For any society, as a percentage of the total active labor force.
[2] For any society, as a percentage of the Gross National Product.

Seen from this perspective, *the health system of any society may be described as that institutional mechanism that transforms or metabolizes what are generalized inputs (legitimacy, knowledge, untrained manpower, and economic resources) into specialized outputs, products, and services of relevance to the health concern of society.* Of these resources, two (manpower and economic outlays) are problematic, scarce and quantifiable, one (legitimacy), is not easily quantifiable though scarce, and one (knowledge) is basically non-finite once generated. The health system, furthermore, 'competes' with other systems for scarce resources. I use the expression 'compete' figuratively rather than literally. And when I say that any society 'allocates' scarce resources to one sector rather than another, I am refererring to both the managerial-political allocative processes of a society such as the Soviet Union, and the processes of a pluralistic system in which market factors of supply and demand co-exist with larger political decisions (such as in the U.S.). But regardless of the nature of this competition for, and allocation of, resources, one can compare one society with another to determine how much of the GNP and the manpower go to health as against other 'competing' systems. By the same token, it is also theoretically possible to compare internal allocations of the health system, among its three major components and among the different services it offers. I might add that there are considerable conceptual and methodological problems inherent in a comparative examination, and that in the final analysis one must compare each society *in its own terms* with other societies. There is, for example, no absolute definition of what a physician or a nurse or a hospital is like. But if society A reports a supply of x physicians per 10,000, and B society y physicians per 10,000, these are the terms of comparison.

The following diagram schematically represents the allocation of resources among competing sub-systems.

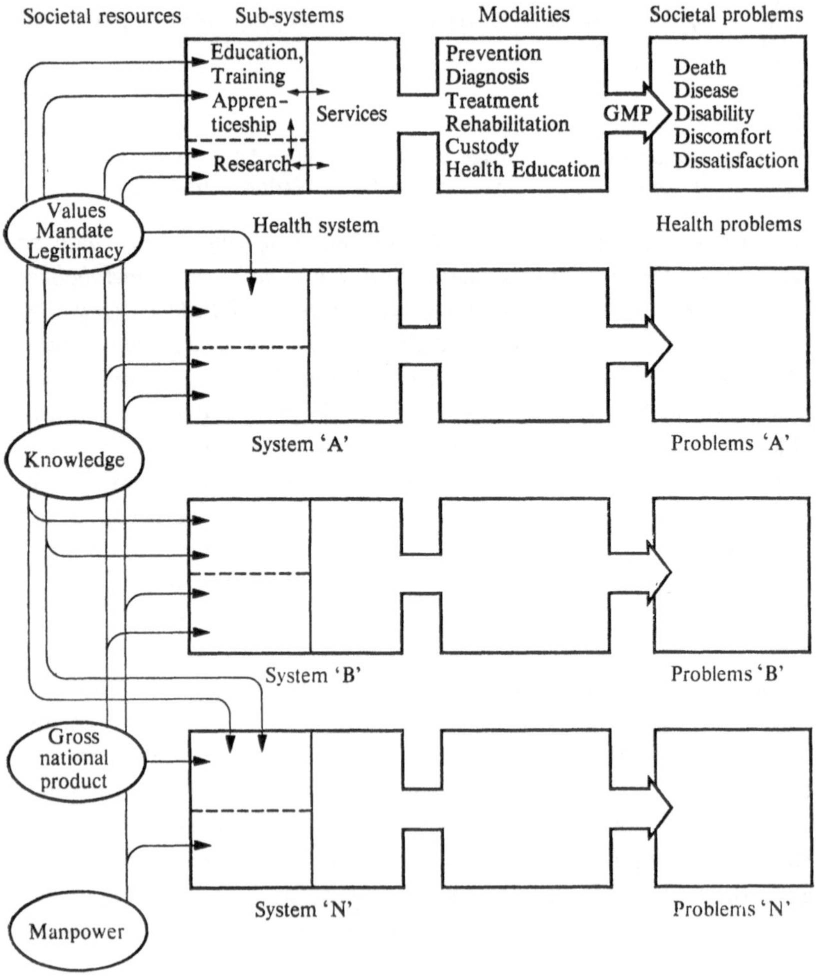

In an attempt to establish a typology of health systems as metabolizers of recources suitable for comparative examination, a major difficulty arises. How shall we tease out of the variety of existing systems a series of *ideal-types*? The following is a most tentative treatment of the subject. Let us, for the sake of argument, limit our examination to the health systems of modern societies rather than developing ones and let us establish the following rules:

1. Our scale of analysis must limit itself to the macro-sociological level, i.e. to an examination of the health systems of *national* societies, rather than regions or communities. The basic assumption is that these set the basic parameters for micro-structures.

2. The approach should be structural-functional in that it identifies a general functional need of society and seeks to identify the aggregate of specific structures that have arisen (or have been devised) to meet that need.

3. The approach should be dynamic in that it should identify these forces (extrinsic and intrinsic) to the health system that affect it and cause it to change (usually from a simple to a complex structure).

4. The scheme should be evolutionary or historical and see the health system today as but the contemporary form of a constantly changing societal mechanism.

At the descriptive level, to go back to the four inputs of resources that support the health system, I assume (generally speaking) that legitimacy and the knowledge components of contemporary health systems, are fairly universal. The variability, to be observed from a comparative analysis, derives from the manner in which the other two resources, manpower and economic inputs, are interwoven with each other and relate to the society, and indeed the manner in which health personnel are controlled and health facilities are owned. I would propose four types of discernible gross national patterns:

(1) The *pluralistic* health system: This system consists of a variety of coexisting institutional schemes for the provision of health and related services. Physicians work in private practice, group practice, or on salaries. Typically, the medical profession enjoys a great deal of autonomy in regulating its affairs and in professional matters. The ownership patterns for health facilities range from the private proprietary, to the voluntary (non-profit), cooperative or group, to public ownership (national,

regional, municipal, etc.). The health system of the United States (sometimes erroneously labelled non-system) best fits that description.

2. The *health insurance* system: To some degree this system resembles the pluralistic one with the exception that most financial transfers, to institutions and to practitioners, are made by third-party agencies, whether these be governmental units or other groups (labor unions, for example). Thus the insurance system, in its pure form, consists only of financial mechanisms, whereby either taxes, dues or contributions are collected from a population or a group, and then disbursed at the time of use, either directly to practitioners or institutions (as benefits) or to patients for part or total reimbursement for their medical and hospital expenses. The fact that third parties are responsible and accountable for disbursements potentially introduces an element of control over practitioners and institutions. However, physicians, as a rule, enjoy the same autonomy as in the pluralistic system. The health system of Western Europe (with the exception of Great Britain) and of Japan fit that definition.

(3) The *health service* system: A system where most facilities are owned outright by the polity (nationalized) and where most physicians, either in private practice (the greater part) or as hospital consultants, are paid from the state treasury in the form either of flat payments based on the size of patient panels (capitation) or salaries or sessional fees. The British National Health Service is prototypical. It should be noted that in this system physicians in community practice consider themselves as private practitioners with the right to choose which patients to accept, and patients have the right to choose their physicians. Physicians enjoy as much professional autonomy as in the previous two systems.

(4) The *socialized* health system: A system where all facilities are owned and managed by the state, and where almost all health personnel (from physicians on down) are state employees, salaried, tariffed, and paid from the state treasury. Physicians are usually responsible for a panel of patients assigned to them on a territorial or occupational basis. The amount of autonomy enjoyed by physicians as salaried state employees, while still considerable, is comparatively smaller than in the other three systems (for example in choosing where to practice). Eastern European and Soviet health systems belong to this type.

There are several issues and questions that this scheme suggests for comparative analysis. The following is only a partial list:

1. Where does the locus of control over the health system reside? By control, I mean here primarily allocative decisions of legitimacy and mandate, the setting of priorities and national policies for the health system, as against other systems, the flow of resources into the system, the management of medical installations, and control over the professional location and activities of health personnel. This then is first and foremost a 'political question'. It might readily be seen that the *pluralistic* system is considerably more difficult to control or manage than the system of *socialized medicine*, with the other two occupying intermediate positions. It is thus practically impossible for American society to control the costs of physicians' services or the aggregate bill the American public pays for these services. On the other hand, in a system where most physicians are salaried, such control is much more possible. It may be quite possible that, in the long run, a pluralistic system is a luxury that will price itself out. By nature, the system of socialized medicine would also be the most bureaucratized.

2. Granted that the health systems of industrialized societies have risen against the background of widely different historical, traditional, cultural, economic, and political conditions, and have given rise to a variety of schemes (four of which I outlined earlier), is it possible that the 'convergence hypothesis', applied to industrial society in general, might also apply to the health systems of that type of society? This would seem to be the case particularly since these systems are subject to the same (though not uniform) universal constraints of increased effective demands for services, fuelled by ideological and political factors and by the increased availability and applicability of bio-medical technology and pressures for their utilization.

3. Do the health systems of industrialized society (regardless of their institutional forms) experience faster growth in size relative to most other sub-systems of society, and do they experience an increased internal differentiation as a result of the explosion of knowldge and technology? Do they as such, increasingly face the problem of the management and the administration of large groups of diverse qualified health personnel, and what are the implications of such pressures?

4. Do the supportive (psychological) pastoral aspects of medical care tend to be squeezed out by the increased application of scientific knowledge and biomedical technology, creating an 'emotional gap' in the care of patients which physicians are increasingly unable or unwilling to fill? What are the implications of this possible trend in societies which are increasingly rationalized (and thereby, increasingly depersonalized) and where the individual is increasingly isolated and alienated? Will this lead to a formal further differentiation in medical roles between scientific physicians and humane physicians? The latter becoming a specialist in generalities, those mandate might not only include the emotional aspects of patienthood, but also the coordination and technical integration of increasingly specialized, narrow and depersonalized services.

5. What is the evolving balance between the health system and other sub-systems in industrial society in view of the rapid growth of the health system, and its increasing claim on scarce resources to perform its mandated tasks? Indeed a comprehensive sociological view must perforce set the health system alongside *other* functionally relevant systems rather than hold it (as health advocates are wont for understandable reasons) as the center of the societal universe around which everything else should revolve. It may well be that in the perspective of the functional needs of modern society, the health system deserves a lower priority ranking than many people are willing to grant it. One must then be aware, at all times, of the 'opportunity costs' involved in investing into the health system, and the importance of trade-offs, whether these be in housing, diet, social welfare, general education, and so on.

In this paper, I have touched only on a few major issues related to the health system of modern society and its relationship to the social system and to other sub-systems. I think these questions are important to an understanding not only of health problems and how they are met, but also to the nature and structure of modern, industrial and industrializing society.

Appendix A

PREVIOUS PERSONAL PAPERS

Technology, Medicine and Society: Effectiveness Differentiation and Depersonalization (Cambridge; Program on Technology and Society, Harvard 1968), 151 pp. mimeo.).

'Allied Health Personnel: The Impact of Technology and Increased Demand', in: E. I. Purkis and U. F. Matthews (eds.), *Medicine in the University and the Community of the Future: Proceedings of the Scientific Session Marking the Centennial of the Faculty of Medicine, Dalhousie University*, Dalhousie University, Halifax 1969, pp. 50–52.

'The Health Care System of Industrialized Society: The Disappearance of the General Practitioner and Some Implications', in: Everett I. Mendelsohn, Judith P. Swazey and Irene Taviss (eds.), *Human Aspects of Biological Innovation*, Harvard University Press, Cambridge 1971, pp. 156–180. Also as: 'The Medical System and Industrial Society: Structural Changes and Internal Differentiation in American Medicine', in: Allan Sheldon, Frank Baker and Curt McLaughlin (eds.), *Systems and Medical Care*, Massachusetts Institute of Technology Press, Cambridge 1970, pp. 143–181.

'Stability and Change in the Medical System: Medicine in the Industrial Society', in: Alex Inkeles and Bernard Barber (eds.), *Stability and Social Chance*, Little–Brown, Boston 1971, pp. 30–60.

'The Manpower Crisis in American Medicine: Analysis and Proposed Remedy', *American Family Physician* **5** (1972) 192–199 (with J. Gershon-Cohen).

'Health as a 'Public Utility' or the 'Maintenance of Capacity' Soviet Society', presented at the *Symposium on the Social Consequences of Modernization in Socialist Countries*, Salzburg, Austria, 1975 (to be published in a book by the Johns Hopkins University Press, 1976).

'The concept of the 'Health System' at the Macrosociological Level', *Social Science and Medicine* 7 (October 1973) 763–785.

'Prospects for the Comparative Sociology of Medicine: An Effort at Conceptualization', in: Margaret S. Archer (ed.), *Current Research in Sociology*, Supplementary Volume 1 to *Current Sociology*, Mouton, The Hague 1974, pp. 147–183.

REFERENCE

* This is not an original paper but a summarization of my work so far and a slightly revised version of my 'The Concept of the Health System at the Macrosociological Level', *Social Science and Medicine* 7 (October 1973) 763–785. Permission was kindly granted by the editors of *Social Science and Medicine*. For greater detail and documentation of previous work, see Appendix A.

THE ADAPTATION PATTERNS OF THE MEDICAL SYSTEM AND SOCIAL CHANGE

ZDZISŁAW BIZOŃ

Department of Psychiatry, Medical School, Warsaw, Poland

In order for a social institution or social organization, or, to put it more generally, any social system, to survive and develop in the changing environment, it must be both functional and adaptive. The term 'functional' means here that the system pursues the goals for the implementation of which it has been established. These goals are defined 'from above', by important needs and values of a broader and superior suprasystem, of which the system is a component part. Because the suprasystem is simultaneously the environment of the system, these goals are for the system external goals. In other words, *functionality* is a kind of a relation [1] between the system and the suprasystem (or, to put it more precisely, between the system and its environment). The '*adaptiveness*' of the system is understood as a certain dynamic quality which resides in the capability of the system to regulate its relations with the suprasystem in time, and correspondingly to the changing goals and functions of the suprasystem as a whole (e.g. in accordance with changing needs and values). To put it briefly, adaptiveness amounts to functionality in time.

All the above statements and definitions apply equally to the *medical system.* [2] The basic unit of the medical system is something referred to as medical action or medical intervention. (A thorough explanation of this concept would exceed the scope of this paper, therefore it has been assumed that its intuitive sense is clear enough for the subjects to be discussed later on.) The basic task of medical action (intervention), that is the primary, traditional, and minimum task, is the 'healing of diseases' and/or the alleviation of pain. With the passage of time these tasks were extending and their current maxima are being formulated differently. The tasks of medical action as the basic of the medical system, are convergent with the external goals of the system as a whole. In our times, the chief agents (actors) of these interventions are medical professionals.

All the same, we know that medical intervention could not for many centuries fulfil the tasks set for it because the means and techniques applied were usually ineffective and sometimes even harmful. Until the 19th century medicine was characterized by an almost complete ineffectiveness in the biotechnical sense. This, in turn, implies that such a system could not fulfil its external goals and was therefore basically dysfunctional (*basic dysfunctionality* is understood here as ineffectiveness in the sense of an elementary incapability of attaining the goals).

In the light of what has already been said, an intriguing question arises: how was it possible for such a basically dysfunctional system as medicine to survive for so many centuries and maintain its social viability? What is more, how could it grow, develop and create a socially powerful profession and other structures within itself? The answer to this question can be found in the specific *adaptive mechanisms* of this system. The system was capable of adaptation and development, despite its basic dysfunction, mainly because of the interaction of two factors:

(i) specific psycho-social defence mechanisms which made it possible to conceal this dysfunction of the system or to make it appear functional, and

(ii) the multi-directional, intensive and effective social activities of these medical groups and occupations which are the actors of medical intervention. These social activities made it possible to counterbalance and compensate for the basic dysfunction of the system.

We shall devote more attention to those two factors since they are of fundamental importance for the maintenance of the system and its adaptive dynamics. They kept the dysfunctional medical system in existence as a part of social reality, and maintained its functional (apparent) image in the social consciousness, and probably also in consciousness of the actors themselves.

As regards (i), *defence mechanisms* protect the system against any threats arising from its dysfunctionality. Thus, they make for the avoidance of external control, and the prevention or reduction of the undesirable results of such control (e.g. criticism). This can be done most easily by concealing the very fact of this dysfunctionality by providing the suprasystem – for example – with inadequate or false information about itself; in other words – by blocking or distorting informational output. Defence mechanisms are, at the same time, system maintenance mechanisms supporting the system as a separate unit and making it appear functional. They play the adaptive role through a pseudo-regulation and not a real regulation of functional relations between the system and the environment. This is, however, a provisional ('emergency') adaptation. i.e. pseudo-adaptation. In the long run they hinder any real adaptation by intensifying the existing dysfunctions of the system or giving rise to new ones.

Most patterns of defence are similar to the so-called personality defence mechanisms which emerge in cases of fear or conflict, and have already been described in psychology. The mechanisms we are speaking about differ from personality defence mechanisms in that they concern not the individual but groups, social organizations or even larger and more complex systems. Here are a few examples of the most common defence mechanisms in the field of medicine:

(a) confusing activities with goals, which leads to cyclic thinking, i.e. activities are assumed to be 'goal-directed'. The most frequent pattern is as follows: 'since what we are doing is being done for the purpose of curing, we do cure'. This is reflected, for example, in various 'therapeutic labels', when an optional or generally useful enterprise is called 'therapy' (balneotherapy, music therapy, occupational therapy, etc.). This is similar to the use of the term 'resocialization' in reference to the presence and work of a prisoner in jail;

(b) reformulating the objectives for action or shifting them to the areas less liable to control (e.g. from the primary task: the reduction of diseases and disabilities, to the less easily defined task: the promotion of health);

(c) giving an exaggeratedly unfavourable prognosis when undertaking medical treatment, so that later on lack of success will be treated as a partial success;

(d) transferring the sources or causes of the diseases, which medicine fails to cope with, to factors outside the human organism or beyond medical control (the environment, 'constitutional factors', civilization). A typical example is the concept of so-called 'civilization diseases' which, at the same time, rationalizes the absence of etiological knowledge and justifies the ineffectiveness of medical control over certain diseases. Moreover, it also fulfils other 'clever' functions: it explains the dysfunction of the system by the faults of the suprasystem and admonishes the supra-system whenever the dynamics of the system lag behind that of the supra-system (in this way it sanctions or justifies the delays of the system).

Obviously the number and variety of defence mechanisms observed in the field of medicine are enormous. They are connected with the various forms of activity practised by the medical profession both in the past and in the present (in order to illustrate this more graphically, present-day examples have been given). They often underlie various manipulative devices and strategies. We shall return to some of these mechanisms further on.

As regards (ii), the danger of being charged with ineffectiveness of medical intervention is of primary importance to medical practitioners. For effectiveness is the foundation or social *raison d'être* of the profession, not to mention the additional advantages gained from it by professionals. Therefore intensive, multi-faceted *activity in the social arena* is of particular importance to them. First of all, it provides an extra safeguard against medical failures by other means, e.g. organizational or political. Secondly, it is a medium for the transmission of various favourable effects of defence mechanisms into social reality. The following main dimensions of this activity can be distinguished: social-organizational and political, ideological, axiological and scientific.

As a result of these activities, the profession managed to counterbalance its ineffectiveness in influencing the natural, biological reality by exerting an effective influence on social reality; to replace the objective dysfunctionality of the medical system with the myth of its functionality in the social consciousness; to substitute for biotechnically ineffective action sociotechnically effective activities. It must be admitted that this was done with masterly skill.

1. SOCIAL AND POLITICAL DIMENSIONS

It would be no exaggeration to say that the history of the profession of medicine has been that of an unceasing struggle for status and power. In this long process the main role was played by various prestige-building activities, such as: seeking support and protection from various persons (princes, bishops, etc.), groups or institutions representing an independent political power; eliminating, subordinating or controlling competing groups of healers, negotiating with the state authorities and getting them formally to legalize the rights, privileges and sphere of competences of medicine as a profession. The profession of medicine owes its successes in achieving and consolidating its autonomy and prestige to the political strategies and tactics applied rather than to the effects of medical practice. The techniques summed up in the present-day term 'social engineering' have always been an object of great concern and attention on the part of medical men. Since the ancient times most of the deontological codes or so-called professional ethics have been for the most part collections of socio-technical prescriptions. The socio-political aspects of the activities of the profession do not have to be described here since they are well known to specialists in the sociology of medicine. They have been discussed and excellently analyzed by some sociologists, in particular by Freidson[3] and Bollough.[4] I should only like to add that political means and activities have met with open approval on the part of contemporary community medicine. In community health programmes, and especially in community mental health programmes, they are recommended and popularized as being among the more important methods to be used. They constitute the basis of social action, consultation work in various fields, etc. Sometimes the suggested practices are given their proper names (e.g. 'political psychiatry'[5]). In these programmes, princes or bishops have been replaced by various community leaders, and local authorities. And it is probably not accidental that such programmes are being developed most intensively in the relatively least effective branch of medical practice, i.e. in psychiatry.

The fact that the profession reinforces its position in the societal arena by socio-political means, cannot but influence the way in which its activities are perceived by others as well as itself. It makes the profession believe that its high social prestige is the result of the effectiveness of its medical interventions. (After all, many dictators have also thought that the respect shown them had its source in their satisfying the most essential needs of their people.) The same fact also shapes indirectly social consciousness and the perception of medical activity. Social consciousness, however, can be influenced directly by presenting suitably favourable picture of medicine to the public, i.e.:

2. PROPAGANDA ACTIVITY

The rich arsenal of propaganda methods and instruments is, of course, very extensive and is not limited to verbal ones. Here are some others:

(a) The creation and dissemination of certain stereotypes of the role of the doctor and his personality traits; presenting him as omnipotent, morally unblemished and embodying all the virtues (altruism, self-sacrifice, wisdom, etc.). This exaggerated, idealized image of a doctor (defence mechanism: sublimation, hypercompensation?) is frequently propagated by the mass media. Its results are often dysfunctional in other respects. They lead to an increased demand for medical help for various non-medical reasons, and easily frustrate the excessive, unrealistic expectations of patients.

(b) Suggesting the importance and absolute necessity of medical intervention by presenting horrifying consequences if medical action is not taken in various situations.

(c) Direct participation by representatives of medicine in the most important and/or tragic situations in life; birth, death, calamities, etc. They strongly stimulate the perception and emotions of laymen and appeal to their imagination. A similar role is played by many other spectacular accessories of medical practice (e.g. the 'teatrum anatomicum' in the past, or the siren of a hurrying ambulance in our own times). There is another process which is also a derivative of propaganda work: that of stimulating medical needs and shaping a particular medical vision of man and the world in the mind of the public, i.e. the process of medical indoctrination. Its effects can often be easily discerned in certain medical concepts and models imposed upon social policies in various fields.

3. VALUE MANIPULATIONS

The role played by this activity can hardly be overestimated. It represents one of the most disabling weapons against external control and criticism. The more common, if at the same time perverse, manipulation patterns include: (a) Blurring the differences between, or identifying general, social or supreme values with the particular values adopted for the use of the profession; identifying the interests of the profession with those of the patient (client) and treatment. This is reflected in the frequently proclaimed thesis that whatever undermines the prestige of the doctor, does harm to the patient as well. As a result of identifying the prestige of the doctor with medical treatment itself, everything which will be recognized as detrimental to the prestige of the doctor (e.g. attempts at criticizing certain oversights) will also be presented as harmful to the patient. (b) Changing the interpretation of some ambiguously worded principles (apparently of a purely moral or ethical type), or using them in different, specific contexts. The fundamental principle proclaimed in medicine, '*primum non nocere*' which is a tribute to its author's circumspection, can be understood not only in moral but also in socio-technical (social engineering) sense. All depends upon which end of the doctor-patient relationship is stressed in a given situation, and the implied 'good of the patient' can easily be used as a screen to protect the 'good of the profession'. For instance in his book *Medicine in Transition*, Galdston[6] devotes a whole chapter, entitled *Primum non nocere*, to... defending the system of private practice and criticizing the harmful idea of a nationalized health service. (c) The inclusion of various values, which have been held either universally or at a given time, but other than health, in the sphere of medical competence, e.g. beauty (cosmetic surgery), sporting achievements (sports medicine), youthfulness, vigour ('rejuvenating' treatment), or sexual satisfaction (sexology as a branch of medicine).

4. 'SCIENTIFIC' MANIPULATIONS

Important defensive functions can also be fulfilled by the manipulation of terms, ideas, notions or figures. This defensive role in the medical system is played chiefly by a subsystem of medical knowledge (obviously this is only one of its functions). The numerous shortcomings of medical knowledge as a science are well known (the lack of operationalization of concepts, the prevalence of logically flawed interpretation models – e.g. '*post hoc ergo propter hoc*', etc.). They result partly from the fact that knowledge plays here, as in other practical sciences, a subordinate and secondary role in relation to practice. In the 'knowledge-action' relation, priority obviously belongs to action. In medicine, the shifting of emphasis onto action is even stronger than in other practical sciences because of the imperative character of the situations in which the action is undertaken, and the values involved in it. The urgent necessity of taking action pushes the question of its rationale into the background and does not favour the development of reliable knowledge (for instance so called 'empirical therapies'). Speculative or ad hoc explanations have many virtues when compared to it. What is more, it can become an inconvenient luxury limiting freedom of action. One might say that one of the 'diabolic' hypotheses formulated by Wilkins [7] in a slightly different context (that 'the amount of information tends to be inversely related to the willingness to take action') has been fully confirmed by the latest tendency to engage in large scale prophylactic programs having no knowledge of not only the causes but even the nature of what they are supposed to prevent (the field of mental health is the best example). They seem to be an expression of the mechanisms whereby certain conceptual models become fixed in those fields in which medicine once achieved its most conspicuous successes (prevention of infectious diseases). Another important fact is that medical knowledge represents, to a high degree, a mixture of cognitive and normative statements, a mixture of information and evaluative interpretations. Therefore, various medical 'theories' are very well fitted for the fulfilment of various defensive functions: for justification or rationalization of the action taken, or of the ineffectiveness of the methods applied, etc.

Occasionally various statistical data and their interpretation are characterized by serious defensive biases. Many apparently documented and popular statements, which ascribe various favourable trends in the fields of health or life (e.g. an increase in the average lifespan) exclusively to medical interventions may often arouse serious doubts; the more so since analyses which take into account the role of control variables are very rare in medicine.[8] No wonder that those diseases with decreasing incidence rates are not referred to as civilization diseases.

* *

*

For nearly a hundred years the relations between the medical system and its environment (at both inter-system and system-suprasystem levels) have been undergoing significant changes which have resulted in serious dysfunctions, thus forcing that *system to seek new adaptive patterns* or dramatic defences of the status quo.

The first really significant successes of medicine at the turn of the 19th and 20th centuries, especially its objectively demonstrated effectiveness in the control of many infectious diseases, had manifold consequences, not only for medical theory and practice but also for the place of medicine in the society. Here we shall note only some of them. First of all people began to expect and demand more of medicine, and that in turn resulted in increased pressure on the medical system. But even more important was the fact that medicine became *the concern of government.* With the possibility of controlling some diseases on a mass scale, it became evident that health has ceased to be a personal matter of an individual and its control the sole business of the medical profession. The vital political, military, economic and demographic interests of the state would not allow it. Therefore, the problem of health became a matter of political significance, first on a national and later on (especially after the Second World War) on an international scale. This situation led to confrontation and conflict between two social institutions, which previously were allies: medicine (strictly speaking the institutional power and interests of the profession of medicine) and the state (political power). In the course of this confrontation the medical profession at first defended itself by making partial concessions to the state (e.g. public health). Where this was not enough the course and solutions of the conflict were different, depending on the relative strength of the two antagonists and their willingness to use it, and on where, when, and in what circumstances the conflict arose, and on many other factors which will not be considered here. As is known, such a confrontation led in some countries to nationalization of the health service. In other countries – the best example of which is the United States – the profession could effectively resist the state's pressure maintaining its institutional autonomy and its traditional free market pattern of practice.

The above-mentioned phenomena and processes were of course but a tiny fragment of more fundamental and global social macro-processes, namely the rapid and profound changes taking place in the entire suprasystem. It would be impossible not only to describe but even to mention all the *effects produced on medicine* by such macroprocesses, as: technological and scientific progress, industrialization, urbanization, economic and socio-organizational development, demographic growth, the expansion of education, the spread of literacy, the changes in ideological orientations and value systems.

The immense changes within the suprasystem constituted the most powerful challenge to the adaptive mechanisms of the medical system. To many of them the system reacted functionally, 'convergently' by means of parallel processes and changes within its sub-systems: by general growth and organizational differentiation (the increasing complexity of organizational structures), introduction and application of new technologies, professional specialization; the development of scientific research and the exponential growth of information; the mass production approach and routinization of services; overconcentration of medical manpower in large urban centres, etc.

Many other changes and elements of the new situation quite clearly were either not recognized or not assimilated by the system. This applies in particular to important changes in the social situation (democratization, the increased significance and power of the mass consumer, the reduction of the intellectual gap between the doctor and the majority of his patients, the higher demands and more critical attitude on the part of consumers, etc.) and in value dimensions.

The system, therefore, reacted to environmental changes in a selective way; assimilated some of them (new technologies, organizational patterns) and rejected the others by giving standard responses to changing social needs, or by remaining completely insensitive to them. This reflected a specific inflexibility of the system which sprang from an overstructuralization and increased autonomy of some of its subsystems, an excessive stability (ultrahomeostasis) gained in the course of the previous process of adaptation, in earlier historical periods. This applies chiefly to the institutional-professional subsystem. Traditional institutional structures of the system were considerably strengthened and consolidated (e.g. the patterns and norms of professional training). Above all the medical profession acquired high status, prestige and considerable autonomy. The moment the process of professionalization was completed, concern for external goals was much less than for internal ones. In addition, the achieved real effectivenes of medical intervention in some fields became a reinforcement for its prestige and status. The medical profession became more conservative and therefore less inclined to make concessions and compromises. A large amount of the professional energy did not have any longer to be focussed on external activity in order to prove its *raison d'être*. Moreover, the *discrepancy* between institutional-professional objectives and general social goals was growing. The system as a whole became not only more rigid but also more self-sufficient than outer-directed. What was changing was the periphery and not the core.

Thus the medical system had to face a new extraordinarily difficult situation. Above all health needs grew considerably, as an effect of the macro-social processes mentioned previously. The demands made of medicine also grew considerably as a result of the greater expectations aroused by the increased effectiveness of medical interventions and the greater publicity accorded to medical successes. The growth of health needs and societal demands were the tasks which the medical system was unable to cope with for many reasons.

This concerns both those factors which acted morphostatically on the system (the stiffening of its institutional-professional subsystem, the traditional pattern of practice, persisting defence mechanisms) and those which were the product of a new dynamism of the system in some of its dimensions according to corresponding macrosocietal processes (new technologies, increasing organizational expansion and complexity). They raised new barriers along the path leading to satisfaction of social demands: e.g. financial (the increased cost of health care) or geographical (inappropriate distribution of medical manpower).

As a result of all these factors, a dramatic gap emerged between social demands and the ability of the medical system to meet them. In this way, in addition to ineffectiveness, another basic disjunction of the system was revealed: its inability to satisfy the health needs of a considerable part of the population. Thus the system demonstrated an unfitness, which was not so much technical as social. This kind of its dysfunction could be defined as *social inadequacy or insufficiency.*

The objective increase in the effectiveness of medical intervention and, to an even larger extent, the propagation of its new possibilities, not only did not help to reduce this dysfunction but made it more dramatic. Besides, many of the previously formed defence mechanisms against ineffectiveness turned out to be inadequate to the new situation. Some of them tended to widen the gap and to increase the insufficiency of the system through positive feed-back loops. The view was generally taken that medicine was potentially able to deliver much more than it actually did, and what is more, that medicine was able to deliver more than it was willing to deliver. So this time the dysfunction of the system was easily detected by the suprasystem.

Where the gap between the theoretical effectiveness of the medical system (parallel to rapid technological progress) and real efficiency in satisfying the health needs of the broad mass of the population was greatest to the disadvantage of the latter, the stronger the pressure of various social forces on the system to seek a solution. This was very characteristic of the U.S. medical system. The previous conflict between political requirements of the establishment and traditional obstructing attitudes of the profession of medicine revived again.

A peculiar social game was undertaken between (a) the establishment threatened by internal social problems and criticism, and (b) the medical profession constantly under threat of an attack by the state against its prerogatives and interests and, at the same time, exposed to severe criticism for being socially backward.

This process was a fairly long one in which both sides used or tried to use various means and tactics, and in which a whole range of defence mechanisms appeared constituting a chain of mutually interdependent actions and counteractions.

This game could be presented in simplified form in the shape of the following quasi-dialogue:

PROBLEM: The extent of unsatisfied health needs anddemands in the general population (as indicated *inter alia* by epidemiological surveys).

STATE AUTHORITIES (GOVERNMENT):

– Medicine is inefficient. The preservation of an anachronistic mode of organization of health care based on practitioners charge fees for individualized services is highly inadequate in coping with health needs on a wider social scale.

– We are doing everything possible to meet your needs and are making increasing financial outlays for this purpose, but your demands are growing incessantly. Our resources, however, are limited. There are other important, competing needs which we have to satisfy.

– Medicine is indifferent to social problems. The medical profession is exclusively concerned with guaranteeing its own interests. The costs of your services are too high and therefore unaccessible to the poorer social strata. We must look after the public interest and protect the health of all, including the underprivileged.

– Health is not a privilege of the chosen few but the right of every citizen. The state is responsible for securing health care to all citizens. This is in the general interest of society and is the business of the state.

PROFESSION OF MEDICINE:

– We could be more efficient and effective if we had the appropriate resources and supplies. The government shows too little concern for health and development of medicine, and the funds it provides are inadequat.

– Effective copingewith many health problems depends on the reduction of social deprivations and unfavourable environmental factors for which the medical profession does not feel itself responsible.

– The solving of social problems is not our business but the state's. Our duty is to care for the interests oj the individual, for the good of the patient. The costs of our services must be high if they are to be of high quality. The state is mainly interested in the quantity of services while we are concerned with their quality.

– Health is the individual's personal affair. A man, as af ree and responsible being, should himself decide about his health and treatment.

– etc

As a result of this social game between the state and the political interests of the establishment on the one hand, and the traditional institution of medicine and interests of the medical profession on the other, a *new adaptive pattern* of the medical system is emerging, which seems to be a compromise advantageous to both sides. It is, of course, no accident that this pattern was initiated and is developing on a broad scale in the U.S.A. Its programme is, I am sure, sufficiently well known in its basic essentials for a description to be unnecessary.

This programme is a compromise for it eliminates such contradictions as: 'health is a personal affair' vs. 'health is a national affair', or 'medicine is responsible for the inadequacy of helath care' vs. 'the state is responsible for the inadequacy of health care' by shifting the burden of responsibility onto local authorities and community resources: '*health is a community affair*'.[9] It relieves the profession of medicine from criticism and moral responsibility for its social dysfunctionality, and acts as a safeguard against central control by the state.

The advantages for the state are also evident: it relieves to a considerable degree the central authorities from the burden of health care; prevents, to some extent, social criticism of the government for shortcomings of social policies (at least in the field of health policy); creates a hope for management of some social problems through an integration of health services with other public services; and also – which is perhaps less important – it frees the state of the necessity of engaging in a dispute with the profession of medicine, with the help of unpopular arguments contradictory to the tenets of prevailing ideology (individualism, free market, etc).

Nor is it surprising that the U.S. Federal Authorities not only declare their support but also offer real help in developing the community health programme (as is seen for example in J. F. Kennedy's support of community mental health centres legislation).

Equally, on the part of the medical profession the new community health care programme met with very little open criticism, at least so far, and there is no comparison with the massive and violent attacks which were once levelled at the idea of nationalization. The absence of sharp criticism might seem surprising because the principles and postulates of community health care appear to present a severe test for the traditional role and status of the profession of medicine, and the proposed model differs radically from previous ones. The explanation for this apparent contradiction is in my opinion twofold: 1. the prospects of benefit for the medical profession are, in spite of everything, very considerable, 2. the new adaptive pattern of the medical system is, to a great extent, an expression of defence mechanisms released by external pressures and conflict situations resulting from the dysfunctionality of the system.

1) The first of these problems will be considered briefly by taking as an example one of the main postulates of community medicine, namely the principle of comprehensive care and team work in the context of its possible advantages and disadvantages for medicine.

The requirement that a doctor participates in a team of representatives of various professions and public services solving health and social problems on the basis of equal partnership, seems to endanger his personal prestige and to be at variance with his stereotyped role. This situation, however, opens up certain advantageous prospects for the profession, such as: the playing of a leading and dominant role in the team; the engagement of other members of the team in the purely medical tasks; the doctor's taking all the credit for achievements of the team, and shifting the responsibility for any failures on other team-members. Thus, the profession of medicine has a chance to subordinate other, partly competing, public services to medicine (as happened with surgeons and barbers in the past). Finally, it enables medicine to enter new, non-medical fields and to rule over them. As we see, these benefits are fairly numerous; whereas the danger of an eventual loss of prestige and power in the new field is more than doubtly. As Anthony F. Panzetta rightly remarks: "...It is within the nature of the powerful to gravitate towards new power. It is therefore quite natural for medicine to see itself as the centerpiece in the broad-spectrum comprehensive care package...".[9]

2) From among the many *defence mechanisms* which have not yet been mentioned and appear to underlie some postulates and practices of community health programmes, I would like to draw attention to the three main ones;

a) '*The setting of over-ambitious targets*"[11] evident in the very large scale plans and multiple objectives of these programmes, which transcend current possibilities and the means available for their realization. This mechanism performs many defensive functions, e.g. by multiplying tasks, it justifies the difficulty of performance, or the lack of present or future success; by safeguarding against a possible charge of inadequate effort and action;

b) '*overdemocratization*' [12] – a tendency characterizing some socio-therapeutic methods and orientations (e.g. the principles of democratization and communality applied in 'therapeutic commuinty' programmes) within the framework of community health care. This seems to be a manifestation of a fear of being accused of domination and autocratic tendencies and, at the same time, a specific kind of 'reaction formation' of the traditional authoritarianism of the medical professionals;

c) '*guilt reducing strategy*' [13] expressing itself in the intensive development of programmes aimed first and foremost at underprivileged groups (the poor, ethnic minorities, black ghettos). These programmes might also be interpreted as "a rapid run from *noblesse oblige* to *mea culpa*" [14] on the part of some professional groups.

Obviously, the process of formation of the 'community health care' model was also influenced by many other factors not considered here. Not all of them are peculiar to the society in which the new adaptive model of the medical system arise, i.e. to the U.S. This problem, however, is a separate topic. It is also possible that community orientation is a minor expression of a more fundamental process of social evolution of the global supra-system from '*complex Gesellschaft*' to '*neo-Gemeinschaft*' [15] of the post-industrial era. It is difficult to make any meaningful judgement in the matter. As it is, it is difficult to answer the simple question: do community medicine and community health care constitute the real socialization of medicine, or rather a 'medicalization' of social problems?

REFERENCES

[1] All structural and functional relations at sub-system level and their regulation will not be considered in this paper.

[2] Most generally speaking, the medical system – as we understand it – comprises: a) institutional norms and organized basic patterns of behaviour; b) occupational or professional groups and organizations of people; c) their activities (patterns of practice and organization of health care services); d) medical knowledge. Such a broadly understood system seems to be a complex of systems rather than a complex system. However, for the sake of simplicity we shall be discussing it in terms of a single system.

[3] Eliot Freidson, a) *Profession of Medicine – A Study of the Sociology of Applied Knowledge*, Dodd, Mead a. Co., New York 1970; b) *Professional Dominance – The Social Structure of Medical Care*, Atherton Press, New York, 1970.
[4] Vern L. Bollough, *The Development of Medicine as a Profession*, Hafner, New York, 1966.
[5] See e.g. Brown and Long, 'Psychosocial Politics of the Community Mental Health Movement, in: F. C. Redlich (ed.), *Social Psychiatry*, The Williams a. Wilkins, Baltimore 1969, pp. 289–305.
[6] Iago Galdston, *Medicine in Transition*, The University of Chicago Press, Chicago 1965, Chapter 12, pp. 188–212.
[7] Leslie T. Wilkins, *Social Deviance – Social Policy, Action and Research*, Tavistock Publication, London 1964, p. 30. One of three hypotheses, which has been raised with respect to research and action in the social field.
[8] E. g. V. Navarro discusses a number of such works concerning the interpretation of mortality in different countries, and writes: "Indeed, except in a very few instances, we do not know the relationship between health services and reduction or control of mortality", 'System Analysis in the Health Field', in: E. O. Attinger (ed.), *Global System Dynamics*, Karger, Basel 1970, p. 292.
[9] 'Health is a Community Affair', Report of the National Commission on Community Health Services, Harvard University Press, Cambridge, Mass. 1966.
[10] Anthony F. Panzetta, *Community Mental Health – Myth and Reality*, Lea a. Febinger, Philadelphia 1971, p. 103.
[11, 12] Such defence mechanisms are described, for the first time – as far as I know – by Cyril Sofer in his study on the process of organizational change, *The Organizational from Within – A Comparative Study of Social Institutions Based on a Sociotherapeutic Approach*, Tavistock Publications, London 1961, pp. 145–170.
[13] The concept of guilt reducing strategy' in the context of community mental health programmes was presented by Panzetta, *op. cit.*, p. 66.
[14] Quoted after Panzetta, *op. cit.* p. 66.
[15] Such a model of societal evolution is presented e.g. by T. R. Young in his book: *The New Sources of Self*, Pergamon Press, Oxford 1972. He writes: "...Societies, like all systems, evolve in order to adapt to their environment as it changes, or they cease to exist. It is our opinion that a more complete model for this evolution is Gemeinschaft to Gesellschaft to complex Gesellschaft to neo-Gemeinschaft...".

APPLICATIONS OF ORGANIZATIONAL THEORY: MODELS OF ORGANIZATION AND SERVICE FOR HEALTH CARE*

ELIOT FREIDSON

Department of Sociology, New York University, New York, N.Y., U.S.A.

Citizens of the United States may think that their country alone is in the grip of a crisis in health care, since those who are Cassandras about medicine in the U.S. use international comparisons of such things as infant mortality rates to show the comparatively low standing of the health care in their affluent nation and, by implication, the lack of problems in others. But the sense of crisis, or at least serious problem, seems to be rather widely distributed, as this very conference suggests. And the character of the problem has shifted.

The contemporary problem of health care is not, by and large, a problem of medical science, as it was when the knowledge and technology for controlling infectious disease and repairing physical damage did not exist. Rather, contemporary concern has shifted from the medical-technical discoveries needed to allow the control of health problems to the means of organizing health manpower to assure that known medical techniques are made available to all the people who need them. An international journal devoted to the problem of delivering health service has appeared, and the World Health Organization is undertaking the development of a new 'Division for Strengthening of Health Services'.

Thus, the problem of health service delivery does not focus on the medical science and technique which physicians learn in medical school, nor do physicians have any special expertise in dealing with this problem. Of course, the problem involves physicians and other health workers. How they think of themselves, what working conditions they believe they need in order to do their work in ways they consider proper, and the social organization of the institutions of practice in which they work are actually part of the problem. But it is their role as *participants* in the problem, not experts *about* the problem which gives these health workers relevance. The scientific variables are primarily psychological, sociological, political and economic, not biomedical. The problem of health care delivery, in short, is a problem of social science and not medical science.

What are the variables of the problem, and how might we consider realistic ways of dealing with them? To answer such a question we need some comparatively parsimonious way of analyzing the issues which does not confuse ephemeral administrative detail for constant problems or patterns. Unfortunately, general public policy positions assert only the most general rationales, and the administrative schemes designed to implement them are created pragmatically in the context of a concrete political and economic situation. But I think that our understanding of the problems of both policy and administration in the delivery of health services can be clarified by systematic analysis based on sociological thinking. In this paper I shall suggest one way such understanding can be gained.

To this end I shall draw on some of the more recent ideas in the literature of organizational theory, and more particularly on the rapidly developing area which might, for convenience, be called occupational theory. Those two areas represent distinctly different ways of looking at the same processes. Organizational theory is preoccupied with the analysis of concrete work institutions, or organizations, their administrative structure, and the performance and productivity of the managers and workers who serve them. Occupational theory is concerned with the reciprocal processes by which tasks are organized into jobs and occupations and by which occupations define, organize and stabilize tasks, whether or not those tasks occur in concrete formal organizations. In the broadest of terms, the former addresses itself to the market for goods or services around which the administrations of work institutions organize labor, while the latter addresses itself to the labor which produces those goods or services and which, by means of occupational organizations, attempts to stabilize and control their work. The former in fact specifies one model for organizing the production and delivery of goods and services, while the latter suggests another. Historically, still a third model was suggested by classical economics. Let us look at them all.

TWO TRADITIONAL MODELS FOR ORGANIZING CARE

Until very recently, only two basic models for organizing the delivery of care were common. Stripping away the details so as to be able to see the basic scheme more clearly, we might call the first, *the free market model*. The classic formulation is represented by Adam Smith and, in the case of health care in particular, some of the remarks of the American classical economist, Milton Friedman. In this model, there is unrestrained competition for patients in an open market among all who wish to sell healing services. Physicians compete freely with hypnotists, witches, herbalists, acupuncturists, homeopaths, diviners, and so on. There is no legal or other constraint placed on any claim to perform or practice any service, medical or surgical or psychological. All are free to compete.

The assumption is that the efficacious service will prosper, and the ineffective service will find no buyers and disappear. That assumption is in turn based on two other assumptions – namely, that the buyer, or customer, can discriminate quality in service and benefit sufficiently well to avoid poor or hurtful service and select only beneficial ones, and that, out of intelligent economic self-interest, the seller will strive to produce the best possible service. Free competition is also presumed to encourage the sellers to keep their prices down. Thus, the free market model is said to produce the best possible service at the lowest possible cost.

The second model is essentially the one on which the health care of many industrial countries is organized, though when one talks about a model one must remember that it is not an entirely faithful representation of the complexity of the world. There would be no point at all to creating a model if it merely duplicated reality. The system in many countries might be abstracted to its essentials as what I shall call *the professional or craft model*. It consists essentially of a protected market for those sellers who have certain agreed on characteristics supported by political authority. In the case of health, the licensed seller – the *bona fide* physician – is allowed to offer his services, and all others attempting to compete with him are prosecuted. Those included within this protected market are, however, free to compete with each other for customers.

When the American Medical Association talks of 'free enterprise', it is not talking about the free market model of the *laissez-faire* economist, but about 'free enterprise' within a carefully protected medical market. The assumption of this particular model is that protective licensing guarantees to the consumer minimal competence on the part of every licensed person. It also assumes that colleague interaction or competition within the protected market in some way regulates the quality of health care and assures an adequate standard of performance for all. And finally, unlike the free market model, it assumes that the layman is not competent to choose or evaluate the care he is to get: consumer choice is limited to approved practitioners only.

A THIRD MODEL

At the same time in history that the professional model was supplanting the free market model, yet another, a third model, was being used for organizing specialized health tasks connected with the control of environmental sources of disease. This model functioned to attack directly the disease-producing aspects of the physical environment as such, and aimed to control disease by the administration of protection from disease to masses of the population. Unlike the two traditional models, which were oriented to consultative relations with individual patients, the public health model was not predicated on the usual ideas of ambulatory care whereby the layman typically sought out care on the basis of his or her own conception of need. Rather, the model was a creation of public policy, aimed at unilateral amelioration and supported by police power. Organizationally, it took the same form as many other agencies of the state, namely that of bureaucracy.

The bureacuratic model, like the others, has its own plausibly attractive rationales. It assumes, first of all, that the workers in any system should be protected from economic pressures and temptations. Competition for fees, for example, is something that corrupts people, so the model says workers should be protected by receiving security and a rationalized career. It also assumes that an effective set of explicit rules and regulations will protect both the worker and the client by specifying the rights, duties, obligations of each. Discretion is reduced and bargaining is minimized. What each can ask of the other becomes not a function of money, or of arbitrary authority, but rather of the rules and regulations. And finally, of course, the model assumes that there will be obedience to these rules, and that predictable performance and a predictable product will result. To assure this aim, the bureaucratic system specifies the necessity of routine, systematic records. Medical reformers, incidentally, are very much concerned with the development of a rational medical record-keeping system, and of course where you have an insurance mode of paying for care, you must also have a record system to sustain it, and where you have a record system, you have the possibility of checking on both the quality and quantity of the services rendered.

THE FAILURE OF TRADITIONAL MODELS FOR AMBULATORY CARE

Both of the traditional models for the organization of ambulatory care have, over the course of time, manifested characteristic pathologies. In the case of the free market model, we all know how, in the events of history, even in the marketplace for material goods, it has developed. While some men do produce the best possible at the lowest possible cost, others compromise quality in order to develop competitive advantage in their prices. While some consumers are able to discriminate quality, others are not. And in health care the problem is even greater, since what is being sold is an intangible service which is more difficult to evaluate than material goods. In the free health markets of the past there was little evidence that the conscientious and learned thrived while the unscrupulous and unskilled found no customers. There was no assurance that self-interest and free competition led to the highest possible quality of care at the lowest cost since self-interest could lead as well to compromising quality for competitive advantage. Recognition of this socially undesirable result, plus belief in the ethical and technical superiority of medicine, led to the gradual elimination of a truly free market beginning even before the nineteenth century, and to the ultimate creation of a protected market by exclusive licensing. Generally, in the history of such changes, the free market model has been replaced by the professional, or craft model.

But the professional model contains its own pathologies. Just as the pathology of the free market stems from its core element of competitive individual self-interest, so the pathology of the professional model stems from its core element, which is protected exclusiveness. That is to say, given the protected market which limits the consumer's free choice under the assumption that all certified parctitioners will posses minimal competence and dedication those who are certified (and protected) have no further worry about attracting clientele. Their major problem lies in controlling the competition among themselves for fees, honors, promotions, etc. which takes place within the protected market. Thus, the main concern of the practitioners becomes the 'ethics' which are designed to prevent one colleague from gaining 'unfair' advantage over another rather than the ethics of service to the client. And so we find preoccupation with 'unfair competition' such as making unusual claims, having secret remedies or techniques, using advertising, and a desire to regulate the disposition of patients almost as a form of property through the formulation of rules against 'stealing' patients.

Apart from regulating the interrelationships among colleagues within the protected market, there is also the issue of maintaining the protected market itself. And so we find members of the profession concerned about the danger to their collective position from the disclosure of individuals' ethical lapses or technical incompetence. Unlike the free market, where each competes freely with the other (and historically each has publically charged the other with all sorts of discreditable behavior), in the professional model we find the cardinal rule among colleagues to be protective solidarity and secrecy. Constraints on internal competition also function to sustain protective solidarity. It is bad manners to talk about whether a colleague is competent or not, even to colleagues one does not know well. It is a virtual sin to raise such questions to the lay public. In effect, there is a conspiracy of silence about erring colleagues, with the consequence that services can be offered in this protected market which are below basic standards, but which are unknown to the public and uncontrolled by the colleague group. Thus, the quality of service is compromised in order to protect the colleague group and to sustain health worker solidarity. Each must protect the other in order to maintain the protection of all from the cold winds of truly free competition, or from loss of freedom within the protected market.

THE EXTENSION OF THE BUREAUCRATIC MODEL

For a variety of reasons, some more important in one national setting than in another, beginning in the nineteenth century but most particularly in the twentieth, the bureaucratic model has been adopted as a superior solution to the problems of delivering ambulatory health care. This trend is now apparent even in those nations which have avoided centralized state planning and control for ideological as well as practical political reasons. Some of the elements of the bureaucratic model are created when the intent is merely to rationalize and humanize the mode of financing the costs of care, for even if all other elements of health care remain unplanned, the creation of a mode of administering payment for care by a central insurance agency automatically creates such essential elements of the bureaucratic model as a system of records, and hierarchical accountability for them.

The problem is, how much better is the bureaucratic model likely to be than those it is supplanting? We all know how bureaucratic systems *can* work out. In a protected position, the worker may be pushed to render service only by a little extra bribe on the side. Or, what may be even worse, workers can lose all motivation to serve because there is security: we all know the stereotype of the bureaucrat who loses all will to work, who simply fills a position and mechanically goes through the motions of work. In addition, we know that the rules can be used conservatively in a bureaucracy, to protect the officials from the outside world. And we also know, even though the people who plan these health systems may have forgotten, that where the production of a personal service is involved, and not something tangible like an automobile, the only evidence that anyone has of anything having happened is a written record. And a written record is the arbitrary creation of those who maintain it, not an object or service in itself. Services can be invented like Potemkin villages, and converted into written records designed to protect the bureaucrat. Indeed, the characteristic pathology of a bureaucracy is that both the needs of the system and its workers are put before the client. It can become an incredible nightmare of forms and rules and regulations which no one outside the bureucracy can penetrate or master to serve individual needs.

CRITICAL ELEMENTS FOR EVALUATING THE MODELS

Clearly, every model I have described has its own difficulties. The pathology of bureaucracy, in which the needs of the system are put before those of the client, is to be contrasted with the pathology of profession, in which the needs of the colleague group are put before those of the client, and the pathology of the free market, in which the needs of the individual seller are put before those of the buyer. The question is, what are the circumstances in which empirical versions of such models are likely to minimize, if not avoid those pathologies? Current work in organizational and occupational sociology suggests that two issues are crucial. These issues are highly interrelated and may in fact be different ways of conceptualizing a single, underlying issue. These issues are, first, the character of the key productive task and, second, the way the work of the key productive worker is institutionalized. Let me discuss them briefly so as to indicate their importance for the issue of organizing health care.

For present purposes, it is possible to distinguish between tasks amenable to routinization and mechanization, the outcome of which is concrete and precisely measurable, and those requiring far-ranging discretion or judgment for their performance, the outcome of which is intangible and difficult to evaluate. The former tasks fit well within the assumptions of the bureaucratic model, and are rather easily created, organized and controlled by formal rules and regulations, and by hierarchical supervision. The latter do not fit in with the assumptions of the model and resist or escape accountability, gaining a kind of autonomy from external administrative supervision which is distintly non-bureaucratic in character.

In contrast to the issue of tasks amenable to classical bureaucratic control and those highly resistant to and perhaps even inappropriate for such control, there is the issue of supervising and controlling workers who have a special status predicated on their task and on their training and skill. The conflict between the 'authority' of the professional worker's presumed knowledge and the authority of the administrative official has been discussed over and over again in studies of civil service agencies, trade union staffs, industrial organizations, large law firms, hospital clinics, and hospitals. The worker with professional status, as opposed to the worker with technician status, is the one who successfully argues that his task is too complex to be subject to evaluation and direction from anyone other than himself or his colleagues. Within the framework of a thoroughly bureaucratized administration of supportive services, he, and those others who work under the direction of his authority, are unusually autonomous of the administration. While hours and wages may be precisely specified and regulated, the task itself, what goes on during those hours for those wages, is neither specified precisely by rules and regulations nor accountable to bureaucratic officials unless they too are professionals.

The position of professionals in such organizations is justified by reference to the character of the tasks they perform, tasks which are said to be complex and irreducible to mechanical operations, requiring the exercise of discretionary judgment and creativity which can be accomplished and evaluated only by those who have gone through long years of special training. But while conceptions of their work justify their autonomous positions, so does their autonomous position grant credibility to their declarations about the nature of their work and allow them to reinforce them. This is why I said earlier that a single issue may underlie the ostensibly separate issues of the nature of the task and the character of the professional worker. It is no mere historical accident that bureaucratization of work has occurred most intensively in industrial and clerical settings where the workers are of low status. In the practical world, rather than in theory, what can be done to organize work autonomously or bureaucratically is a function of the interaction between the task as such, and the social characteristics of those who perform it.

TWO TYPES OF HEALTH CARE

What has all this to do with health care? In assessing the proper model of organization for delivering health care this analysis points to the necessity of examining the nature of the tasks to be organized and the social organization of the occupations who perform them. And in separating out the two variables, one must recognize how interactive or dialectical is their relationship. One way to sort them out, however, is to avoid using the same holistic conception of task advanced by those who perform it, for while a job is almost always composed of a *bundle* of tasks which have quite heterogeneous characteristics, those who perform the job are prone to characterize their work by the most dignified and impressive of the tasks and omit mention of or deprecate the others. Health care in fact involves a variety of tasks, and should be divided into those which are sufficiently concrete to be bureaucratized, even mechanized, and those which are amenable only to the appearance but not the substance of bureaucratization.

Exact delineation of the corpus of tasks to be assigned to one classification or another is a medical rather than sociological matter, but bearing in mind the bureaucratic criteria of detailed rules and regulations governing procedure, it seems that most work in public health, much in preventive medicine (particularly that dealing with infection and communicable disease for which management is virtually standard), much in curative practice in clinical medicine and some in surgical repair belong in this category. Indeed, mechanization would even be possible, were the population amenable to diagnosis and treatment by machines. But with or without mechanization, real bureaucratic control over such work is possible because the rules for work can be specified and the outcome of the work itself can be evaluated comparatively simply. That those tasks are not bureaucratized in many industrial countries is not explained by their 'objective' characteristics so much as by the historical development of the division of labor for health care, political policy, and the professional standing which has helped medicine to define and organize health care work non-bureaucratically.

In contrast to those bureaucratizable health tasks, there are those which involve so many considerations as to defy standardization or routinization both of procedure and of evaluating outcome. Some of these tasks are not standardized merely because of their rarity or complexity, but to my mind the most significant group of unbureaucratizable tasks are those which emerge in advanced industrial societies after the fatal or crippling communicable diseases are virtually wiped out and the population expects to live long enough to age. What remains are chronic conditions connected with aging, and a broad assortment of biological, psychological, and social disabilities, none of which can be treated with 'magic bullets', and most of which involve many more subjective than objective elements in evaluation of progress and outcome. They are 'beyond the germ theory'.

HEALTH TASKS AND THE BUREAUCRATIC MODEL

The conclusion to be drawn from these distinctions should be clear – that the bureaucratic model is appropriate for some kinds of task, but not others. In reality, of course, the tasks are not and probably cannot be so neatly divided and allocated to different modes of organizing care.

The difficulty exists in part because health workers are organized into occupations, professional or technical: they do not gain and maintain jurisdiction over tasks on purely functional grounds nor are they passive pawns of formal administrative planning. Nonetheless, it is possible to say that the bureaucratic model is more likely to be useful in societies whose stage of development is such that the most widespread problem lies in health care tasks of the first order, tasks involving the application of comparatively straightforward techniques for the prevention and cure of clear-cut disease entities. The bureaucratic model is appropriate even when the status of the primary healer is professional, though both cost and efficiency are likely to improve if the worker has technician status.

The problems are different in most of the advanced industrial societies of Europe and North America where the most conspicuous need for health care lies in tasks of the second order, in the chronic diseases and various disabilities. True bureaucratization, particularly but not solely when the key workers have professional status, is not likely to prove an adequate answer to the problem of 'health services delivery' in such cases either for advanced industrial societies which have created a new system in answer to newly perceived needs (like the United States), or for societies which try to transform a bureaucratic system developed for earlier requirements to meet new needs. While the system will give the *appearance* of bureaucracy by virtue of the forms and records it produces, it will not be able to function successfully as a true bureaucracy. Such a system cannot meet the bureaucratic requirement of standardized procedures amenable to precise supervision and accounting, nor can it measure 'output' directly. While true bureaucratization may occur for the organization of the financing and logistical support of health care, only mock bureaucratization is likely with respect to the actual health care itself.

A CONSUMER MODEL

If the bureaucratic model cannot solve the problems of delivering adequate health care to the entire population of advanced industrial societies, what can? Few of us would propose a return to the free market model, for we are inclined to feel that the public welfare requires some limitation on the freedom of consumer choice in such a critical and complex area as health. Most would probably be inclined to preserve the professional model, with some reform by means of externally imposed requirements for 'peer review', by bureaucratic control over appropriate tasks, and by careful fiscal control – in essence, a blend of professional and bureaucratic models. But this does not seem to me to be an adequate solution either, because it does not have built into it any means of avoiding the characteristic pathologies of both of the models – putting the needs of the colleague group and the system before those of the client. What is perhaps even more important, it contains no recognition of the special problems of management which health care in advanced industrial societies entails. Indeed, it seems to me that if we face the character of those problems, we are led to visualize ways of dealing also with the pathologies of the traditional models.

In essence, I suggest that a model which includes within it an untraditionally active role for the patient, or consumer, is both appropriate for the typical health problems in advanced industrial societies, and for discouraging the characteristic pathologies of professional and bureaucratic systems. In the case of health care for chronic disease, disability, and other modern problems, a number of analyses have shown the necessity of gaining the active cooperation of the patient, indeed, the necessity of his becoming an active, involved participant in the therapeutic process itself. Such participation is not merely one of assent to professional recommendations, but informed discussion of options, and genuine choices. Both the therapeutic process and the outcome are interactional, with the patient's evaluation constituting a critical outcome in itself. The consumer's 'subjective' reaction becomes as 'objective' an element of outcome as his 'behavior', 'functioning', and other crude operational measures, since much of the latter is *produced* by the former.

Similarly, it is possible to conceive of a health delivery system in which the consumer is an active participant. Unlike both professional and bureaucratic models, a consumer model is not organized on the basis of preconceptions of what is to the benefit of the health consumer and then allowed to run itself with, perhaps, formal consumer representation built into governance, and periodic review by policy makers. A system which is created as an institution deliberately *insulated* from consumers virtually encourages the development of autonomy and self-protectiveness. A consumer model is instead one based on a system open at a variety of points to continuous consumer intervention and participation, demand and choice.

Obviously, complex matters are involved here, and space forbids lengthy discussion, but if I had to characterize the basic rule for such a system it is the rule that consumer choice be maximized, and that professional and bureaucratic secrecy or confidentiality be minimized. In concrete terms, such a rule means allowing the patient free access to his own medical record and administrative file, the right to enter his own opinion on the record, or to question the validity of what is on record. Furthermore, such a rule means keeping staff meetings open to the interested consumer, and preserving significant elements of choice by the consumer among practitioners and their practices. The essential assumption of such a system is that when, within the broad limits established on the basis of reasonable administrative and technical considerations, the health consumer has the maximum range of choice open to him, and access to most of the information circulating within the system, his activities will at once discourage bureaucratic and professional pathologies while at the same time advance the effective accomplishment of the tasks of health care in advanced industrial society.

REFERENCE

* Helpful comments on an earlier draft by Arlene K. Daniels are gratefully ac knowledged.

Direct reprint requests to: Eliot Freidson, Department of Sociology, New York University, New York, N. Y. 10003, U.S.A.

CONSUMERISM AND HEALTH CARE

EUGENE B. GALLAGHER

Department of Behavioral Science, University of Kentucky, Lexington, Ky., U.S.A.

In this paper, I will analyze health care by drawing upon relevant conceptual resources in the social sciences. I will approach this task from my sociological background, using sociological concepts primarily, but I will look also toward social psychology and economics for their contribution. My analysis will be conducted not solely as a disinterested dissection of health care institutions but also with a view toward current issues in health policy and practice.

In applying to health care a set of concepts from the stock of the social sciences, I shall move to the *terra incognita* of health care from a *terra firma* of social science which is, relatively speaking, better known. This analysis of health care will depict it as an area of contemporary social life which is in a state of rapid change and expansion. The systematic study of health care is an endeavor of recent origin paralleling the growing importance attached to health services in society. The characterization of health care as a *terra incognita* stems precisely from the fact that health care is in flux, with no accepted analytical framework for assessing its structure and its directions of change. Health care has the momentum and loose delineation found in many contemporary social processes. It is a conspicuous, and altogether typical, example of William Ogburn's concept of cultural lag, that the bioscientific vocabulary for describing human disease is profuse and precise, while the vocabulary for describing the situations, roles, and attitudes of sick people is weak, imprecise and tied cumbersomely to the traditions and language of our culture.

Questions of how to provide, distribute, staff, and support health services are increasingly in the arena of public controversy and policy.

There is a great need to rethink health objectives and to develop new concepts of health care. I suggest that contributions which social scientists can make to the analysis of health care will play an important part in the formation and resolution of issues in health policy. My attention in this paper to consumerism will help to focus problems concerning the patient role and the utilization of health services which run as a common thread in various health care systems.

HEALTH CARE

Health care, as a category of human endeavor, embraces a multitude of activities. It includes the complex processes of diagnosis, treatment, management, care, and rehabilitation performed by physicians, dentists, nurses, physical therapists, pharmacists, and many other professional workers. Health care is a very ancient enterprise, but its effectiveness has vastly increased within the last hundred years with the application of advances in the biological and physical sciences. The social structures and institutional processes for providing health care have concurrently become more ramified and more highly differentiated.

The person who benefits from health care and for whom the apparatus of health care is established has traditionally been designated as the *patient*. This is a social role which is firmly rooted in the common understanding of people in society. Children learn about the patient role through the multifarious cumulative social influences which constitute the socialization process. The patient role is enacted when a person becomes sick and receives health care. Social scientists have systematically studied the patient role, the conditions of role entry and exit, its social contexts, the effects of patient role assumption upon self-concept, and the interaction between the patient and health personnel.

Contemporary concern with health care provides a new role-concept to identify that person for whom the health care apparatus functions – namely, the health care *consumer*. This role is presently ill-defined; its essential parameters have not been clearly delineated. 'Health care consumer' lacks the fund of common understandings associated with traditional roles such as patient, teacher, father; and although social scientists devise thorough and ingenious methods for studying their subject matter, their formulations and findings gain cogency only as they approach matters in common experience and culture. Of course, it is equally true that culture does change, and that social scientists and other intellectuals assist change processes by conceptual innovations which link up with broad sociohistorical trends. For example, pre-Socratic Greece had no concept of citizen, as distinct from member of a tribe or clan. With the formation of the city-states, the concept of citizen evolved, assisted of course by philosophic insight.

The role of health care consumer is in an important sense incommensurable with that of patient. I do not mean that a person cannot be both a patient and a health care consumer, or that he can hold both roles only with a heavy burden of role-conflict. Rather, I mean that our terms for understanding the situation and world of the patient are sharply disparate from those for understanding the health care consumer. The health care consumer is a species of the economic genus, consumer. A consumer relates at arm's length to economic types such as providers, producers, sellers, and insurers. The patient, by contrast, can be described in terms drawn from psychology and sociology. He has dependency needs and anxieties; he undergoes alterations in body image and self-concept. He has his characteristic individual ways of responding to, and coping with, his illness – he may accept it, deny it, exaggerate it, cling to it, or reject it. In the hospital or clinic he may be viewed as a cooperative patient or a demanding, difficult patient. In a more sociological vein, he can be seen as a member of a particular family, social class, or community.

I will examine these roles in greater depth, to exhibit their contrasting features. Following that, I will discuss consumerism as a contemporary movement in health care with manifold implications for the structuring of health services.

THE PATIENT

In a study of mental patients' conceptions of the mental hospital and their illness, Daniel Levinson and I set forth the idea of *patienthood* – the state of being a sick individual within an institutional structure.[1] Although our notions of patienthood were developed around mental illness, they apply as well to the patient with a somatic disease or disability, and it is the latter category I wish to focus upon here. Patienthood is, internally and subjectively, a category of existence which creates distance between the patient and his world. Patienthood is also a comprehensive social role which, when a patient is incapacitated by severe illness or is institutionalized, transcends his other social roles – he is a patient first and only secondarily a family member, breadwinner, and citizen. The totalizing character of his role is related to the disabling nature of his disease and the need to receive treatment in order to cope with it.

Passivity is a second characteristic of the patient role. In a strictly etymological sense, 'patient' means he who suffers and is acted upon. A patient is at the receiving end of his disease or health problem and also of the treatment and care directed to him. He responds but does not initiate; he is the opposite of 'agent'.

A third characteristic is that it is an affective, rather than a cognitive, role. The patient responds to his illness and his situation with affect more than cognitive appraisals and decisions. To be sure, he has awareness of his illness and the means of ridding himself of it, but basically he reacts to his condition and situation in terms of emotion. The emotions associated with illness and injury are of course negative; there is the distress of pain, and fear of loss of bodily function or life. Health problems also cause him to deviate to a greater or lesser degree from his usual life course.

A fourth characteristic is dependency. It may be distinguished from passivity in that dependency refers to the patient's social relationships and performances, while passivity refers to his inability to control his illness and to do more than react to it. The patient's illness renders him dependent and alters his network of social relationships. People cannot count upon him to bear his usual responsibilities; they must, instead, help him. He depends upon technical professional help, deferring to the judgment of doctors and others. The increasing base of biomedical knowledge about disease and treatment tends greatly to enhance the patient's dependence and reliance upon the health care system.

These four characteristics – totality, passivity, affectivity, and dependence – are the essential elements of the patient role as I outline it here. I would emphasize that these are, in my view, *role* characteristics and not personality characteristics of the person occupying the role. It is an open question, the extent to which a dependency-inducing role such as patient draws upon deeper-lying dependency needs. That is to say, how do the emotional resources and various adaptive-defensive mechanisms of the patient come into play as he reacts to the social expectations of his role? This is a prototypical problem for social-psychological research.

No one will accept the foregoing sketch of the patient role without serious reservations. I will revise it so that it more fully encompasses changing tendencies and trends, some already quite far advanced, in health care. The revision will also serve as a prelude to a consideration of the health care consumer.

This sketch fits best one class of health problems, namely, the acute illness or accident which immobilizes a person and renders him totally the object of health care for a specific, usually brief, period of time. It does not fit the situation of the person with a *chronic* illness who may, with medical support, function in society with varying degrees of impairment. Such a person may be completely reliant upon medical care, but if he maintains a range of social functions, then patienthood is scarcely the categorical condition of his existence. Another major exception arises around *preventive* medicine – all the protections and fortifications a person can acquire, while in health, to decrease the likelihood of illness. There is also *elective* health care, in which the person with an existing need or problem prudently has it solved in advance of undesired or potentially damaging and painful developments. Familiar examples of elective care include: medically supervised contraception; hernia repair; varicose vein ligation; early management of hypertension, gastric ulcer, and diabetes; prenatal care; and orthodontia. Also included would be the taking of many drugs, such as tranquillizers, which require medical surveillance. The category of elective care shades off, in one direction, to interventions of a highly technical and professional nature which can prolong the life or maximize the comfort and function of persons who are critically ill and, in a full sense, patients; in another direction it becomes preventive, embracing elements of personal life-style, such as diet, non-prescription self-medication, and exposure to environmental risks, which are relevant to health but outside the sphere of professionally provided, individual health care.

Chronic, preventive, and elective care together comprise a very large part of contemporary health care. They reflect changes in societal expectation and advances in biomedical science which are of more recent origin than the traditional cultural concept of patient. In an earlier day, most people with chronic illness lived less happily and died younger, without benefit of much health care. Effective preventive and elective modalities were unknown. Contemporary medicine offers a range of technique which distorts and obsolesces the traditional concept of the patient as the recipient of its benefits. Whether this concept can be modified, in a best-fit sense, to fit the new situation, or whether it has been substantially invalidated is a moot question. If it has been invalidated, then role-concepts must be constructed to fit the new situation, but this is an order of cultural change which is never very rapid, direct, or deliberate.

THE CONSUMER

Let us turn to the role of the consumer and then to the health care consumer. In the history of Western economic thought, earliest attention focussed upon the trader, the person who is impelled by the strong economic logic of buying cheap and selling dear. Somewhat later, the role of the entrepreneur was conceptualized – the person who mobilizes and processes raw materials to produce a marketable product. Then the idea of the consumer as the focal point, whose needs, desires, appraisals, and decisions set into motion all the activities of an economy, was developed.

The role of the consumer contrasts sharply with that of patient. We have spoken of patient*hood*, but it would be apt to speak of consumer*ship*, implying that the consumer conducts his activities in considerable autonomy and independence. He goes forth into the marketplace and, with the money in his pocketbook, he has purchasing power to command the goods and services of his choice. It may of course happen that he enters the market at a disadvantage. With many wants and with little money at his disposal, he may be forced to make purchases at high prices. Whether the consumer is in a strong or a weak position, the very structure of the market situation evokes active, evaluative, decision-making behavior from him. His stance is skeptical. He does not believe everything he hears regarding the worth of goods presented for his consideration. He may well develop trusting relationships with certain sellers and suppliers, but in general he maintains an attitude of vigilant self-regard.

The consumer role thus diverges sharply from that of patient. The consumer's critical judgment is unfettered by the burden of illness. While sellers may compete for his attention and attempt to induce brand loyalty, there is no general cultural presumption that he should entrust his welfare to their claims. Health personnel and institutions, on the other hand, implicitly assume that the patient will trust to their good intent and their competence in judgment and performance.

THE HEALTH CARE CONSUMER

The foregoing characterization of the consumer role applies generally to the situation and orientation of the consumer. While admittedly too general for the task set here, it nevertheless serves as an initial indication of the profound difference between the patient and the consumer, as recipients of health care.

Two specifics apply more particularly to health care: the overwhelming extent to which it consists of personal *services* rendered to the recipient, and the element of *uncertainty* attached to the need for services.

Economists divide objects of economic value into goods and services. Most health care is provided in the form of professional services which are based upon valid scientific knowledge, and which adapt this knowledge to the clinical status of the individual recipient. Particularly in his role as dependent patient, the recipient is entitled to confidence that the health care professional is knowledgeable, skilled, and dedicated to his well-being. The worth of a personal service does not 'speak for itself' as fully as does a material object.

In modern societies, health professionals are socially recognized through various kinds of licensing and through the formal approval of the institutions where they learn to practice. Such recognition means that not anyone, but only those duly qualified, may provide services. This amounts to a curtailment, in the public interest, of the right of unqualified persons to practice. Scarcely anyone finds this objectionable nowadays, though it is interesting to recall Rudolph Virchow's advocacy, in the early period of scientific medicine, of an open approach permitting almost anyone so inclined to practice medicine. Virchow believed that an enlightened public would recognize what was best for it, without the need for coercive law. [2] While legal restrictions upon health practice seem reasonable, they impair the freedom of the consumer to seek disallowed services, and this seems somewhat more questionable. That is, if a person wants a certain medicine or a certain kind of practitioner because he believes it will help him, on what grounds is he denied this option? The sociohistorical answer, convincingly expounded by Eliot Freidson, is that scientific medicine achieved, during the nineteenth century, a sufficient doctrinal hegemony among dominant elements in society so that practice based upon alternative and competing belief systems concerning disease was gradually excluded. [3] While there may be little contemporary sentiment for deregulation of the health professions, policy questions about the optimum form and degree of regulation are becoming ever more critical. Regulation can serve not only to protect the recipient of service but also to protect and advance the political and economic advantage of health professionals, and of particular professional groups within the health field, to the disadvantage of the public.

These questions revolve around the relative importance of services in the total complex of health care. Goods, that is, tangible commodities, are by no means unimportant. The material paraphernalia of health care is constantly increasing, both the equipment and supplies which professionals use with recipients, and those which recipients themselves use directly. Medicines are the most venerable material adjunct of health practice. New pharmaceutical products are being developed at a pace which taxes the ability of prescribing physicians to understand and master their uses. The growing contemporary list of other 'goods' includes prosthetic equipment of many kinds to replace or supplement bone, nerve, muscle, and sensory function, contraceptive devices, surgical suture materials, apparatus for home renal dialysis, cardiac pacemakers, incubators, intravenous feeding equipment and substances, and many others. Even biological transplantable tissues such as blood, bone cornea, and kidney have obvious significance as material objects which, but for legal and professional controls, could easily ripen into the status of a marketable commodity. Many countries do, of course, permit economic traffic in blood components.

It may be argued that a paramount professional service element lies concealed within the rising material apparatus of health care. No one takes medicine simply as he takes food, that is, with no concern beyond a reasonable assurance that it is wholesome. With medicine, however, there is an implied service commitment that it is pure, non-toxic, effective against the health problem encountered, and competently prescribed in view of the particular clinical needs and psychosomatic function of the recipient. Even the placebo effect – scarcely a new feature in the history of medicine – can be seen as a limiting case in which the material significance of the medicine vanishes and the whole of its efficacy is due to the skill and art of the prescribing physician.

The dual goods-service aspect of medical materials was clearly demonstrated in a recent American health controversy. Commercial blood banks sought to have blood declared a commodity, so that it would be subject only to superficial surveillance by an agency of the national government which regulates advertising and marketing practices of private, commercial enterprises. Blood, so ran their claim, is a marketable economic entity no different from automobiles, chairs, and pencils. Professional groups favored regulation by another national agency, which would impose much stricter controls on blood banking, similar to the controls on the production of pharmaceutical products. They argued that it is the professional skill and technique in gathering, storing, typing, and fractionating blood which impart worth to it. This view won out in the end. The distribution of blood is regulated in the manner of a professional service, rather than a market commodity.

Emphasizing the particular importance of services in health care consumption leads to the further observation that many of the services are direct and highly personal, oriented to the problematic organic status of the consumer. The services are rendered in the context of relationships between the professional and the consumer. Through the medium of the relationships established, the skeptical, autonomous stance of consumership is transmuted into a compliant, uncritical patienthood. If the recipient harbors misgivings and doubts about the services rendered him, he feels less free to raise questions or to seek an alternate source of care than he would in most consumer contexts. In addition to the niceties of the service relationship, there are, it may be suggested, psychological mechanisms at work which produce this general inhibition: if the consumer is able to choose the occasion for seeking care and also to select the physician, hospital, or other source of care, then his own decision may generate a commitment which silences the expression of doubt. In other parlance, the phenomenon would be that of the self-fulfilling prophecy and cognitive dissonance reduction. That is, in regard to matters so personally important as health and illness, the consumer's initiative itself generates confidence and trust in the worth of professional services received.

The other aspect of health care as a consumable economic entity which we wish to emphasize here is its uncertainty of incidence. The waywardness of health problems is notorious; many come to the consumer as crises or emergencies. From the standpoint of service, the health professional is trained and experienced to handle calmly the problems the consumer brings to him. The consumer wants, along with remedy for his problem, some relief from the task of coping with it on his own. However, the disparity between the professional's knowledge and competence, and the health consumer's ignorance and urgency generates a deep gap, not easily bridged, between the two.

The unpredictability of health problems makes also health care a difficult matter to rationalize within family income and budgeting processes. This consideration applies most forcefully to acute care but also to much elective and chronic care. The social economist, Kenneth Arrow, observes: "The most obvious distinguishing characteristic of an individual's demand for medical services is that it is not steady in origin as, for example, for food or clothing, but irregular and unpredictable. Medical services, apart from preventive services, afford satisfaction only in the event of illness, a departure from the normal state of affairs. It is hard, indeed, to think of another commodity of significance in the average budget of which this is true".[4]

The feature of unpredictability, coupled with increasingly high costs, has had the effect of removing a great deal of health care out of the realm of individual market purchase. In many societies, health care is completely or largely a governmental function. There is a central ministry of health, and health professionals work for the ministry, either as civil servants or on a contractual basis. Health care is then available to citizens as a politically-determined benefit; the citizen may be represented in the legislature, but the consumer does not directly enter the marketplace. In such systems of health care, the consumer role remains implicit within the general political context, and consumer demands are perhaps less likely to coalesce into a relatively articulate ideology of consumerism.

CONSUMERISM

As a concept in health care, consumerism has over the past ten years come to command considerable attention in the United States. For clarity, I wish to distinguish *consumerism*, as an ideology and critique of health care systems, from the *consumer role* and its associated concepts.

As an ideology, consumerism defines the situation of the health care consumer and attempts to improve it. Like most ideologies, consumerism accents elements of conflict within a problematic situation and espouses a program of reform which may be simplistic or utopian in relation to the existing realities and the possibilities of change. The analysis of the consumer role, in contrast, simply delineates an important component in the structure of an economy and social system. This analysis is, in the sense of Max Weber, value-neutral. [5] By analogy, one may contrast feminism, as an ideology and social movement for the improvement of the status of women, with the more dispassionate study of the female role in society.

It is a fact of interest and significance that the ideology of health consumerism has, thus far, remained an American phenomenon. Many of its claims and concerns have revolved around the limited access of poor people to adequate health care. Given the fact that the American health care system, more than in most other modern societies, functions through direct purchase of services (or of health insurance), it is not surprising that this important problem in health care is conceptualized in consumer terms. One solution to the problem lies in supplementing the income of poor people, so that they will be able to purchase health care. Because it aims to increase purchasing power, such a solution is strongly consumer-oriented. It preserves the structure of the market-place in which professionals make health services available and consumers utilize them. It relies upon the economic forces of supply and demand to correct problems such as the shortage and maldistribution of professional personnel.

Another solution to the American problem of health care for poor people has been to allocate public funds for the establishment of so-called 'health maintenance organizations'. Such an organization hires doctors, nurses, and other personnel and directs their services to the low-income families of a particular geographic area. The organizational policies and procedures are established by a governing board which includes representatives of the health professionals who provide the services and also of the families who receive the services. The important point, for purposes of our discussion here, is that the consumer role in such an organization extends somewhat beyond sheer economic capacity to command health services – it also goes into questions of *how* the services are provided. Consumer representatives are concerned, for example, with whether the professionals are courteous in rendering services and whether records remain confidential.

The earlier observation that health consumerism is, for the present at any rate, of no great importance outside the United States may be accounted for on the basis that the American health care system remains strongly tied to the fee-for-service, private practice of medicine and upon the consumer's entry into health care through the purchase of services. It is my contention, however, that while the foregoing characterization may be correct, consumerism addresses important problems which are present in all health care systems, extending well beyond the urgent problem of access to care by poor people in the United States. Consumerism, I suggest, offers a thoroughgoing critique of contemporary health care.

What does the health care consumer want?

This is obviously a difficult question to answer in general terms, because the individuality of consumer preference, the influence of subcultural and group norms, and many other particularizing forces come into play in health care, no less than in the consumption and utilization of services in recreation, education, and other fields. For the discussion here however, we may trace out an answer against the backdrop of prevailing trends and tendencies in health care. To make this formulation of the consumer's stance more vivid, I will phrase it in first person terms.

"When I am sick, I want may illness to be treated by a doctor who is superbly trained, natively gifted for his profession, humane, sensitive, patient, and wise. I want him to tell me as much as I want to know about my sickness and about his measures for dealing with it. If my sickness is serious, and he recommends drastic treatment – potent medicines or major surgery – then I want to have the immediate and the long-term effects of such treatment explained and I want to decide for myself, applying this explanation to my own life and situation, what will be done. I realize of course that the doctor's knowledge is limited, but I would like to control the course of my treatment in the light of that knowledge which he does possess. Since I am not medically qualified myself, I expect him to communicate this information in terms which I understand but with no compromise of essential material.

"I want my doctor to provide the full range of services I need, so that my care will not be referred or delegated to others. I expect him to be both primary care physician and specialist. If, as a last resort, he finds it necessary to have others deal with me, for a limited time and for specific purposes, then I expect him to direct this arrangement himself and to manage everything for my benefit.

"I want my health care to be paid for by taxes or insurance, in such a manner that my expenses will be no greater when I am receiving it than when I am not. Unless there is a compelling reason for me to be treated either at home or in hospital, I desire to be treated in the setting of my preference. In general I want my health care to be readily available at times and places which are convenient to me, in view of my activities, responsibilities, and general mode of life."

The foregoing statement articulates consumer interests in two different, though interrelated, directions.

It states a consumer position, first, in regard to access to care, which is to be free, easily available, and responsive to consumer demands for continuity, comprehensiveness, and freedom from bureaucratic complexity. By rather direct extension, consumer requirements for access bear upon considerations of health manpower production and training, geographic distribution of practicing professionals, financing, and other factors which directly and indirectly determine whether consumers can obtain the health care they want and need.

Most public discussion has centered on problems of access, as do debates over the merits of socialized medicine, private health care systems, health insurance schemes, and similar issues.

The second direction of consumer interest embodied in the statement is, I suggest, of equal importance. It deals with the communication processes and role-relationships established between the consumer and health professionals. In general, it favors a strengthening of the consumer's capacity for a more autonomous participation and decision-making in his relationships with professionals. Much of the present structure of health care is distinctly inimical to such a role for the consumer. The increasing weight of biomedical knowledge makes more difficult the task of conveying clinically relevant information to the consumer. The traditional cultural conception of the patient also predisposes the doctor and other health professionals toward paternalistic and autocratic, albeit benignly autocratic, styles of behavior.

Frequently, the doctor must communicate not only across an ignorance barrier due to the consumer's lack of medical background but across an anxiety barrier because of the unpredictable and highly personal nature of health problems. It does not come easily to health professionals to attempt this kind of communication, nor to become proficient at it. Freidson states: "Characteristically, the professional does not view the client as an adult, responsible person... The client lacking professional training, is thought to be unequipped for intelligent or informed cooperation with his consultant".[6] The health professional in his dealings with the consumer is not strongly supported by official or formal authority, but there is a cultural presumption of professional superiority which intimidates the consumer and deters him from raising questions and seeking information concerning his treatment. The thrust of scientific medicine, as imparted in medical education and subsequent professional practice, runs toward decisive intervention against disease and the establishment of definitive formulations concerning pathology. The doctor, along with other health professionals, is not expected to develop skills in communication. Indeed, communication may be viewed as an extraneous, defensive activity, to be conducted only when consumer demand becomes insistent or effective action is impossible. The consumer, conceived by the professionals in the role of passive patient, becomes the compliant appendage of scientific medicine. This development in general curtails autonomous decision-making and cooperation, creating the basis for consumer alienation and malaise; in relation to the entire field of chronic disease, its effects can be particularly adverse.

Two other obstacles to optimum health care which are significant from the perspective of consumerism lie first in the complex organizational structures which administer and provide health care and, second, in the preference for 'high' technology as against simpler, more personal methods for dealing with health problems. Social scientists since Karl Marx have catalogued and analyzed the depersonalizing effects of large-scale organization in industry, education, housing and many other fields. While in health as elsewhere there are benefits to be realized from specialization and the economy of scale, it nevertheless appears that a rationalizing, organizing daemon is at work among health professionals, which intrinsically prefers the complex to the simple and the automatic to the human, without any criterion of comparative effectiveness. Multiphasic diagnostic screening may be cited as an illustrative current example of a high technology approach to the important task of medical diagnosis and early screening. I do not doubt the effectiveness of the various automated components used to monitor bodily function; the point is that, as frequently used, multiphasic screening displaces physical diagnosis as an important modality in the doctor-patient relationship. Moreover, it can be used effectively only in an organization which is of considerable administrative complexity.

We have endeavored to codify some of the grievances and demands of consumerism, and to show how organizational, technological, and professional forces have generated the faults in health care to which consumerism addresses itself. It is one thing to articulate a program of reform and quite another to translate it into actual change in health care. Sociologists can contribute their expertise both to the delineation of problematic situations and to the analysis of the deep structures and traditions in health care which offer a formidable inertia.

REFERENCES

[1] Daniel J. Levinson and Eugene B. Gallagher, *Patienthood*, Houghton Mifflin, Boston, Massachusetts 1964.

[2] Erwin H. Ackerknecht, *Rudolf Virchow*, University of Wisconsin Press, Madison, Wisconsin 1953.

[3] Eliot Freidson, *The Profession of Medicine*, Dodd, Mead, New York 1970.

[4] Kenneth J. Arrow 'Uncertainty and the Welfare Economics of Medical Care', *American Economic Review* (1963) 941–973.

[5] Max Weber, *The Methodology of the Social Sciences*, Free Press, New York 1949, translated and edited by Edward A. Shils and Henry A. Finch.

[6] Eliot Freidson, *Professional Dominance*, Atherton, New York 1970.

THE BRITISH NATIONAL HEALTH SERVICE: MODERNISATION AND CHANGE

D. G. GILL

M.R.C. Medical Sociology Unit, University of Aberdeen, Aberdeen, Scotland

THE BRITISH NATIONAL HEALTH SERVICE: MODERNIZATION AND CHANGE

The tripartite structure of the British National Health Service arose out of conflict and schism via disagreements not only between the profession and the State, but also between the three main branches of the profession – the specialists, the generalists and public health practitioners.[1,2,3] Power and prestige were and still are differentially distributed between these three groups, with specialists maintaining their dominant position, public health practitioners the least influential[4] and general practitioners occupying the middle ground of the medical pecking order. As a consequence, the structure of the National Health Service which emerged in 1948, was most acceptable to and reflected most clearly the interests of the hospital consultants – favourable conditions of service, freedom to continue private practice (a privilege also enjoyed by general practitioners, but which has never attracted more than a handful of private patients per G.P.) and control of the merit awards system. While the State took note of and acceded to some of the requests of general practitioners, the desire of public health practitioners for a completely integrated and locally oriented service was rejected.

The restructuring of the National Health Service in May of 1974 is intended to achieve an integrated service in which the three arms of the medical care system will come together to provide a holistic approach to perspectives on health and the problems of illness with the overall objective of improving patient care. To what extent is this broad aim likely to be achieved?

In a number of Government publications [5-11] considerable emphasis has been placed on improvements in managerial and administrative efficiency for achieving unification in the Health Service. The philosophy underlying the Management Arrangements for the Reorganised Health Service is best summarised by a phrase taken from Appendix II of the White Paper ..."there should be maximum delegation downwards, matched by accountability upwards. [12] Thus the Districts will be accountable to the Area Authorities, the Areas to the Regional Health Authorities and the Regions to the Department of Health and Social Security and ultimately to the Secretary of State.[13] Nevertheless... "Accountability in the Health Service is not easily determined, because consultants and general practitioners are primarily accountable to their patients" [14] and ... "Both general practitioners and consultants exercise clinical autonomy and are consequently their own managers".[15] These two statements, if they are true and if they have practical consequences, are of considerable significance for assessing the extent to which the reorganisation of the National Health Service will achieve its major objective of an improvement in patient care by providing a unified and integrated service centred upon the needs of the patient and of the community.

It is proposed to comment upon the second of these two statements first, since a clear understanding of the concept of clinical autonomy is necessary before we can agree or not that a consequence of its existence *is* that medical practitioners *are* their own managers.

CLINICAL AUTONOMY

Both primary and secondary physicians, specialists and generalists have to come to terms with failure. Death is, of course, inevitable, but the science, some would argue the art, of medicine is sufficiently imprecise to ensure that all practitioners are bound to be faced with diagnostic and/or treatment failure at some stage of their careers. Moreover, the clinical approach, the clinical mentality as Freidson describes it, seeks to apply the best available scientific knowledge to a given disease condition, but in a way which allows the doctor to aplly his own experience to the situation. The uniqueness of each individual patient is emphasised. When scientific and medical technology is inadequate for the condition at hand, the physician can utilise his clinical experience to try to do at least something for the patient. Whatever the outcome, the physician has done his best. Even when a treatment regime is indicated by reasonably objective criteria the argument still holds that the physician's clinical experience may suggest variation from the usual procedure or an alternative course of action. Variability of treatment is legitimated by the tradition of the clinical method and by the concept of functional autonomy which characterises not only the relationship between the profession and the State but also the doctor-patient relationship.

Clinical autonomy almost certainly arose because of the high degree of uncertainty, to put no finer point upon it, associated with the practice of medicine in the nineteenth century. McKeown[16] has shown that the intervention of medical practitioners on the process of disease (with the possible exception of smallpox vaccination) during the nineteenth century was not responsible for the improvements in morbidity and mortality which were characteristic of the second half of the century. Indeed it is not really until the twentieth century that the scientific revolution and improvements in medical technology created the circumstances whereby doctors could intervene effectively in disease conditions. In these circumstances it is not surprising that clinical autonomy, clinical judgement became an accepted part of the doctor's *modus operandi*. An individual doctor's diagnosis and treatment was as likely as not to be effective as the next man's and since failure rather than success was the normal outcome it became even more important for the individual doctor to know that his judgement would not be called into question by his colleagues. If a patient or his relative demanded an explanation of the doctor's failure, then a retreat into the esoterics of medical language erected an impenetrable barrier between the profession and the laity.

ACCOUNTABILITY AND DECISION-MAKING

Today in at least some spheres of medical work conditions are very different. Members of a team working in an operating theatre are clearly exposed to each other's scrutiny and judgement. The judgement about what is to be done and how it is to be done becomes a collective one. In obstetrics the limitation of clinical autonomy is even more clearly demonstrated. Many departments convene a meeting of staff to discuss the circumstances surrounding a still birth oı first week death. Here the doctor or doctors concerned give an account of their management of the situation and collective opinion is brought to bear on the problem with a view to determining what caused the fatality. In this procedure errors of judgement are exposed to the scrutiny of all. Moreover both epidemiological and clinical research have indicated mechanisms for identifying women likely to be at high risk during pregnancy and parturition. As a consequence techniques for the management of pregnancy, such as induction of labour at post maturity and elective caesarian section for cephalo-pelvic disproportion have been routinely introduced. In effect the area of clinical autonomy, of clinical judgement has been reduced as a result of the success of research studies which have identified and explained previously ill-understood circumstances during parturition which were responsible foı reproductive failure and the introduction of a specific set of management techniques had reduced the element of individual judgement to be applied to each pregnancy. In these ways the individual clinical autonomy of physicians and surgeons, while they still remain responsible for their own patients, has clearly been limited. Indeed their accountability to each other has been increased. The analysis of the statement "...both general practitioners and consultants exercise clinical autonomy and are consequently their own managers..." can now be extended.

An increase in the degree of accountability of hospital doctors to each other has been demonstrated. Is this also true of general practitioners? More and more general practitioners are now members of group practices or health centres. One of the possible consequences of this form of primary care provision is that more patients are likely to be treated by more than one doctor since 'their' doctor may be on leave, on a refresher course, or manning—say a family planning session or assisting in hospital. In this way the members of the practices or health centres are likely to become aware of each other's diagnostic and treatment habits which way in turn influence their own patterns of behaviour. The monitoring of prescription costs already exposes the prescribing habits of general practitioners to the judgement of other employees of the National Health Service.[17] If 1974 does lead to a closer integration across the present three arms of the Health Service then it would seem almost inevitable that all medical practitioners are likely to experience a greater degree of interaction with their colleagues and acquire greater knowledge of their pattern of behaviour as well as releasing information to others on their own pattern of diagnosis and treatment.

This is not to suggest that clinical autonomy will disappear, rather that it is becoming collectivised. What implications does this have for the statement... "general practitioners and consultants exercise clinical autonomy and are consequently their own managers"? One consequence would be that management itself becomes a collective enterprise and an enterprise which is increasingly subject to influence if not control by advances in scientific and medical technology. In this sense a unit in a hospital setting, such as an obstetric department discussed above, begins to manage itself. Routine procedures for induction of labour and elective caesarian section are laid down and any one of the clinicians could undertake the responsibility for drawing up work schedules specifying periods of duty time. Where clinical uncertainty persists (leaving aside for the moment the problem of functional uncertainty, e.g. whether or not to inform a dying patient of his condition) then all members of the department, doctors, technicians, nursing staff and trainees, may have opinions on what regimen is appropriate. In these circumstances all treatment regimens need to be kept under constant review and again this becomes a collective enterprise. Where functional uncertainty exists, again, in all logic, decision-making must be shared. All members of the ward or unit are likely to have views on what is or is not appropriate and in the absence of 'hard' data some agreed decision about procedures is all that can be expected.

In group practices and health centres some of the problems of management and administration are inevitably different. The primary care team involves health visitors and social workers as well as doctors and nurses and the concerns of the medico-social or socio-medical workers are different from and often ill-understood by the medical staff. Nevertheless these efforts are complementary to those of the doctors and nurses and with the shift from acute to chronic illness conditions and an increased concern for prevention and/or early treatment of disease the role of the health educators and social workers becomes an even more important part of the health team's activities. In the case of the elderly, nurses, health visitors, social workers and home helps are probably much more important than the doctor. Doctors are still imperfectly trained in the medical aspects of primary patient care and their understanding of social problems is limited, to say the least. While some medical schools in the United Kingdom are providing some instruction in the behavioural sciences, there is much debate about what should be taught, but above all what is the overall purpose of such instruction. If a collective orientation does emerge in general practice, then members of the team will become accountable to each other and share responsibility for decision making. Indeed it is difficult to see how any other mechanism would be possible. A hierarchical system, placing overall responsibility in the hand of one of the doctors would involve him indirectly in controlling his medical colleagues and nurses, and also the social workers about whose jobs he can know little. Mutual accountability and shared responsibility for decision-making is surely more practicable.

A UNIFIED APPROACH

A team approach is also dictated by the changing pattern of disease which in turn induces a shift in medical practices and priorities. Rising rates of morbidity and mortality due to various cancers, respiratory and circulatory diseases, require that the health care system place more emphasis on preventive and screening services which, if they cannot eliminate the predisposing conditions, facilitate early diagnosis and treatment. Health education, whether directed at attempts to change patterns of behaviour to reduce the risk of illness or injury or to persuade people to utilise screening and other preventive services is always a long-term procedure. Moreover the success or failure or health education campaigns is notoriously difficult to assess and attempts to do so must include an examination of the context in which health advice is provided with particular reference paid to accompanying service provision. The fall in legitimate fertility in the city of Aberdeen in recent years provides an opportunity to examine, at least in part, the relationship between service provision and health education.

In 1970 there were 2414 live births to married women in Aberdeen, a reduction of 602 compared with 1965 (Registrar General's figures). Of this short fall approximately 23%–141 was due to therapeutic abortion. Assuming that migration has had little impact upon fertility, then the remaining 461 'missing' births are to be explained by the influence of sterilisation[18] and contraception. Now it is logically possible that the reduction in legitimate births could be due to a sudden increase in sexual abstinence in the population. No direct evidence is available to confirm or deny this statement, but Illsley and Gill[19] have argued that sexual activity has almost certainly increased among married and single people and it would seem reasonable to assume that abstinence as a mechanism for controlling fertility is unlikely to have played much part, especially in recent years.

In 1970 a total of 240 married women were sterilised compared with 192 for 1965, with a rise in the number of sterilisations over the 6 year period giving an annual average of 220. Sterilisation will, of course, have a cummulative effect over the 6 year period, but sterilisations which were performed in the 40s and 50s will also affect the numbers of births occurring in this later period. While it is not possible to calculate the number of 'missing' births which are attributable to sterilisation it would seem evident that this form of fertility control or rather absolute limitation of reproductive potential has made a very significant contribution to the reduction of births other than by therapeutic abortion. Nevertheless some of these sterilisation are substitutes for contraceptive techniques rather than women choosing this method for the first time to avoid further pregnancies. Thompson in her 1969 article[20] states that by the end of 1967, a few women, after three or four years of oral contraception, were requesting tubal ligation. It is possible that this demand by women for a complete and final cessation of their reproductive careers may represent an increasingly large proportion of the sterilisations carried out in the recent past. A preliminary analysis of the sterilisation data suggests that women sterilised in recent years had had fewer children than their equivalents in previous years.[21]

The dramatic increase in the number of new attenders at the City's family planning clinics (from 388 in 1964 to 1632 in 1971) would suggest that women in Aberdeen are becoming increasingly interested in contraception and this increase is not limited to married women. The number of unmarried new attenders has increased even more noticeably in the last two years. Both women who attend the clinics and those who get contraceptive advice and devices from their G.P.s now readily accept the Pill and its popularity may be associated with the real advantages this contraceptive technique offers compared with other methods. Various authorities and organisations in Aberdeen have followed a vigorous policy of proselytisation of family planning and the management of pregnancy and maternity service has been designed not only to reduce rates of reproductive loss but also to improve the quality of human life by enabling women to avoid excessive childbearing. Sterilisation was available to the debilitated grand multiparae over three decades ago and a closely integrated and rationalised system of maternity care has been the end product of co-operation between hospital doctors and public health practitioners, particularly since the formation of the N.H.S. in 1948. Nearly all births which take place in Aberdeen are hospital confinements and all three branches of the medical profession and support staff co-operate closely under the general control of the Department of Obstetrics and Gynaecology throughout ante-natal care, parturition and post-natal care. Anecdotal data suggests that the city's population has gradually become aware of the facilities available for controlling fertility. The staff of the maternity unit report that some women request sterilisation as a result of coming into contact with relatives, friends or neighbours who have had or know of the operation. Over a cup of tea the question is sometimes raised: – "Have you had your operation?" – and from such conversation the impetus for another request is generated. At the very least mothers are aware of sterilisation through such informal information networks and are perhaps less taken aback if the subject is subsequently raised at a later stage by maternity unit staff.

The city's health visitors under the direction of the Medical Officer of Health and his staff are required to discuss family planning with their clients whenever it seems advisable to do so or whenever the clients themselves either raise the topic or hint that they would like more information. The family planning clinic has sub-branches operating in the larger housing estates, they are open outside normal office hours, provide advice and services free, and any procedure for referral is accepted. This last point may be particularly important since many women may be reluctant to go through the normal referral channels, particularly via their own G.P. The ability to walk into or to be able to telephone for an appointment at a family planning clinic located conveniently close to one's own home may be particularly conducive to utilisation.

The city has also pioneered the development of sex education programmes in schools (part of a wider and growing emphasis on general health education) and in collaboration with the local independent television company and Dr. John Dennis, formerly of the Department of Obstetrics and Gynaecology, a film of human sexuality has been produced which is shown to the city's school children in eight episodes. In Aberdeen it would seem that the integrated programme of maternity care, family planning and fertility control has created a climate of opinion in which women are very happy to exercise a high degree of control over their reproductive behaviour.

While sterilisation and abortion are very important features of the over-all system of care, contraceptives, particularly the Pill, play an important part. The rise in new attenders at the city's family planning clinics coincided with the introduction of the oral contraceptive. No data exists on why women have apparently been happy to accept the Pill, but some hypotheses can be attempted. Once the decision to control conception has been taken the Pill is perhaps the easiest contraceptive to use. It is completely dissociated from the act of intercourse reducing to a minimum the need to anticipate individual sexual episodes. Once the routine of pill-taking is established ingestion is habituated, but even if a woman forgets to take her Pill for up to 4–5 days, contraceptive efficiency is hardly impaired. The oral contraceptive is entirely in the control of the woman. She may, if necessary, indemnify herself against the risks od conception without her partner's agreement or even knowledge. A number of authorities, particularly obstetricians and gynaecologists, have suggested that many working class women have been reluctant to use a diaphragm because this requires them to handle their genitalia. Both Rainwater's[22] and Kinsey's[23] findings suggest that working class men and women find barrier methods of contraception unseemly and certainly unpleasant to use. Squeamishness over the use of – say – a diaphragm may be enhanced in a working class household where storage space and a degree of privacy for fitting the device may be difficult to achieve. The Pill, as well as being virtually 100% effective, overcomes these difficulties and, so long as side effects are minimal, is an attractive contraceptive technique.

Notwithstanding these advantages of oral contraception the popularity of the Pill may owe something to the attitudes of the clinic doctors.

The staff of the clinics are reluctant to fit IUDs except when strong contra-indications for the Pill are present. Their reluctance to fit IUDs is justified (by them) on rather poor experiences with various forms of the device and the general view that this form of contraception is relatively inefficient. However, in certain clinics in the South West of England IUDs are fitted to 70% of the attenders. Moreover the Pill tends to be prescribed for middle class women who are thought to be more capable of handling a 'self-controlled' device. Working class women are much more likely to be fitted with an IUD.[24] Clearly the influence of family planning clinic staff on contraceptive habits is worthy of further investigation.

The reduction of fertility in Aberdeen was therefore the product of a multi-pronged approach in which the provision of services had, by far the largest part to play. Technological innovation in the form of the oral contraceptive was also important, but these changes were accompanied by a changing climate of opinion in favour of family planning and family limitation and by a gradual spread of information among the population on the availability and type of fertility control services. Health visitors clearly played an important part in the dissemination of information. Public Health practitioners, general practitioners and hospital staff were all involved in the overall programme, some rather more passively than others, but it should be stressed that these developments took place when there was no formal mechanism available through which co-operation across the three arms of the service could be achieved. Indeed some of the changes and improvements on the public health side took place without even the prior knowledge of the hospital staff. Hopefully, post 1974, such examples of collaborative activity will become more commonplace.

Part of the success of the fertility control services was attributable to the fact that attempts were made to take the service to the target population. Health visitors were instructed to raise the subject of family planning in clients' homes and the siting of family planning clinics over the city was determined by the distribution of population. Other preventive health measures and screening campaings are often under-utilised, particularly by those groups who are likely to be at high risk to actual or potential morbidity. Many studies have shown that rates of under-utilisation of preventive and screening services tend to rise with falling social class. If high rates of under-utilisation are to be reduced then the most practicable mechanism would seem to be ..."to change the system of medical care so: that it is more fitted to the attitudes and styles of life of those who currently underuse its services... Although not all under-utilisers are social class V and although not all those in the lower income groups are underusers of preventive services, the *concentration* of under-utilisers in social class V indicates that a re-structuring and reorganisation of screening services which took explicit account of the predilections and preferences of the deprived would be the most promising path towards increasing the take-up rates for preventive and screening services".[25] One of the major roles of the new speciality of community physicians will be to monitor the operation of health services and to identify the health care needs of the populations of Regions, Areas and Districts. As information builds up the identification of high risk groups will, presumably, become more exact. Under-utilisation seems to be associated with certain cultural features of the life styles of the deprived, ..."first, through the foreshortened temporal prespective of the deprived which militates against forward planning of their lives, and, secondly through a dislike of 'bureaucratic' and impersonal relationships compared to personalised and informal relationships".[26] Even when high risk groups or individuals have been identified it is still unlikely that they will present themselves for further screening and treatment at centrally based, bureaucratically controlled premises. At least the initial stages of the screening process, therefore, needs to be taken to the potential client; early investigations need to be completed in the proto-patient's home. In short, medicine has to become more home-centred, but it would clearly be very costly if doctors were to spend more and more time on house calls. Fortunately, however, a number of factors in combination, are beginning to show that alternative methods of diagnosis and treatment other than the utilisation of expensive and expensively trained doctors are practicable. The continuing success of the Feldsher system in Russia, improvements in simplification and routinisation of diagnostic procedures as scientific medicine increases, are leading to the utilisation of medical assistants in both the developed and the developing world. In Great Britain in Cheshire health visitors are already being utilised to conduct screening tests in patients' homes.[27] Once an actual or incipient illness is suspected or detected it is then much easier to persuade the patient or proto-patient to see a doctor. A secondary advantage of this technique may be the de-mystification of medicine, medical practitioners and medical procedures. The physician's assistant may be a less distant and less frightening figure than the white-coated, auro-shrouded doctor.

The changes in the practice of medicine discussed and proposed here, the development of mutual accountability, shared responsibility for decision-making and greater co-operation between doctors, other para-professional staff and social workers etc. represent, as Sokołowska has suggested, a shift from an individualistic to a collectivist orientation in medicine.[28] This collectivist orientation underlines what perhaps should always have been the case, the social responsibility of the medical profession and systems of health care. Nevertheless Goode has argued[29] that one of the characteristics of a profession is that ..."The practitioner is relatively free of lay evaluation and control". Hence consultants and general practitioners are *not* primarily accountable to their patients, at least not in any direct sense. As Freidson has so ably demonstrated, the medical profession did achieve functional autonomy – a virtual monopolistic position over the treatment of disease ..."the exclusive competence to determine the proper content and effective method of performing (its) task".[30] Yet as early as 1911 in Britain the functional autonomy of the medical profession was, in fact, limited. ..."In 1911 and again in 1948, the State decided that the freedom of doctor and patient to reach whatever agreement they could achieve in relation to treatment and payment needed to be constrained."[31] Since then the accountability of the medical profession to the State has certainly been maintained if not increased. The profession is not, however, accountable to the public except indirectly, i.e. through the State. The most obvious shortcoming, indeed the tragic irresponsibility, of the current proposals for the re-organisation of the National Health Service is that no provision has been made to make the profession directly accountable to the public. Even the community health council will not be directly elected[32] and since their powers are only advisory this sop to the need for public representation and accountability is derisory. Given the relative powerlessness of the patient in the individual doctor-patient relationship this lack of public accountability at the collective level is even more regrettable. An increase in the degree of accountability of doctors to each other is perhaps the best safeguard that the patient has that his treatment has been or will be appropriate and effective. Most patients possess insufficient medico-scientific knowledge to evaluate for themselves the efficacy of the treatment recommended for them. Nevertheless mutual accountability of doctors is likely to be enhanced if the health care system is subjected to public scrutiny since the doctors will be encouraged to attract the support of their colleagues and thus present a united front to the scrutineers.[33] Public accountability for the allocation and distribution of resources, planning for the future health requirements, the determination of priorities, establishing, maintaining and improving co-operation between medical and social systems of care, etc. is an obvious necessity if the views of the laity are to play an effective part in the development of an integrated health service. Indeed, without the involvement of consumers in planning etc. the danger that reorganisation will further most the interests of doctors and others working in the health service rather than those of patients is a real possibility.

ACKNOWLEDGEMENT

I wish to thank my colleague, Mr G.W. Horobin, Assistant Director, M.R.C. Medical Sociology Unit, for his comments on an earlier draft of this paper.

REFERENCES

[1] A. J. Willcocks, *The Creation of the National Health Service*, Routledge and Kegan Paul, London 1967.
[2] D. G. Gill, 'The British National Health Service: Professional Determinants of Administrative Structure', *Int. J. Hlth. Serv.* 1 (1971) 342.
[3] Sir J. Brotherston, 'Evolution of Medical Practice', in: G. Mc Lachlan and T. McKeown (eds.), *Medical History and Medical Care*, O.U.P., London 1971.
[4] D. G. Gill, 'Status and Prestige within the Medical Profession: Some Speculations, paper presented to the British Sociological Association's Medical Sociology Group Meeting, Blackpool, November 1970 (mimeo).
[5] H.M.S.O. The Administrative Structure of the Medical and Related Services in England and Wales (First Green Paper), 1968.
[6] H.M.S.O. Administrative Reorganisation of the Scottish Health Services (Green Paper for Scotland), 1968.

[7] H.M.S.O. Report of the Working Party on Management Structure in Local Authority Nursing Services (Mayston Report), 1969.

[8] H.M.S.O. The Future Structure of the N. H. S. (Second Green Paper, England), 1970.

[9] H.M.S.O. N.H.S. Reorganisation: Consultative Document (England), 1971.

[10] H.M.S.O. Management Arrangements for the Reorganised N.H.S. ("Grey Book"), 1972.

[11] H.M.S.O. Report of the Working Party on Medical Administrators (Hunter Report), 1972.

[12] H.M.S.O. N.H.S. Reorganisation: England. Cmnd. 5055 (White Paper), 1972.

[13] In Scotland there will be no Regional Health Authorities.

[14] "Grey Book", *op. cit.* p. 17.

[15] "Grey Book", *op. cit.* p. 68.

[16] T. McKeown, *Medicine in Modern Society*, Allen and Unwin Ltd., London 1965.

[17] D. G. Gill and G. W. Horobin, 'Doctors, Patients and the State: Relationships and Decision-making', *Soc. Rev.* **20** (1972) 505.

[18] For the period 1965–70 male sterilisation was exceedingly rare in Aberdeen's hospitals and can be ignored for all practical purposes.

[19] R. Illsley and D. G. Gill, 'Changing Trends in Illegitimacy, *Soc. Sci. and Med.* **2** (1968) 415.

[20] B. Thompson *et al.*, 'Some Aspects of Oral Contraceptives and Married Women, *Med. Offr.* **121** (1969) 93.

[21] I am grateful to Miss Susan Teper, Demographer, M. R. C. Medical Sociology Unit, for this information.

[22] L. Rainwater, *And the Poor Get Children*, Quadrangle Books, Chicago 1960.

[23] A. C. Kinsey *et al.*, *Sexual Behaviour in the Human Male*, W. B. Saunders and Co., Philadelphia–London 1948.

[24] I am grateful to R. Snowden, Ph. D. of the Family Planning Research Unit, Department of Sociology, University of Exeter, for this information.

[25] M. J. Bloor and D. G. Gill, 'Screening of the Well Child: A Discussion of Some of the Problems Involved, *Med. Offr.* **129** (1972) 135.

[26] Bloor and Gill, *ibid.* p. 135.

[27] Dr. B. G. Gretton-Watson, County Medical Officer, Cheshire County Council. Personal communication.

[28] M. Sokołowska, 'Two Basic Types of Medical Orientation'. Paper presented to the Third International Conference on Social Science and Medicine, Elsinore, Denmark, August 1972 (mimeo).

[29] W. J. Goode, 'Encroachment, Charlatanism and the Emerging Profession: Psychology, Medicine and Sociology, *Amer. Soc. Rev.* **XXV** (1960) 903.

[30] E. Freidson, *Profession of Medicine*, Dodd Mead and Co., New York 1972, p. 10.

[31] Gill, *op. cit.* (1971) 352.
[32] P. J. M. McEwan, 'Consumer Participation in the Health Service', *Comm. Med.* **129** (1972) 189.
[33] Doctors might be tempted, by such a system, to protect each other from adverse criticism by 'covering up' for each other's mistakes. Indeed Freidson has argued that this is, in fact, the case today. The subjection of the process of mutual accountability to public scrutiny is perhaps the best defence against this form of medical solidarity.

SHIFTING SOCIAL POWER IN THE CANADIAN HEALTH SYSTEM

ROBIN F. BADGLEY, CATHERINE A. CHARLES AND GEORGE M. TORRANCE

Department of Behavioural Sciences, University of Toronto, Toronto, Canada

As the nature of social control shifts in a nation's health affairs, basic, and often unintended, changes can occur in established health institutions and in how health care is seen by the public. The structural changes which have taken place in Canada as a result of the introduction of national health insurance are a national case study of trends which may be occurring elsewhere. Part of a comparative study on the impact of health insurance undertaken with Odin W. Anderson of the University of Chicago, changes in two components of the health system, the role of private health insurance and the social structure of the medical profession, are reviewed here.

THE HISTORICAL SETTING

Initiated by one western province, Saskatchewan, and then for the nation, state health insurance is now administered by the country's ten provinces, but financed through joint federal-provincial cost-sharing arrangements. While several provinces had introduced hospital legislation in the late 1940s, the federal scheme was not completed until 1961 when all provinces endorsed the national program. Subsequently, the socialist government of Saskatchewan's 1962 medical care insurance legislation triggered a broad national debate and culminated in a 23-day doctors' strike. Triggered by a minority government situation, the 1968 federal program was based on Saskatchewan's medical care plan. By 1973, all of the country's provinces had met the terms of the federal Medical Care Act.

Each province now operates, either separate or combined health insurance programs (hospital and medical care) which adhere to four conditions necessary to obtain federal fiscal support. These legislative criteria require each province's health plan to provide: (1) universal coverage, i.e., for all residents; (2) comprehensive basic hospital and medical care services, a program available regardless of an individual's ability to pay or his health status; (3) the portability of health care benefits for individuals moving between provinces; and, (4) program operation under public administration.

The intent of the federal program was to remove all direct economic barriers for Canadians in the obtaining of health care. Unlike Saskatchewan's legislation upon which it was modelled, the federal program did not seek to initiate sweeping changes in the social structure of the nation's health system. It is now apparent a few years after their introduction that the impact of these measures has extended beyond initially intended economic consequences. As Odin W. Anderson has observed in *Health Care: Can There Be Equity?*, one aspect of health services cannot be manipulated on a piecemeal basis without effecting the whole institutional web of the health system.

The Canadian health system is a complex mosaic of private and public enterprise with multiple sources and levels of power in decision-making. Gauging the full impact of a major innovation such as health insurance requires a review of the whole range of institutions which have been affected in unanticipated, and often subtle, ways. While each provincial health program is almost a mini-health system reflecting the particular imprint of a province's cultural and political history, emergent social forces resulting from recent social security measures are restructuring the nation's health institutions in many similar ways. Health insurance has intiated or accelarated broad changes in the focus of voluntary health insurance plans, restructured the role of government in health affairs, and changed the established functions of professional associations.

Taken together, these changes reflect wider trends: a gradual rationalization and bureaucratization of health care; the emerging dominance of public over private initiative; and, a displacement of local community autonomy and established professional powers by central control public accountability and civic responsibility.

THE HOSPITAL SYSTEM

Because of growing public demand, but limited by government during the depression of the 1930s and World War II, the country's hospitals had for many years faced serious economic difficulties. They were not adverse to proposals for more extensive government support. By 1958 four provinces had a variable form of government hospital insurance. By this time provincial political support for a national program had become widespread. For its part organized medicine had anticipated national hospital insurance. While opposing specific legislative provisions, the profession generally supported the new federal scheme.

The new provincial hospital plans were designed as cost-sharing mechanisms. They had two secondary, but less visible policy aims: to raise the quality of hospital care and to develop an integrated hospital system. Each provincial program, it was anticipated, would have rationalizing and standardizing effects on hospital financing, operations and planning. Implicitly recognized, but not then stated, was the intent that these changes would require a substantial transfer of power and responsibility from the private to the public sector.

Since its introduction hospital insurance has let to an across-the-board rationalization and standardization in accounting and operating procedures. Previously, each hospital had developed its budget in terms of its special needs and priorities. To obtain financial reimbursement from government, hospital budgets are now scrutinized by a provincial agency. Accounts must be uniformly defined to permit comparison with other hospitals of the same size in terms of their requirements for personnel, salaries, days of service, equipment and general operating costs. Unlike the post World II period, hospitals no longer face economic uncertainty. Major deficits can now be avoided or minimized and major expense items predicted in advance.

Current review procedures illustrate the trend toward a growing bureaucratization of the hospital system and the flow of power from local to central units. Complex government administrative machinery has evolved to monitor these massive public programs. Budgetary review procedures allow for a centralized evaluation of local costs and of operating efficiency on a comparative province-wide basis. Individual hospital budgets can and are cut down or expanded in line with broader standards. In Saskatchewan for example where budgets were limited in 1973 to a nine per cent increase, the province's Minister of Health with some disbelief cited one hospital's 1974 estimates which sought a 56 per cent increase.

Because hospitals are now directly dependent on the public purse, fiscal control is a significant but not yet fully used social lever for effecting organizational changes. This dependency is exemplified by the provincial government enquiries into medical staffing procedures, legislative modification of prevailing hospital acts and the initial steps by government to eliminate the costly duplication of services and facilities to foster the development of district hospital planning councils. Central consultant services are made available to local hospitals concerning their operations and administration.

There is now a limited margin for private enterprise in the development of Canada's provincial hospital systems. To a limited extent certain capital costs can and still are financed independently. Since the start of health insurance, major construction projects have been undertaken by parochial hospitals, certain centres with a national service reputation, individual municipalities or physician entrepreneurs relying on private capital. The controversial One Medical Place and Medical Inns, Ltd. in Ontario are examples of this limited private enterprise. The construction of these new hospital facilities does not quarantee their continued financial solvency for operating costs. Unless provincial governments back up these privately started facilities with legal and financial support, these ventures may fail, or alternatively, rely on private philanthropy.

How effective these public controls have been in improving the level of patient care is unknown. Like many other social innovations, new institutional forms may have a limited impact in alterning their centrol aim, in this case, the delivery of good medical care. Some observers in Canada contend that recent government fiscal ceilings and cutbacks in hospital beds have had an adverse effect on the hospitals' ability to maintain high quality patient care.

Stringent controls on operating costs are emerging at a time when the hospital labour force is becoming unionized and increasingly restive. Recent examples of this changing mood are the strikes of hospital workers at the Toronto Western Hospital, of paramedical workers in New Brunswick and work-to-rule campaings by interns and residents in Ontario's teaching hospitals. Although these service workers have traditionally espoused professional ideals, centralized planning and its by-products are fostering union membership which will have predictable consequences. Strikes and walkouts by health workers until now relatively rare, are becoming a more common means (e.g., some 40 since 1972) to extract higher wages and better working conditions.

Community involvement in hospital affairs has changed little since the introduction of government health insurance. With the exception of Quebec whose hospital boards are elected, elsewhere as in the past, hospital trustees are appointed to hospital governing boards. Avowedly made to involve special administrative skills or to represent the community, these appointments to hospital boards are made on a political basis to maintain the *status quo* of business and professional interests. At no time has their membership genuinely represented a broad cross-section of the community.

Some of the traditional powers of hospital trustees have eroded under hospital insurance. Responsibility for final budget review and major fund-raising activities has been ceded to provincial authority. While government at this level ostensibly represents the public interest, the direct voice of the public in hospital affairs is now in fact one step further removed from the major site of decision-making.

Historically, Canada had a strong network of voluntary religious hospitals. These institutions were permeated by a firm sense of institutional pride. Members of religious nursing orders who assumed managerial and patient care functions received little or no remuneration. Their moral statisfaction derived from a sense of special calling. This situation has now changed as high operating costs and a decline in recruitment have forced many religious orders to close the doors of their hospitals. In some cases, these hospitals have been taken over by government. What is unknown is whether the introduction of a secularized labour force into these institutions has displaced the sense of intrinsic reward for economic gain or altered qualitatively the nature of patient care.

Voluntary associations in the hospital field have been reshaped by public health insurance plans. The chief aim of the Canadian Council on Hospital Accreditation (C.C.H.A.) established in 1958 was to improve hospital standards through the administration of voluntary survey procedures. To forestall further government intervention and to maintain a voluntary system of surveillance at the local level, its programs were extensively overhauled in 1972. But as in the past the Council's review measures focus on physical plants and facilities of a hospital, not in depth on patient services, such as quality control and the actual use of hospital services.

Economic restraints and control review procedures will significantly influence the future nature of hospital care, determine the volume of patient admissions, and shift the fulcrum of health care from the hospital to the community. During the present period of transition, few viable community alternatives have emerged. Nor have hospitals been compensated or motivated by incentives to realign more efficiently their existing programs.

The geographical distribution of doctors and hospital facilities has not been substantially altered by state health insurance. Some rural and outlying areas in a province like Ontario have held their own in the supply of doctors. This fact reflects the impact of special incentive programs for underserviced areas rather than being a consequence of medicare. Despite their mandate to develop an integrated hospital system, public agencies have not fully exercised their legal power to introduce a coordinated and balanced hospital service. Public initiative has centered on *ad hoc* and uncoordinated measures to impose bed cutbacks, operating fiscal ceilings, or to reduce patient utilization patterns. Neither voluntary inducements nor mandatory cost controls have yet significantly altered the existing pattern of distribution of hospitals relative to the population.

Publicly financed programs for nursing and home care are evolving in some provinces as alternate sources of extended health care. In essence, these programs seek to change the health seeking behaviour of the public rather than fundamental shifts in the distribution of facilities or personnel. The degree to which these innovations represent add-on services as opposed to viable alternatives in health care is as yet unknown. It is apparent that the result of grafting a public program such as health insurance to an established private enterprise has proven to be a costly, temporary measure in Canada, one which by leaving the public purse open to be billed by physicians paid by fees is generating growing public pressure than either government or the health professions anticipated.

VOLUNTARY PREPAID PLANS

The profession-sponsored medical plans and commercial/voluntary hospital insurance programs fluorished after World War II. The effects of government medical and hospital insurance varied for these two private enterprise measures, and as well, from one province to another.

The physician-sponsored prepaid medical plans were successful until the introduction of the federal government Medical Care Act in 1968. In 1967 Trans-Canada Medical Plans, a national association coordinating these programs, covered nearly six million people, or some 29.2 per cent of the population.

The prepaid plans introduced the concept of a third party paying agency which directly remunerated physicians for their services and verified submitted accounts. The centralized paying agency represented a new form of health bureaucracy which intervened in the lives of physicians and between them and their patients. Medical associations took on new functions related to voluntary health insurance such as the development of fee schedules and the review of claims.

These changes reduced the autonomy of the individual physician. They imposed on him new legal, ethical and financial responsibilities. For the first time across Canada, as contrasted with the western provinces' municipal doctor programs or Ontario's Medical Relief Program of the 1930s, physicians in private practice signed letters of agreement with paying agencies which committed them to specified contractual conditions. These contracts required adhering to financial and accounting procedures to obtain reimbursement of claims. Provincial fee schedules evolved which were set by professional associations rather than as before at a local level. In some cases, extra billing by physicians was disallowed. Disciplinary procedures were established to discourage the potential fiscal abuse of the private plans.

In exchange for the loss of local autonomy, the medical profession as a whole in each province gained unilateral control over the administration of the prepaid plans. It assumed responsibility for their financial solvency. A strong vested self-interest was built up to maintain the voluntary principle. Opposition to government encroachment evoked a firm ethos of professional loyalty and/or selfdiscipline which accounted for the viability and financial success of the private plans.

During this era of professional dominance, the medical profession gained certain new occupational privileges. Facilitating legislation and the absence of direct government involvement allowed it to strengthen its virtual monopoly in the field of medical care insurance. Two prime tenets of the prevailing medical ideology, physician control and voluntarism, were reinforced in the structure of doctor-sponsored prepaid plans. Occupational competitors such as chiropractors and osteopaths were excluded from the mainstream of insurance coverage. Also, because they lacked physician sponsorship, hospital prepaid plans covering medical benefits were for several years excluded from membership in a national association of medical plans.

With the advent of medicare, the profession mobilized its considerable resources to oppose certain terms of medicare proposals put forward by government. The prime issues at stake were the right of physicians to opt out of public programs, and to maintain professional control over the setting or modifying of medical fee schedules. Because of this defensive position, a potential source of continuity in administrative leadership stemming from the more than twenty years of experience by the profession with prepaid medical plans was for the most part lost in the transition to a publicly financed health insurance program. In their fight to preserve their professional interests, medical spokesmen in many parts of the country abandoned their leadership roles in these plans. With a few exceptions, the majority of the doctor-sponsored plans either ended their activities or revised available insurance benefits to cover extended care programs. The Trans-Canada Medical Plans Association went out of business in 1969, one year after the federal program was started.

An immediate consequence, then, of the introduction of government medical care insurance was to end the direct control and administrative leadership of the medical profession in the health insurance field. What subsequently happened was that these pervasive powers of the profession were displaced into more informal channels which proved to be equally effective in delaying structural changes sought by government, such as in revising fee schedules, controlling physician immigration or imposing regional health manpower quotas.

The experience of hospital insurance programs under national health insurance contrasts sharply with the demise of the physician-controlled plans. Several provincial hospital programs initiated in the late 1940s pre-empted the development of voluntary plans. With the introduction of the government scheme in British Columbia for instance, Blue Cross terminated its insurance activities in that province. In contrast, the 1958 fledgling public program in Ontario drew heavily on the experienced administrative cadre which had been built up by Blue Cross (Ontario). No less than 500 former Blue Cross employees, including the director, moved into government jobs. Despite this exodus, Blue Cross in Ontario, and in several other provinces, by moving into fields left uninsured by government schemes, has survived the introduction of public hospital insurance. Those voluntary plans which now remain provide benefits such as selected extended care provisions, semi-private and private hospital accommodation, private duty nursing and dental care. In effect, they have survived and fluorished as private competitive options which complement government measures.

One unanticipated effect of the introduction of public medical care insurance in Ontario was to ensure expanded business for Blue Cross. This program had an enrollment in 1973 of over four million people (almost half of the population) covered through a diversity of private health care plans. The comparable figure in 1959 during the first year of operation of the government's hospital scheme, was 1.75 million individuals. This remarkable comeback reflects the fact that despite the soaring costs of health insurance to the public treasury, in Ontario accounting for 28 per cent in 1974 of provincial budget expenditures, many Canadians were still willing to spend more money on health care than the level of basic coverage provided by government.

Blue Cross is developing new schemes to meet these accelerating demands. This situation, while providing institutional flexibility and options in the private sector, sharply erodes the concept of social justice and equity which were embodied in universal government health insurance schemes. It is apparent that fewer of the poor enroll in these private programs than to the affluent, a point underscored by the fact that high income groups now spend four times the amount of money in out-of-pocket expenses on health than do the poor. As long as the voluntary sector remains solvent, and offers more extended health benefits than are available under government plans, an individual's income, job security, type of employment and occupational affiliation in Canada still determine selected aspects of the type of service which he receives, his life changes, and the conditions under which he obtains health care.

THE MEDICAL PROFESSION

Government health insurance ushered in a period of complex new relations between the medical profession and the state. In earlier decades government health policies developed through an informal entente between medical leaders, public administrators and legislators. While the medical profession lost its direct control of physician-sponsored plans with the advent of medicare, this informal arrangement still persists but in some ways has become more formal. Certain key documents or statistical reports prepared by government are circulated to a privileged 'short list'. In a few instances such as a major report on ways to reduce health costs in Ontario, or the impact of deterrent fees in Saskatchewan, government has withheld the distribution of reports to the public in deference to the opinions of leaders of the medical profession. In this way the profession still exercises considerable control on decisions made by government, on the fate of new planning proposals or in terms of public accountability.

Public health insurance is slowly changing these comfortable 'behind-the-scenes' arrangements and in most Canadian provinces, more formal procedural channels of negotiation have evolved as a basis of a routine exchange of views and as a means of anticipating, and possibly avoiding confrontation. In Ontario for instance, the health minister meets on a monthly basis with the executive officers of the provincial medical and hospital associations. This tacit recognition of who holds social power in the health system is underscored by the fact that such meetings are not regularly scheduled with representatives of other groups of health workers such as non-professional personnel.

A sharp division of labour has emerged between the administrators of government programs who monitor health insurance measures and the physicians and other health workers who provide these essential services to the public. This change is in how each group performs their work, and in the case of the civil service, its recruitment and its composition of personnel.

As a consequence of the bureaucratization of health insurance, the power of the medical profession has declined within the civil service. Men trained as physicians no longer hold key positions of power in departments of health. Because of non-competitive incomes with private practice and the changing of basic job functions, the role of doctors has been downgraded in filling senior administrative posts. Today new skills are needed, especially administrative expertise. New medical men have come in, but most senior appointments are now made to non-medical specialists such as accountants, business administrators, or systems management experts. As recently as 1955 in Ontario for example, 12 of the senior 19 administrative officers in the Department of Health were physicians; 10 of these posts were held by public health physicians. By 1970, there were 27 men at the level of branch director or above. Only 14 of these individuals were physicians, of whom five had public health training. Public health's representation dropped from more than half of these posts to less than one-fifth (52.6 to 18.5 per cent).

Under the existing open-ended financial system, there are few or no incentives to encourage local cost controls. The medical profession now has no direct responsibility for the solvency of government plans, a stake which it previously had in its own plans.

This separation of responsibility has had predictable consequences for raising medicare costs. Inevitably, more stringent controls on physicians' incomes have or are now being implemented in several provinces.

As more formal controls emerge, the established functions of provincial licensing bodies and voluntary associations have been extended by government. In several instances these groups have been given quasi-official status as bargaining and policing agents of the government programs. Changes in the structure of the medical fee schedule are now partly determined by negotiation, although government has not developed alternate fee schedule models as a counter bargaining strategy. Several provincial licensing bodies have appointed medical review committees to assess the practices of physicians and their income profiles. This process has been facilitated by the use of computer technology applied to the accounting of fee-for-service bills.

The question of fee schedules and how they are established has brought the medical profession into the front row centre of the political arena. Anxious lest government revoke or limit their powers, provincial medical associations are more than before organizing themselves as collective bargaining units. In Quebec for instance, a number of separate syndicates were formed in the late 1960s for this purpose. Professional political activities have become more important: collective bargaining procedures, public relations programs, negotiations with government over specific principles, and even strikes, the ultimate political weapon, attest to this fact. Despite its fundamental antipathy to the political arena, medicine in Canada has become inescapably bound with politics. A process of 'learning the ropes' is going on as can be seen by some of the rather maladroit adjustments which medical associations have made to certain public programs, and the dilemmas in self-image with which the profession across the country is now preoccupied.

The field of medical economics has expanded so greatly over the past twenty years that the national and provincial medical associations have appointed a wide variety of committees to study and bring forward recommendations on a range of controversial economic issues. Many of these recommendations eventually find their way into official medical policy. Given the tempo of change in the health care system, a pace accelerated by government insurance and the growing bureaucratization of professional associations, it is becoming more difficult to achieve broad policies on which there is consensus within the profession. Individual physicians may well find themselves at variance with the official pronouncements of their associations, and in the future, they may be even farther removed than they now are from the centres of medical decision-making. In this respect, the physician is caught between two powerful bureaucracies, the government and the profession. Neither of these groups may adequately express his personal concerns or his frustrations with emerging health policies.

TOWARD A PUBLIC SERVICE SYSTEM

What these numerous changes represent is a national health system which has been going through a period of rapid transition. The mandate of medicine in Canada as one of the traditional 'free professions' has been curbed, but doctors have not become attuned to their role as career public servants. In the context of the Canadian experience, their emergent status is that of professional entrepreneurs with certain privileges sharply defined by the state. In this evolving status, private and public interests will co-exist which will challenge a rigid specification of their work functions, and in turn, contribute to a sense of adaptability and continued challenge by medicine in the face of social change.

In this case study of one nation, health insurance has been a fundamental catalyst of social change in the health system. While its intent was economic in nature, the program has stimulated broad structural changes in the system as a whole. These changes have led to sharp modifications in the status, power and social mandates of particular groups or institutions and the evolving relations between them.

The balance of social power in health affairs in Canada is now more equally balanced than in the past between the private and public spheres. This situation ensures certain universal benefits while social disparities still persist as in the case of the regional distribution of services. While central health planning along the lines achieved by some socialist or communist nations is still far on the horizon, the newly reached private-public balance of power in the Canadian health system allows for institutional flexibility, innovation and an emergent public accountability which is unusual for many nations.

What remains unknown as these changes occur in Canada, as for other nations, is their direct impact on raising the level of health of the Canadian people, how the social definition of health and illness has been altered, or how the altruistic dedication traditionally attributed to the healing professions may have been affected. In this respect from the Canadian experience, the structural changes in the health system and the shift in social power from the private to public arena may demonstrate a social truism, namely, that multiple social means can accomplish similar social ends.

DEPRIVATION AND HEALTH CARE PLANNING IN THE U.S.

GEORGE G. READER

Department of Public Health, Cornell University, New York, N.Y., U.S.A.

In every society there is a segment that has few of the good things of life and a number of people who must struggle even to maintain themselves. These are the deprived members of society. The Oxford Dictionary defines deprivation as the taking away of something enjoyed. In our usage of the term, it means the inability to enjov whar is available to the rest of society. Some never achieve what the majority take for granted, so that it is not as much a matter of loss for them as of being left out altogether. Deprivation may be considered absolute when referring to those below a subsistence income level. In the United States the poverty level is presently considered to be an income of $3,500 for a family of four, which is the point in most states at which people are eligible for public assistance. Another form of absolute deprivation is lack of access to resources. Because of maldistribution of personnel and facilities, needed services may be unobtainable or access may be difficult to those that are available. Deprivation may also be relative, in that the 'revolution of rising expectations' may create dissatisfaction with availability of services at a faster rate than delivery can be improved. Therefore, even the relatively well-to-do individual may feel deprived when he cannot obtain wanted services or services he was led to believe were necessary. This paper will address itself to an exploration of how the deprivation of health services functions as a stimulus and modifier of health planning, particularly in the United States.

Social planners in the health field must take into account both relative and absolute deprivation, and must try to determine what is necessary to maintain health as well as to acknowledge demands above that level. Identifying fundamental needs is a difficult process. It is often carried out by official agencies such as public health departments. These agencies usually view basic needs in terms of such universalistic health measures as pure food, safe housing, immunization and sanitation. On the personal level, needs and demands are often intertwined and impossible to separate. The individual with a common cold may not actually need to see a physician but by doing so many occasionally prevent further complications, such as pneumonia. Demands stem from the cultural values and the level of education of a community as well as expectations of what should be available. In a democratic society, the social planners must also consider the satisfaction of the consumer in judging the success of their work. For the consumer to be satisfied, he must feel that his demands and expectations are being met reasonably well.

HISTORY OF SOCIAL WELFARE PLANNING IN THE U.S.

The experience with social planning in the U.S. has emphasized the values placed on individualism up until very recent times. During the colonial days, there were few efforts at public control of health and illness except those designed to protect the community from epidemics. Physicians cared for the indigent as a personal charity. Some cities established poorhouses where the sick poor might find rest and sustenance, but most charity was personal rather than public. Health facilities were founded by public subscription through voluntary contributions. Benjamin Franklin and Dr. Thomas Bond raised funds from the citizens of Philadelphia for the first hospital in America, The Pennsylvania Hospital. Similarly, Dr. Samuel Bard and Sir Henry Moore solicited contributions from the citizens of New York City for the second, The New York Hospital. Sir Henry Moore who was Governor General of New York, personally contributed and also induced the New York Legislature to vote an annual stipend for the Hospital. This stipend continued for many years, but represented only a small fraction of the Hospital's support. Eventually, municipal and even federal hospitals were founded, but the tradition has remained to this day that the majority of U.S. hospitals are supported by voluntary contributions, rather than by taxes. This stands in marked contrast to the United Kingdom and the countries of Western Europe where the majority of the hospitals have been publicly owned from fairly early times.

The frontier had a profound influence on American thought during most of the 19th century. Those who were dissatisfied could go westward to find a new life, and the virtues of individualism and self-sufficiency fostered by frontier living were constantly reinforced. Making one's own way came to have a high value; and health care, like most benefits, was a privilege to be earned rather than a right. It was generally believed that the poor did not strive hard enough, and consequently got what they deserved.

At the beginning of the 20th century, the second great waves of immigration from Russia, Poland and Southern Europe began. The immigrants constituted a large part of the poor for many years. Many of the majority felt they did not really belong and, therefore, that society had no particular responsibility for them. They could prove themselves worthy of full membership in society only by making their own way. Negroes, too, until very recently, were not allowed to participate in social life. They have always contributed a large segment to the poor, but because they were not considered full members of the body politic, were not, therefore, particularly deserving of public concern. The focus of public and official efforts through most of U.S. history was on protecting the community, not in helping the individual.

Up to quite recent times, the American Medical Association has argued that health care is a privilege and not a right. Many members of the AMA, however, have expressed the belief individually that no one should suffer for lack of care. The discrepancy seems to lie in a belief strongly held by many American physicians that their delivery of medical care is a kind of private monopoly, and that they want to provide it themselves to those who cannot pay as an act of personal charity. Making it publicly available invades their autonomy and robs them of the chance to do a good deed. Fortunately, today many physicians and particularly the younger members of the profession can see the pattern of delivery in economic perspective especially to the underprivileged, and they welcome efforts by government to see that distribution of services is made more equitable. Even so, there still remains a strong feeling in American medicine that payment should be by means of fee-for-service, and that government reimbursement should follow this pattern. In Europe, physicians, particularly those serving the indigent, have traditionally been salaried or paid on a capitation basis. As a consequence, the European primary care physician is usually a generalist who decides when and to whom he should make a referral. In the U.S., the physician cares for his patients both in his office and in the hospital. The hospital is the workshop of the community physician, in contrast to Europe, where it is the domain of the salaried specialist. Patients in the U.S. tend to choose their own physician and often even their own specialist. It can be seen, then, that U.S. medicine is highly individualistic and exemplifies a free-enterprise economy, compared with the organized system available to all levels of society in Western Europe. Medicine in the U.S. is pluralistic and diversified, which inevitably produces fragmentation, but on the positive side, perhaps more readily accepts innovation.

Darwin Palmiere identifies three types of health planning in the U.S. [1] Chronologically they are: (1) Dispersed, in which each provider, consumer and financing organization does its own planning; (2) Focused, in which voluntary associations of persons and organizations join together in an attempt to solve common problems; (3) Central, in which the planning unit can force other individuals and organizations to use their own resources in accordance with its plans. All three types function today, reinforcing and supporting one another; their existence emphasizes the diversified decision-making that characterizes U.S. health planning.

The growth of the health insurance industry in the U.S. reflects the same pluralism in delivery of services and, in fact, in itself reinforces it. Health insurance began with the stimulus of the depression to provide coverage for the most expensive feature of illness, i.e. hospitalization. From its beginnings in the 1930's, it has grown today to be a $14 billion industry. Nevertheless, health insurance does not cover everyone but primarily serves the employed middle class and is of little help to the deprived. The poor, until recently, have been almost entirely dependent on individual physicians' charity or on public clinics for their medical care. The rest of American society, however, is also relatively deprived because of the built-in limitations of private health insurance. Senator Kennedy has pointed out: [2]

> In 1969, of the 180 milion Americans under 65 years of age, 18%, or 34 million had no hospital insurance; 21%, or 38 million had no surgical insurance; 35%, or 63 million, had no outpatient X-ray and laboratory insurance; 52%, or 94 million had no insurance

for prescription drugs; 57%, or 103 million, had no insurance for physician office visits or home visits; and 95%, or 173 million had no dental insurance.

IDENTIFYING THE HEALTH PROBLEMS OF THE DEPRIVED

The poor in all countries are more likely to suffer illness. They are often malnourished, subject to overcrowding in housing, exposed to accidents and infections and frequently have difficulty finding adequate medical care, sometimes because of their own apathy but often because it is not readily available to them. In the U.S., as Ashley Weeks states:[3]

> Ten to 12% of the U.S. population live in poverty as defined by the U.S. Census Bureau. Groups that show an especially high incidence of poverty are the aged, with greater than 20% of both men and women below the poverty level; female heads of families, with 29% below the poverty level; non-whites; and the poorly educated, 21.4% of those with less than a sixth-grade education having poverty incomes. Studies of health care in infancy in the rural South indicates the relationship poverty has to both physician utilization and illness. Although 5% of the sampled population experienced no well-child care, 17% of non-whites and 21% of children whose mother had only a grade school education had no physician visits. These groups also showed the highest percentage of people having one or more chronic diseases. The relationship between poverty and illness is an ever-widening dynamic circle in which poverty contributes to illness and illness brings out further poverty.

A study of the New York City Welfare population carried out by us from 1960–1965 and reported in *Welfare Medical Care: An Experiment*,[4] indicated that the sample of New York City Welfare clients we studied were a good deal sicker than were people situated in a random sample of the entire population of the City of Baltimore. Tuberculosis, malignant neoplasms, anemia, kidney disease, and other urinary disorders all exceeded the Baltimore rates by a wide margin. Arteriosclerotic heart disease was five times more prevalent in the New York City Welfare clients than in the Baltimore population. Psychiatric conditions, however, showed the most dramatic difference. The rate of psychosis was 106/1,000 in the New York City Project compared with 6/1,000 in the Baltimore study. Alcoholism, mental deficiency, and behavior disorders all showed much higher rates in The New York Hospital Project. Differences for psychoneurosis were less marked.

It is also well known that poverty is associated with increased infant mortality. A study done on the U.S. population by the National Center for Health Statistics[5] found that infant mortality rates were highest in families who measured low on family income, education of mother and education of father. Increase in socioeconomic status as measured by anyone of the variables was associated with a decrease in infant mortality rates.

These then are some of the special health problems of the deprived: chronic illness, psychiatric conditions, and high infant mortality. Some of them are obviously likely to be responsive to general improvement in the quality of life, better income, improved housing, and education and employment opportunities. Social planning for health must certainly take these factors into account. Now let us turn to what has been done specifically in social planning for the deprived.

CURRENT STATUS OF HEALTH CARE PLANNING

As has been noted, the depression of the 1930's was a major stimulus for social reform in the United States. The elderly and the disabled were the first target for assistance, and the Social Security Act of 1935 was the beginning of what has been a slow evolutionary process. In signing the Act, President Roosevelt, called it:

> A cornerstone in a structure which is being built, but is by no means complete – a structure intended to lessen the force of possible future depressions, to act as a protection to future administrations of government against the necessity of going deeply into debt to furnish relief to the needy – a law to flatten out the peaks and valleys of deflation and inflation – in other words, a law that will take care of human needs and at the same time provide for the United States an economic structure of vastly greater soundness.

The Social Security Act provides continuing income maintenance for most families if the breadwinner retires because of age, becomes disabled or dies; except for general financial support, however, in its original form, it did nothing directly for the health care of the people covered.

Free milk stations for poor children were established about the turn of the century by charitable agencies and these gradually evolved into child health centers supported by municipal government. But it was not until 1936 that the Federal Government began to supply funds for child care. Since then, the States have received annual grants to extend and improve maternal and child health services and crippled children's services, especially in rural and low-income areas. The amounts appropriated are apportioned among the States according to formulas that take into account child population, number of births, income and other factors. The States are required to match half the funds granted with their own funds. After 1963, several new maternal and child health programs were established by amendments to the Social Security Act in response to serious shortages of services for low-income families. One such program of Maternity and Infant Care Projects provides comprehensive care to high-risk mothers and their infants.[6] Fifty-six projects serve urban areas that had above-average rates of infant mortality. The 1965 amendments to the Social Security Act also authorized grants for projects providing comprehensive health care for children of school and preschool age in low-income areas. There are now 59 Children and Youth Projects serving 475,000 children, 2/3 in inner city areas. A series of projects in dental health for children in low-income areas was begun in 1971 with an emphasis on continuous dental supervision, beginning in the preschool years. Thus far, 18 projects located in rural countries as well as urban areas have been started.[7]

The first federal effort to confront health problems of the deprived directly was the Kerr–Mills Act of 1960. It provided matching grants to states for medical care of the indigent aged. Many states failed to implement it, and some required such rigorous eligibility that an aged person's near relatives had to prove they were destitute before the beneficiary himself could be declared eligible. Its inadequacies, however, served to alert the Congress to the need for better legislation.

In 1965, therefore, despite the bitter opposition of the American Medical Association, Congress amended the Social Security Act to provide for health insurance benefits to all over age 65 covering both hospital and nursing home charges, physicians' fees and home care, and direct benefits to the medically indigent. The latter section was a revision of the Kerr–Mills Act that was intended to require all states to participate and to forbid a 'means test' except for the beneficiary himself. Nevertheless, Medicaid, as it is called, is a welfare program and each state is free to fix its own eligibility levels. Some states have required actual poverty, i.e. income below the subsistence level, for eligibility.

Wilbur Cohen, former Secretary of Health, Education Welfare, points out that by 1967, the Social Security program, as a whole, was releasing $20 billion a year to some 23 million men, women and children, or one out of every nine persons in the country.

There is no question that this has had an enormously beneficial effect on the health care of the deprived, and particularly the elderly. But it has limitations too, and many deprived persons find they must delay medical attention because of the costs of co-insurance or the barriers to eligibility.

One of the unexpected consequences of Medicare and Medicaid has been the inflationary effect on health care costs. It was thought that many older people would rush to obtain care for their illnesses and thus would swamp the available facilities. This did not happen; the elderly were found to be no more eager to enter hospitals than they had been, and there has been little over-utilization. Injection of large amounts of money into the U.S. health care system, however, without expansion of the numbers of health personnel or facilities inevitably resulted in higher costs. Reimbursement to hospitals under the legislation was based on true costs and, for physicians, was based on prevailing and customary fees. Hospitals immediately began adding equipment and personnel because they could be justified as costs of operation. Blue collar workers in the hospitals, who had been seriously underpaid compared with similar jobs in other industries, began to demand more equitable pay, and unionization, in some cases, reinforced their demands. Hospital-based health professionals such as nurses and interns also won increases, and physicians in practice sought higher fees. The result has been that hospital costs have reached levels of $150 a day per bed in some parts of the country and have risen dramatically everywhere.

About the same time as the passage of Medicare and Medicaid, another national effort was mounted to deal with the specific problems of the poor and deprived. This was the Economic Opportunity Act of

1964. It established the Office of Economic Opportunity in the Executive branch of the government, and provided funds for development of community action programs in deprived communities across the land. A unique feature of the effort was a directive to allow 'maximum feasible participation' by the poor themselves. This was interpreted to mean that the deprived should share in planning for services and in distribution of government funds. The community action groups quickly identified lack of access to health services as a major problem for the poor, and after considerable thoughtful planning, the Office of Economic Opportunity outlined the form of organization through which health services might most effectively be delivered. This has come to be known as the Neighborhood Health Center and has the following characteristics: [8]

1. Focuses on the needs of the poor.
2. A one-door facility, readily accessible in terms of time and place, in which virtually all ambulatory health services are made available.
3. Intensive participation by and involvement of the population to be served, both as policy-makers and employees.
4. Full integration of and with existing sources of services and funds.
5. Assurance of personalized, high-quality care and professional staff of the highest caliber.
6. Close coordination with other community resources.
7. Sponsorship by a wide variety of public and private auspices.

Except for the emphasis on consumer participation, one can recognize that the model followed is quite similar to the urban polyclinic common in Eastern Europe as the main source of primary care.

Besides the Office of Economic Opportunity, the Public Health Service sponsored the development of neighborhood health centers. Starting with only three OEO centers in 1965, by 1973 there were 117 centers throughout the country serving over a million people. Most were to be found in urban settings but a few have been successfully started in rural areas.

A major attempt to apply social planning principles to health also began in 1966 with the passage of the Partnership in Health Act. The aim was to relate the federal government to local communities by establishing state-wide health planning agencies in each state and then relate to them a network of local planning agencies with one in each community. The law mandated a minimum of 51% consumer representation on each of the planning bodies and directed that planning grant applications "must show that preventive diagnostic, treatment and rehabilitative programs shall include special attention to the health needs of high risk population groups in terms of age, economic status, geographic location, or other relevant factors".

Community health planning agencies may be expected eventually to have a profound effect on delivery of services and identification of the special needs of the deprived. They are just getting underway in most localities, however, and it is too early to tell what their impact may be in the near term.

A parallel program designed to speed delivery of services to those in need of them was the Regional Medical Programs Act. Local agencies were organized composed primarily of providers, who were directed to use federal funding to improve the organization and delivery of services in their local region. Some regions encompassed several states, but the larger states usually had a number of regions within their borders. Although some useful programs were developed with this stimulus, it was the judgement of the Nixon Administration that this was a wasteful and inefficient arrangement for disbursement of federal funds, and the program began to be phased out in the Spring of 1973.

SOCIAL PLANNING FOR HEALTH IN 1971–1972

President Nixon in his Health Message to Congress in February 1971, spoke of building a national health strategy.[9] He proposed that it be built on four basic principles:

1. Assuring Equal Access – by removing racial, economic, social or geographic barriers.

2. Balancing Supply and Demand – by improving the health care system.

3. Organizing for Efficiency – by emphasizing health maintenance and preserving cost consciousness.

4. Building on Strengths – by accepting diversity in our system and encouraging better cooperation and coordination.

His statement suggested a form of national health insurance to be paid for by employer and employee contributions. A new family Health

Insurance Plan would replace Medicaid and would be fully financed and administered by the Federal Government. It would provide health insurance to all poor families with children headed by self-employed or unemployed persons whose income was below $5,000 for a family of four.

Despite considerable effort to encourage Congress to pass such legislation, nothing came of these recommendations in 1971, and the thrust was lost in the preparations for the election of 1972. Since then, the initiative seems to have swung away from the President to Congress, and the Administration has now retreated to cutting back almost all of the present governmental programs dealing with health problems of the deprived as an economy measure supposedly to check inflation.

PROPOSED LEGISLATION

Polls indicate that both physicians and patients believe there are serious inadequacies in our health care today, even though most would not go so far as to declare there is a crisis. Congress is responsive to such opinion and various Senators and Representatives have themselves developed proposals for change. The leading contenders at present are the Health Care Insurance Act, the Health Security Act, the National Health Care Services Act, the National Health Care Act, and the Catastrophic Health Insurance Act.

The Health Care Insurance Act, also known as Medicredit, is supported by the American Medical Association. It would provide tax credits for health insurance premiums, and for the poor, the government would pay the premiums. It would not change the present system otherwise at all.

The Health Security Act, also known as the Kennedy–Griffiths, is supported by organized labor. It would replace Medicare and Medicaid and be financed through social security taxes and general revenues. The country would be divided into regions which in turn would be subdivided into health service areas. Funds would be allocated to each region. Health providers would have to operate under an annual budget approved by the government. Physicians could choose to be paid by salary, capitation of fee-for-service, but fees would be regulated by fee schedules. It is the most wide-ranging and the most expensive of the proposals, estimated at $59 billion a year.

The National Health Care Services Act is supported by the American Hospital Association. It would set up health care corporations to provide services organized by the providers and subject to state regulation and national standards.

The National Health Care Act is supported by the insurance industry. It provides for a three-part voluntary health insurance plan: an employer-employee part, an individual plan, and a plan for the poor and uninsurable. Tax credits would be offered to both employers and individuals. General revenues would pay the premiums for the poor. There would be no other change in the present system.

The Catastrophic Health Insurance Act may have the widest appeal to legislators at present since it only reinsures against catastrophic illness. It would be relatively inexpensive and require no change in the present system. It would, however, be of little value to lower middle income persons who might be wiped out financially by an illness before the insurance could come into effect. Health activities oppose it because if accepted it might delay development of more effective legislation.

All current proposals except Kennedy–Griffiths and the American Hospital Association bills depend on better ways of paying for care without changing the system of delivery. They might help to solve the important problem of financial disability but would do little for the other barriers to access. Both the absolutely and relatively deprived in the U.S. require a new and better system to provide equal access for all members of the population, and to end fragmentation. If this can be accomplished while still preserving diversity and pluralism in American health care, it might come within the next few years. If the only solution is a new and monolithic system, however, the prospects for a significant change soon in health care of the poor are relatively dim.

REFERENCES

[1] S. Palmiere, *Community Health Planning*, pp. 59–82. L. Corey, S. E. Saltman and M. F. Epstein, *Medicine in a Changing Society*, C. V. Mosby Co., St. Louis 1972.

[2] E. M. Kennedy, 'Changing the Face of American Health', in: L. Corey, S. E.

Saltman and M. F. Epstein, *Medicine in a Changing Society*, C. V. Mosby Co., St. Louis 1972, pp. 105–116.
[3] A. Weeks, 'The Pathology of Poverty', in: L. Corey, S. E. Saltman and M. F. Epstein, *Medicine in a Changing Society*, C. V. Mosby Co., St. Louis 1972, pp. 8–21.
[4] C. H. Goodrich, M. Olendzki and G. G. Reader, (eds.), *Welfare Medical Care: An experiment*, Harvard University Press, Boston 1970.
[5] National Center for Health Statistics, 'Infant Mortality Rates: Socieconomic Factors', *Vital and Health Statistics*, Series 22, No. 14 (1972) 2–7.
[6] U. S. Department of Health, Education, and Welfare, *Promoting the Health of Mothers and Children: FY 1972*, Rockville, Maryland: Health Services and Mental Health Administration, 1972.
[7] V. E. Weckwerth, 'Progress Report – Assessment of Child Health Care Delivery and Organization', *Comment Series*, Systems Development Project, No. 0–7 (29).
[8] L. B. Schorr, 'The Neighborhood Health Center – Background and Current Issues', in: L. Corey, S. E. Saltman and M. F. Epstein, *Medicine in a Changing Society*, C. V. Mosby Co., St. Louis 1972, pp. 138–147.
[9] 'Health – Message from The President of the United States: Relative to Building a National Health Strategy', *92nd Congress, 1st Session, February 18, 1971*, House Document No. 92–49, Washington, D. C., U.S. Government Printing Office, pp. 2–4.

PROFESSIONAL HEALTH PLANNING AND THE HEALTH PROFESSIONS

ERIK HOLST

Institute for Social Medicine, University of Copenhagen, Copenhagen, Denmark

As an observer over a number of years at close quarters of interprofessional interaction in the health field and its impact on decision-making, I have been tempted to set down – no doubt prematurely – some impressions of this phenomenon in relation to planning.

I have in my approach drawn heavily on inspiration from ideas put forward by Mark Field, Eliot Freidson and Magdalena Sokołowska, to whom I am thus indebted.

1. THE CONCEPT OF HEALTH PLANNING

Where health planning used to denote the planning of a multiplicity of programmes for organized combat of specific diseases or for the protection of specified risk-groups, it has lately developed into a more comprehensive concept, becoming a means for the systematic promotion of health of the total population on a rational medico-socio-economic basis. The reasons for this development could be seen as a result of the general tendency towards more comprehensive socio-economic planning in a field which is rightly or wrongly considered to be well-defined and is of natural public concern. It might also be due to the realization that the improvement in health conditions is stagnating or even being reversed in spite of present efforts. Or, it may be due to concern over the rapidly increasing financial and human demands on society by the health care system in a highly urbanized/industrialized society.

Along with this tendency towards a more comprehensive planning of health care there is a growing realization of the need to see health planning as an integral part of general socio-economic planning (WHO, technical discussions, Geneva, May 1972).

In spite of this there is still a noticable reluctance to let the concept of health planning transgress the traditional boundaries of the health care system.

2. RESPONSIBILITY AND COMPETENCE IN HEALTH PLANNING

Traditional competence and responsibility relative to health planning have been a prerogative of the health professions, more specifically of the medical profession. This competence and responsibility was early invested in public health authorities concerning health programmes aimed at combating sanitary problems or infectious agents. The administration of such programmes was considered a technicality which could be handled by the health professions themselves with the aid of minor clerical and technical assistance.

The primary health services were also – as a matter of course – administered by the helath professions themselves, and only the growing size and complexity of the specialized hospitals introduced independent professional administrators and gradually also advanced technologists into the staff structure of modern hospitals. Parallel to this development, the increasing sophistication and specialization of individual care brought new clinical professions into the medical organization: clinical psychologists, logopeadics, physiotherapists, ergotherapists and social workers, as well as laboratory technicians to take care of the increasingly complex diagnostic examinations.

In the planning of new services and especially in the building of new hospitals, more professional competence was involved in the form of systems engineers, economy analysts and operational analysts. These new professions demanded better basic information concerning the expected demands on and functions of the hospital and gradually emphasized the need for improved medico-statistical and epidemiological services. This again brought the demographers and the health statisticians into the center of the picture.

Finally, the behavioural scientist appeared on the scene, together with sociologists and social psychologists, to plead the case of the recipients of modern medical care: i.e. of the patient, who was somehow the last to be asked about his views on the services planned.

Politicians and voluntary organizations have been considered responsible for representing public opinion, i.e. collective interests of the citizens. And these representatives of non-professional opinion were normally those responsible for financing the operation of health care institutions and programmes. This would normally ensure a strong influence on planning or at least in implementation of any plans, but there are some indications that non-professional control of health care planning and health care operation is not terribly effective, and this may be due to the nature of the objectives.

In the field of primary health care, where this has remained a market for free enterprise, the patient as a consumer retains a similar influence as a non-professional controller of the services supplied again with a very limited impact on the planning and operation of these services.

3. PROFESSIONAL BIAS IN HEALTH PLANNING

As long as health planning was considered an aspect of medical care that could be left to the discretion of the health (medical) professions, problems of professional bias, scientific outlook, and ethical attitude were not too obvious determinants of development.

As other professions moved into the health field their professional bias, their scientific outlook, and their ethical attitudes became apparent through their criticism of prevailing traditions and procedures in the organization of medical care.

Questions like the formulation of the ultimate purpose of the operation of a health care programme may have seemed quite clear to the classical health profession bred in the Hippocratic tradition, whereas new professions might introduce concepts with a different kind of emphasis than that of preserving life at all cost. Not only was there a difference of opinion regarding ultimate purpose, but also in the likelihood of achieving optimal results by sticking to a purely natural-scientific approach to illness. And finally, there was the challenge by new professions to the traditional health professions to give up their claim to a virtual monopoly of the latter professions over all health care issues.

In this connection it is worth noting that the concept of the role of other members of what has come to constitute the health care team, is probably very often a rather simplistic model. This may lead to the new professions adopting, and the classical health professions accepting, a delimitation of their role in the team which is rather less than the actual capacity of these professions might warrant. It might seem as if such a conscious or unconscious relative underrating of the capacity of nurses and doctors were a necessary step in the introduction of new members to an established organization.

The medical profession has been more than willing to accept the claim to superiority in scientific excellence by natural scientists of various disciplines. The profession has however been much more reluctant to accept a similar assessment of scientists from the behavioural and social sciences – even though these sciences are also considered 'basic sciences' compared to the 'applied sciences' represented by the health professions.

This acceptance of the natural scientist among the health professions has long been witnessed by the presence of natural scientists on the staffs of medical schools. Behavioural and social scientists are much harder to find in this capacity but are gradually being introduced, often headed by the clinical psychologist, followed by the biostatistician and the sociologist. The integration of these scientists into the medical school is facilitated by the fact, that everybody at the university runs through an identical career pattern and that the role of university teachers is only marginally dependent upon professional background.

In the traditional area of medical care, however, the new professions are finding some difficulty in obtaining an equal share of responsibility and influence. It is perhaps significant that most of the professional analysis of medical care operations is concerned with the framework of the institutions rather than with the essential processes of medical care, i.e. the decision-making concerning diagnosis and treatment, including the evaluation of these activities.

I think the alternative approaches represented by the medical care professions and the social care professions may be used to exemplify the kind of interprofessional conflict I am trying to elucidate. Both groups have well-defined ways of assessing a case and both offer a number of treatments that will be of benefit to patients/clients representing typical medical or social problems. The increasing realisation by both professions, that human beings are biological as well as social entities, has called forth a demand for integration of medical and social care in primary as well as in specialized care. The professions involved have consequently entered into an uneasy cooperation, each group with a deep-rooted professional bias, each group having problems with the dominance of the traditional professions in the health and social care sectors respectively. In a segregated system patients/clients are divided into categories dominated by health or social problems respectively. The experience of professionals from each sector is therefore dominated by cases requiring (or seeming to require) the expertise of the traditional professions of that sector. This becomes the basis for a mistaken generalization that all or most cases needing social and/or medical care represents the same relative distribution of medical and social problems as the selected case-population that that profession is used to handle. This again, brings about a natural overestimation of one's own professional role and capacity within the integrated care team and a complementary underestimation of the role and capacity of other professions in the team.

Instead of leading to fraternal cooperation, these confrontations between professions in the socio-medical team may cause some to have recourse to a formal distribution of power within the team backed up by the professional organizations of the various members of the team.

What was originally a question of emphasis in the evaluation of a patient's/client's need for care develops into a struggle for supremacy among several professions. And as the issues are not seen as organizational problems but as the basic right of each profession to exert its professional skill to its full extent—it may also develop into disputes between the scientific societies built around the disciplines involved.

The strong professional bias demonstrable in such attempts to establish multidisciplinary health teams would clearly suggest that the development of the health care system is influenced strongly by the health professions along lines that would be challenged by other professions were they in a position to exert any influence.

It is obvious that such a modifying influence on developments is necessary when the scope of health care is extended beyond the traditional limits of the health care system into the social care sector. But this also applies wherever stronger emphasis on the socio-psychological aspects of health care is desired. So health planning must as a minimum be based on the coordinated opinion of all the professions involved in the care of human beings within the health care system. And no single profession can demand supremacy in this task. Apart from the professions directly involved in the care of patients, the technological and administrative professions responsible for the operation of health institutions and programmes have vital contributions to make to health planning.

4. PROFESSIONALIZATION OF HEALTH PLANNING

A special role in health planning is played by the various analytical professions studying the health care organizations from the organizational, economical, sociological and psychological viewpoints. These professions are partly called upon by the health services to help improve existing services or to plan new services. Partly they enter the health field for academic studies of the health care organization with a view to describing the social or interpersonal relationships and the basic concepts existing in this field.

These groups provide a new means of evaluation of the organizational, economic and human aspects of the health services untainted by the professional bias of the health professions. Naturally enough the health professions take a rather defensive attitude to this kind of evaluation by outsiders, seeing it as a potential threat to their freedom to pursue their professional goals as they see them. It is interesting to observe the way health professions handle the eventual absorption or rejection of new professions being transplanted into the health field. But basically it is only a variant of the situation which arises when new people are introduced into established groups.

An initial superficial demonstration of hospitality, a realization of the threat to the system's integrity, a sharp delimitation of the intruder's field of operation, conscious or unconscious attempts to downgrade his competence or at least his relevance to the health field. If, at this point, the system has reasserted itself sufficiently to take a milder view of the risk involved in the intruders' activities, some form of working coexistence may develop and the intruder is thus assimilated.

If, on the other hand, the intruder seems to threaten basic concepts, a professional conflict develops and the intruder is rejected by the system. In this situation the intruder is likely to try to further his course through appeals to public authorities, politicians or public opinion through the mass media. This is normally up-hill work, but may be somewhat easier in the health field due to the extensive public interest in problems of health.

The outside influence on the health services will in this case often be effected through a reevaluation of the issue by the health professions themselves, but this does not mean that the health professions have given up their monopoly over the services – only that they have decided to exercise this monopoly in a slightly different way.

This is what makes it necessary to establish within the health sector, and preferably among the health sciences proper, multiprofessional centers which may develop the appropriate tools for a continuous analysis of the health care system from within making use of the expertise of all the professions involved.

A development along these lines may eventually provide health planning with adequate and so far as possible unbiassed information about the operation of health services.

There is, however, an inherent risk that overall planning for health will be prejudiced by the very refinement of our analysis of existing health services and programmes. Attempts to extend health planning beyond the medical care services involves a break-down, not only of a traditional professional monopoly, but also of the concept that health is achieved primarily through medical care. In an attempt to widen the scope of health planning, the interprofessional problems are almost reversed insofar as in such planning the health professions will be the intruders into areas like production, transport, education and housing.

The traditional division of labour among the various professions dominating each of these sectors is becoming a barrier to comprehensive planning and the implementation of community action. At least planning itself and the creation of a sound, unbiassed basis for planning, must therefore be developed into a crossprofessional discipline in its own right with its own ethical standards and its own scientific basis.

As has been pointed out by Magdalena Sokołowska, medical ethics are applicable only to the doctor/patient or nurse/patient relationship—not to health issues on a macro or societal level. This does not mean, however, that the professional health planning team does not require among its members persons with a solid medical background, but it means that a professional training in the science of health planning must be added to professional training in health care. In this respect, however, the health professions will be joined by professionals from other disciplines, who must undergo special training in order to be able to apply their basic training to health planning on a professional level.

5. NON-PROFESSIONAL CONTROL OF HEALTH PLANNING AND THE ROLE OF THE PATIENT

With improved health planning services and a multiprofessional assessment of needs and programmes, political decisions concerning health issues will come to rest on much sounder foundation than the professional-pressure-group/type of direction hitherto available has allowed. The individual citizen/patient/client as the recipient or consumer of services, however, should be given a prominent position, side by side with the professional health planners, as the other important advisor to political decision-makers.

SUMMARY

For a variety of reasons health planning has conceptually developed out of planning a multiplicity of programmes for the ogranized combat of specific diseases and the protection of specified risk-groups into comprehensive planning for the systematic promotion of health. There is also a definite trend to see health planning as an integral part of overall socio-economic planning.

Traditionally, competence and responsibility with regard to health planning have been a prerogative of the health professions, the planning and administration of health institutions and programmes being considered secondary and purely technical or clerical functions. Various forms of non-professional control of the health professions in the role of planners and administrators have been exercised by political bodies, public authorities or private voluntary organizations, but such control may not have been very effective in directing development.

The professionalization of planning on the community level has brought a host of new professions into the health field, primarily in connection with the building of new medical centres, and the running of these complicated organizations has turned over to other professions the administrative, economic and technological responsibility hitherto handled by the health professions.

The more comprehensive concept of health care has involved professions operating in sectors normally considered outside the health field in the planning and operation of health-promoting activities. The conflict inherent in the necessity of bringing the knowledge, with its attendant biases, of widely different professional groups to bear on the task of comprehensive health planning is an obvious difficulty which may bar developments which would otherwise be possible. This conflict is based not only on professional traditions – which are strong and long established in the health field – but as often on differences in basic ethical attitudes, in scientific schooling and in the concept of the roles of existing and new professions and their respective claims to represent an informed opinion on planning for health.

This is not only an inherent conflict at the local level, but also between professional organizations and scientific societies. The role of the patient in health planning is still conspicuously small and should also be considered as a necessary development in the future shared responsibility which the health professions must accept in this field.

V. TEACHING

FROM LEARNED PROFESSION TO POLICY SCIENCE: A TREND ANALYSIS OF SOCIOLOGY IN THE MEDICAL EDUCATION OF THE UNITED STATES

SAMUEL W. BLOOM

Mount Sinai School of Medicine, The City University of New York, New York, N.Y., U.S.A.

INTRODUCTION

> "The reconstruction of our medical education... is not going to end matters once and for all. It leaves untouched certain outlying problems that will all the more surely come into focus when the professional training of the physician is once securely established on a scientific basis. At that moment the social role of the physician will generally expand, and to support such expansion, he will crave a more liberal and disinterested educational experience." (Flexner, 1910)

During the first half of this century, medical education in the United States was preoccupied with the establishment of scientific medicine as the basis of the professional training of physicians. In the process, the populist, Jacksonian-democracy spirit of the frontier gave way to the elitist, science-oriented standards of the English and German universities, and the independent proprietary medical schools of the nineteenth century were almost totally replaced by university medical schools.

At mid-century, this process was substantially completed. The American medical schools, with remarkable unanimity, presented the same curriculum and standards for admission. From the parochial, clinical, and socially open institutions which they had been in 1900, they became a wholly different type of organization. Dominated by the laboratories of a federation of basic biological scientists and research oriented clinical specialists, (Stevens, 1971, pp. 348 ff.) their recruitment was highly selective, producing a competitive situation for aspirants that implicitly favored students from advantaged backgrounds in social class and education.

It was at this point, about twenty-five years ago, that American medical educators began to seriously consider new directions for the training of physicians. Much as Flexner predicted, they waited until the scientific basis of their professional training was secure, and only then reached out toward the expansion, in more liberal intellectual terms, of their teaching. As part of this shift in orientation, the social sciences were invited, at first with caution and some skepticism, to join in medical education. It was also at this point historically that medical sociology, as an organized field, was born.

Today, the role of sociology as a collaborating discipline in the training of physicians is established. Although the extent and stability of sociology's position in medical education should not be over-estimated, the fact of its existence is unquestionable (Hyman, 1967; Kendall and Reader, 1972; Freeman *et al.*, 1972). After a quarter of a century of active trial, medical sociology is part of American medical education.

The current acceptance in medical school faculties, however, carries with it role expectations which are quite different than those which sociologists themselves sought at the beginning of their relationship with medicine. They entered the medical school as behavioural scientists, in a posture much like that of physiology seventy-five years earlier (Cameron, 1952; Reader and Goss, 1958; Stainbrook and Wexler, 1956). At that time, the role demand from medicine was a close fit to the self-perception of sociologists as members of a scholarly, academic profession. More recently, however, a shift has occurred. Increasingly medical sociology has come under pressure to apply its knowledge, to become a 'consulting' profession.

It is this trend toward professionalization, as Freidson defines that process (Freidson, 1971), which is the subject of this paper. Within this general problem, I am most interested here in the *development of knowledge*. The types of research, the theoretical emphases, the selected emphasis of the questions asked in the major published achievements in this field, and why medical sociology has chosen certain patterns of concern over others—these are the preoccupations of this discussion. The focus, in other words, is on the sociology *of* medicine, but this is not taken to exclude sociology *in* medicine (Straus, 1957). These two facets of development, knowledge and work role, through not always related in development, are, in the final analysis interdependent. Indeed, one of the purposes of this paper is to show how knowledge and role in medical sociology can be brought into alignment.

More precisely, I will be concerned with a series of linked trends in medical sociology which appear to direct knowledge development as follows:

FROM	TO
a social psychological frame of reference	institutional analysis
small scale social relations as the main subjects of research	large social systems
role analysis in specifically limited settings	complex organizational analysis
basic theoretical concerns with classic social analysis of behavior	policy science directed toward systematic translation of basic knowledge into decision making
a perspective of human relations and communication	power structure analysis

I will discuss these patterns of knowledge development with two major questions in mind. On the one hand, I am applying the sociology of knowledge to medical sociology. What are the sources of the professionalization of medical sociology? The second question inquires about the effects of this trend. What is the meaning to sociologists who have been working in this field of the shifts in demand from typically 'basic' problems of scholarship to 'relevant' research problems? Does the trend include the germination of some form of organized practice for the skilled application of sociological knowledge?

I. THE PATTERNS OF KNOWLEDGE: THE DEMONSTRATION OF THEORY

At the outset of its relationship with medicine, sociology was in a stage of its own history in which the central, preoccupying concerns were those of academic legitimacy. It was a time when the liaison between the heroic European theories and the empirical social research methods of American positivists was most passionate.

Medical sociology was born, therefore, in the university and its early primary drive was toward the development of knowledge. A profession only in a limited sense, it did not perceive itself as responsible for the organized application of knowledge in the service of a constituency of clients. It was colleague-oriented, not client-oriented. Its primary responsibility was as a field of scholarship and therefore to knowledge development rather than to the application of knowledge in the solution of problems. In these terms, sociology came into medical education much the same as various biological sciences had done earlier. Moreover, just as an independent subject like physiology, upon entrance into medical education was grouped with other biological areas like anatomy and chemistry, and the group renamed the 'biomedical' or 'basic preclinical sciences' so did medical sociology find itself joined with a group of disciplines called 'the behavioral sciences of medicine' (Badgley and Bloom, 1973).

The pattern of its first accomplishments reflects these strong roots of medical sociology in the university. Typically, the first 'medical' sociologists were individuals who already had secured and established credentials in the mainstream of general sociology. Each pursued his intrinsic theoretical interest, seeking in medicine only the data to demonstrate propositions which were derived from previous analysis of other or more general social phenomena. Examples which come quickly to mind include Faris and Dunham, Talcott Parsons, Everett Hughes, Robert Merton, and August Hollingshead.

Robert E. L. Faris and H. Warren Dunham (1939) conducted in the early thirties what is probably the best known of the basic studies in the social epidemiology of mental illness. Followers of Burgess, they conceived their research as a means of testing the urban sociology identified with the University of Chicago Department of Sociology of that time. It was but one of a variety of field researches designed to test and develop theories of social ecology.

Talcott Parsons, during the thirties and forties, worked steadily at the construction of the comprehensive theory of society which he published in 1951 (*The Social System*). Medicine as a social institution and illness as social deviance were used to illustrate this theory. In Chapter X of that work, his functional analysis is applied to health in society. The following passage is illustrative:

> "... The problem of health is intimately involved in the functional prerequisite of the social system... Certainly by almost any definition health is included in the functional needs of the individual member of the society so that from the point of view of functioning of the social system, too low a general level of health, too high an incidence of illness is dysfunctional. This is in the first instance because illness incapacitates for the effective performance of social roles. It could of course be that this incidence was completely uncontrollable by social action, an independently given condition of social life. But insofar as it is controllable, through rational action or otherwise, it is clear that there is a functional interest of the society in its control, broadly in the minimization of illness."

The essence of this view is that the social relationships within the social institution of modern medicine are *patterned* and therefore contain predictable regularities. They are, in other terms, part of man's culture, a social heritage which provides sequences of behavior which each culture member learns and which are controlled by the structure of social institutions.

Parsons' analysis of the social roles of patient and professional is a key influence in the history of medical sociology. Parsons, himself, is best known, however, as a general theorist, as a great teacher of a generation of sociologists at Harvard University. He never, except for a very brief period of field observation, actually worked in a medical setting.

Everett Hughes began his studies of medicine within the frame of reference of occupational sociology. His research on work was well known as part of the continuing intellectual heritage of Robert Park. With his former students, Howard Becker, Anselm Strauss and Blanche

Geer, this line of inquiry culminated in the case study of a medical school (Becker *et al.*, 1961). Again however, the focus was theoretical, with Hughes, Becker, and Geer continuing from that point to build their careers less as medical sociologists than in a more generic concern with the analysis of social deviance.

Robert Merton's studies in the sociology of medical education are contemporaneous with the studies of medicine by Hughes and Parsons. Although younger – he had been a student of Parsons at Harvard – Merton was, like them, already established as a sociologist. At Columbia University, he taught and wrote as a theorist and, in collaboration with Paul Lazarsfeld at the Columbia Bureau of Applied Social Research, he sought to apply his theoretical ideas in a variety of empirical inquiries ranging from mass communication and housing to modern bureaucracy. Medical education was first chosen for study on the basis of a university's seminar on the professions which Merton conducted together with William S. Goode. He saw medicine as the archetype of the modern professions. Medical education, therefore, was hoped to yield the model for a general theory of socialization for professional role behavior. Like the others above Merton no longer is active in medical sociology. His current work is more in the sociology of science, a continuation of early studies in that area.

Hollingshead, prior to his research on mental illness (Hollingshead and Redlich, 1958), was already a senior member of the Yale University faculty and well known for studies of social class. His work on class and secondary education (1949) was standard required reading in American sociology. Of all those sociologists whom I have discussed in this section, Hollingshead went on to become the most intensely involved and identified with medical sociology. Nevertheless, like the others, his pattern of interest and commitment was primarily to general academic sociology. Social class was his central theme.

Medicine was therefore the subject area of inquiry, but not a vital problem focus in itself, for the major scholars in the early history of medical sociology. The testing of knowledge, establishing the validity of concepts, propositions, or developed theories, these were the main tasks. Essentially, none of these individuals sought to join medical institutions; nor did medicine seek to recruit them as other than consulting scholars. As research scientists, they asked and were given access to study and collect data. Throughout the entire period, to this very day, they retained, with little or no thought to change, their prior status in the sociology departments of their universities.

Changes were gradually occurring, however, and especially for the new recruits to medical sociology during the decade of the fifties. The results represented a striking new pattern, both in knowledge and work role.

II. THE DEVELOPMENT OF COLLABORATION: SOME EFFECTS OF NATIONAL PRIORITIES IN SCIENCE AND FEDERAL POLICIES OF SUPPORT

The sociology of medicine is a field in which research has been conducted for at least three-quarters of a century. It is only as the organized field of both inquiry and work called 'medical sociology' that it is barely twenty-five years old and, at the same time, one of the most rapidly expanding sub-fields of sociology (Riley, 1960; Suchman, 1963). McCartney (1970), in a survey of the full range of topical fields of sociology (19 categories), found that in the decade 1895–1904, the sociology of medicine (including mental health and gerontology) ranked 9 in the per cent of articles published in the three leading sociological journals.[1] The actual number was small, 3.1 per cent, compared with 'social theory, history, and change' which contained 30.6 per cent and ranked first. The sociology of medicine continued as a low-ranking, but continuously visible area until the decade following 1955 when, with 7.5 per cent, it became the fourth ranking area of sociological publication.

McCartney was interested in questions about the influence of both funding and styles of scientific work on the history of sociology. He found that the pattern of development was toward increasing support and the increasing use of statistical presentations of data in the published articles of most fields. In the decade after 1895, for example, none of the articles in the survey sample cited any support for the work reported. By 1955–64, the per cent citing support was 45.9.

The change is equally striking in the styles of inquiry. Empirical research was the basis of 27.6 per cent of the articles in 1895–1904, and 72.5 per cent in 1955–64. The presentation of statistical data, over the same period, changed from 16 per cent to 60 per cent.

Further data strongly suggest that these two trends are directly linked: articles based on supported research are shown to use statistical analysis distinctly more than unsupported research. The most significant point in time clearly was 1945.

Funding for sociological research was minor until after World War II, and the base of funding has never been broad. The major source is the federal government, through the National Institutes of Health (NIH), and it was primarily the National Institute of Mental Health (NIMH) which supported sociological research. Relatively few private foundations were involved.

Medical sociology closely follows this general pattern. Most of its reported work was supported and used statistical analysis. Indeed, during the two decades following 1945, McCartney's data rank medical sociology second only to the sociology of education in the per cent of published writing that is supported.

The special advantages of medical sociology, within the general framework of sociological research since 1945, are obvious. The National Mental Health Act of 1946 gave a broad mandate to both training and research on issues of health and not simply disease. The National Institute of Mental Health (NIMH) which the Act created and formally established in 1949, built upon that mandate a variety of research and training grant programs for which sociologists were eligible.

Although the NIMH programs were open to various types of sociological research, there was an advantage to health-related proposals. It might be expected, and it was common for social scientists to believe, that at least some of the subsequent research effort was directed 'where the money is'.

I have already argued that the motives of the major early figures in medical sociology were not 'external', or in response to influences like government requests or supportability, but rather can be clearly linked with long-standing intrinsic interests among the prime investigators. The patterns varied, however, and during the fifties, two types of trends emerged which show an important effect of government priorities in science and policies of support. The first was a development of collaborative research joining medical researchers with sociologists in relatively large-scale team studies that could only be carried out with the newly available financial sources; the second was a movement toward the creation of new full-time roles for sociologists that were in medical institutions primarily rather than in university sociology departments. Both trends, I believe, were important intermediary steps toward the professionalization of medical sociology.

The research collaborations include studies of the social etiology and ecology of disease, social components in therapy and rehabilitation, and the sociology of medical education. Space allows me here to cite just some of the outstanding examples.

Following the line of inquiry of Faris and Dunham, several teams of investigators were formed soon after World War II to study the 'total prevalence' of mental illness. They were designed specifically to document the degree of untreated illness and thus to correct the errors of estimate which were inherent in previous studies, all of which were based on reported prevalence (i.e., diagnosed cases extant at a given time). The best known of this research category are the Midtown Manhattan Study (Srole and associates, 1962; Langner and Michael, 1963), and the Stirling County Studies of Nova Scotia (Leighton and associates, 1959, 1960, and 1963). Another of this type which combines total prevalence research design with analysis of cultural influences on illness is the Hutterite study by Eaton and Weil (1955). In their report to the Joint Commission on Mental Illness and Health, Plunkett and Gordon (1960) cite eleven community studies which were designed to study the total prevalence of mental illness.

Both the Midtown Manhattan and Stirling County Studies were conceived by physicians but designed and conducted by social scientists. The operational approach of the research work involved close and continuous collaboration. The financial requirements were of a scale which, except in wartime, had previously been rare for social science research. Studies of this type would not have been possible without the new policies of the government and large private foundations toward social science research, and when such research clearly involved a high priority national problem like mental health, the willingness to commit such resources was more readily forthcoming. In other words, there developed after 1945 new policies for the support of empirical studies of human behavior with reference to important social problems. Health and illness were high on the list of priorities for such problems. A collaboration between physicians and sociologists emerged to take advantage of these policies.

That the motivation and direction of such research was different than the earlier research discussed in this paper seems clear. The institutional position and professional roles of the sociologists were also very different. Whereas the earlier generation of studies derived from senior established figures in the university, who remained in departments of sociology during and after their major research contributions to medical sociology, the sociologists who joined in the new collaborative health research were, for the most part, employed in medical schools. In the beginning, they were full-time research associates, assuming the risk of academic positions which were based entirely on research grants. From their numbers, many gravitated toward the academic positions which gradually were established for sociologists in medical schools, Leo Srole, for example, was for many years, in a special research status at Cornell while the intensive work of the Midtown study was being conducted. On his staff was Thomas Langner. Both moved from research staff positions to appointments in medical schools; Srole is currently a Professor of Sociology at Columbia University at their Psychiatric Institute, and Langner is at the Columbia University School of Public Health, Similarly, Charles Hughes, one of the senior authors of the Stirling County volumes, became a Professor of Anthropology at Michigan State University School of Medicine.

I am not suggesting an invariable pattern but only a trend. Some of the sociologists who began their work in medical collaborations returned to departments of sociology as a matter of strong preference. Eliot Freidson and David Mechanic are examples. Even in these cases, however, a continuing involvement in the field of medical sociology persisted. It is interesting to note that most, if not all, of the physicians who initiated the important collaboration of the 1950's have continued strong associations with medical sociology, including working partnerships with social scientists. George Reader, for example, has continued to work with Goss, for whom he created a full-time position in Cornell Medical School. Redlich, after his early collaboration with Caudill, has worked with Hollingshead and others. Stanton, George Silver, Leighton and others, provide similar examples.

A third important development from the national priorities in science represented by NIH and NIMH were the research training programs. Specifically intended to provide the recruitment and training of young Ph.D. sociologists into health research, training grants were offered to departments of sociology throughout the country. Although these grants were to become very broad in their definition of types of supportable training, the relevance of medical sociology to their basic mandate produced a network of training centers at universities throughout the United States. Reinforcing the effect of these programs were specially created efforts to aid medical schools to provide teaching position for social scientists. The NIMH grants for the teaching of human behavior in psychiatry, initiated in July of 1960, is but one example.

As medical sociology entered its third decade, therefore, it was building upon the following distinctive foundations for knowledge:

(1) A body of published research derived from the theoretical interests of a group of highly respected sociologists. The result was 'basic behavioral science' in the traditions of the mainstream developments of the field of sociology as a whole.

(2) The experience of interdisciplinary research collaboration with medical scientists in a variety of types of inquiry. The orientation of these studies was toward medical relevance in problems of etiology of illness, reforms in medical education, and the evaluation of social components and their influences in therapy and rehabilitation.

(3) The further experience of active teaching of medical sociology to both medical students and graduate students of sociology. Thus, the task of the synthesis and communication of basic knowledge in the field had been faced and a series of texts and reports of teaching models were published.

III. THE EMERGENCE OF COMMUNITY MEDICINE: SOME EFFECTS UPON THE KNOWLEDGE AND TEACHING OF MEDICAL SOCIOLOGY

As medical sociology expanded its knowledge base and its role in medical education, it found itself, within what was called the behavioral science movement, participating in several differing types of teaching. These types may be categorized in a fourfold table which combines two major dimensions: (1) the orientation or approach to knowledge as basic or applied; and (2) the type of content which is emphasized in the definition and presentation in education of behavioral science. Four types emerge as follows:

Content Emphasis		Orientation: Basic Science	Orientation: Applied Science
	Bio-Psychological	(A) Basic Science of Behavior e.g. Michigan	(B) Clinical Behavioral Science Preclinical Psychiatry e.g. Cameron
	Socio-Cultural	(C) Social Behavioral Science e.g. Kentucky	(D) Behavioral Components of Community Medicine

FINAL SECTION

The concluding section of the paper develops the fourfold table immediately preceding and outlines the proposed approach to teaching medical sociology. The latter is summarized in the table on the next page. This discussion will be completed in writing subsequent to the Conference where its elements will be presented.

REFERENCE

[1] *American Journal of Sociology*, *American Sociological Review* and *Social Problems*.

A TYPOLOGY OF HUMAN RELATIONSHIPS AND RECIPROCAL MEDICAL THEMES

TYPES	DEVELOPMENTAL FRAMEWORK OF HUMAN RELATIONSHIPS	THEMES UNDERLYING THE PHYSICIAN'S ROLE
I	– The human individual – the internal organic environment.	– *Disease* expressed in doctor-patient dyad. Goal: containing the disease; curing
II	– The human individual – significant others (e.g., the human family)	– *Disease* as primary cause, but conceived as being influenced by *psychological* and *sociological components* expressed in doctor-patient treatment group.
III	– The human individual – institutionally organized significant others (e.g., the school, the hospital).	– *Disease in context*. Theoretically expressed in the host theory of disease. In professional practice expressed by: milieu therapy; the life island; surgical intensive-care; comprehensive care.
IV	– The human individual – categorically identified populations (e.g., socioeconomic strata, cultural origins).	– *Social ecology*. Emergence of *prevention* as status equivalent of care. Goal: identification of populations at risk. Major method: epidemiology.
V	– The human individual – as a member of plural institutions organized as a community (e.g., neighborhoods, ghettoes).	– *The community*. An organic-whole conception of professional-client relationships. Goal: optimizing social functioning of the client as a necessary part of treating pathology.

SOCIAL SCIENCE TEACHING IN MEDICAL EDUCATION: AN OVERVIEW OF THE SITUATION IN GREAT BRITAIN*

MARGOT JEFFERYS

Bedford College, University of London, London, England

INTRODUCTION

In 1965, a Royal Commission representative of doctors, social administrators and the lay public was set up in Great Britain to review the current state of medical education, including the methods and type of recruitment to medical school, the content, length and focus of the curriculum, and future manpower recquirements for generalists and various kinds of specialist. It reported in 1968 and recommended, among other things, that all medical students should be introduced to the basic principles of medical sociology during the first two years of their studies.[1] It envisaged sociology as well as psychology as essential disciplines whose relevance for medicine needed to be understood as much as did the biological sciences which were already an accepted part of the preclinical learning experience of students.

The main reason which the Royal Commission on Medical Education gave for its recommendation was that the medical student should be aware

> "Why patients and families behave as they do in situations of illness; of the social and cultural factors which influence the patients' expectations and responses; of the problems for doctor, patient, and family in management of illness and handicap in the community; of the social, ethnic, occupational and psychological forces which can hinder prevention and treatment; and of the difficulties of communication and other problems which arise from established expectations about the way a person in a defined situation will behave, particularly in hospital".[2]

The commission further thought that such teaching would contribute to the general education of the student by "demonstrating to him the cultural relativity of his own environment and its values, and by enabling him to acquire objective methods of observing and analysing human behaviour in relevant medical care settings". [3]

IMPLEMENTATION OF THE RECOMMENDATION

Despite the strength of this recommendation, some medical schools in Britain have done very little to implement it in the five years which have followed the issuing of the report. Other schools have made efforts to act but have been discouraged by what appears to them to have been the lack of conspicuous success for their efforts.

An account of the experience of the thirty-six medical schools in Great Britain would show that in only a few of them are there courses in medical sociology as such. In most, the discipline, if it is taught at all, is either part of a course in social medicine or part of the behavioural science course for which the department of psychiatry is usually responsible. In such courses, it is not uncommon to find that medical sociology occupies less than five hours of a student's contact time with staff (faculty). In the University of London, where there are twelve medical schools, the new model syllabus for the M.B., B.S., includes proposals for fairly extensive teaching and examination in medical sociology; [4] but each school has considerable freedom to devise its own curriculum and set its own college-based examinations, and only three of the twelve schools have so far begun any systematic course work and the examination requirements are not stringent. In Scottish and English provincial medical schools the input is usually greater; but at least two of the schools which have the most solid commitment – Bristol and Edinburgh – had developed their courses well before the Royal Commission recommended that they should become universal.

What accounts for the slowness in introducing social science teaching into the medical curriculum? What is likely to enhance the chances of faster progress in the future? These are the questions to which I propose to address myself in the rest of this paper. While I shall be drawing on the situation in Britain because I know it best, I believe that parallels can be found in most of the capitalist societies of Western Europe and

North America as well as in the developing countries of Southeast Asia and Latin America which have been much influenced by the patterns of medical education of the former imperialist nations.

BARRIERS TO THE DEVELOPMENT OF SOCIAL SCIENCE TEACHING IN MEDICAL SCHOOLS

The comparative failure of the medical schools to implement the Royal Commission's recommendation cannot be attributed to a single cause. A number of factors of greater or lesser importance have influenced the situation, eroding the influence of other countervailing forces which were seeking to promote the social sciences in medicine. While these factors interact and thus either reinforce or diminish the significance of each other, for purposes of this paper, I propose to analyse them as though they were discrete, independent factors under the following headings:

1) Factors reflecting the influence of the structure and focus of the health care system.
2) The influence of the power structure within the medical school.
3) The influence of the medical student culture.
4) The influence of the social scientists.

1. The Influence of the Health Care System

The past one hundred years, and at an accelerating pace the last 25, have seen a disproportionate growth of specialist, hospital-based medical practice and services as against those delivered by generalists in the community.[5] This development has gone further in the U.S.A. and some European countries than it has in Britain where the general practitioner is still responsible under the National Health Service for the care of patients in 90% of all their illness episodes. Nevertheless, the trend is reflected in Britain where the proportion of doctors in hospital-based specialities increased between 1950 and 1970 from about 33% to about 50%.[6] Over the same period, hospital costs rose from about 55% to over 60% of all health service expenditures.[7]

The growth of specialism in the delivery of medical care was accompanied by the exponential growth of knowledge about the normal and abnormal functions of body organs and tissues, the effect of particular disease vectors on them, and the ways (chemical, physical and surgical) in which pathological processes and states could be prevented, reversed or arrested. Much of this knowledge was the product of successful laboratory research which utilised the methods and findings of the natural sciences in the fields of biochemistry and microbiology. To such research was attributed much of the spectacular success in dealing with some of the diseases which were major causes of mortality and morbidity in industrial, urbanised societies. While the discovery of sulphonomides and penicillin was very important in the reduction of mortality from many infectious diseases it must also be remembered that the greatest reduction in such mortalities occurred as a result of improvements in environmental sanitation and nutritional standards, a process which began long before the advent of science in clinical medicine. It was not surprising, however, that those responsible for the delivery of medical services, who are not trained as statisticians or epidemiologists, should atrribute the successes to medical technology and should hold it essential that doctors in training acquire a profound knowledge of the basic biological sciences and of the findings to which they gave rise.[8]

The assumption was made, in my view wrongly, that if mortality and morbidity were to be further reduced, all doctors in training needed to acquire a knowledge of the growing mass of esoteric information concerning body systems. From the Second World War medical schools in Britain almost without exception began to recruit only students who had already specialised in secondary school in pre-medical sciences (biology, chemistry and physics) and had shown by their performance in nationally set examinations that they could master these subjects successfully.[9] The fallacy lies, I believe, in assuming that modalities and the human qualities which led to success in extending the frontiers of knowledge in microbiology and laboratory-based scientific work, were also necessary for success in diagnosing, treating and managing illness in the community. Indeed, some of the scientific discoveries with the greatest potential in the health field – for example the discovery of the association between heavy cigarette smoking and many pathological conditions – could be applied successfully without skills in medical intervention of any kind.

Nevertheless, despite the comparative smallness, when viewed objectively, of the contribution of much 'high-powered' scientific research to improvements in health status or longevity, the fact remains that those who used the scientific method began to acquire high prestige among their peers and, through them, among the lay, consuming public, who were ready to believe in miracles performed by the contemporary alchemists – the scientist physician – or even better by the contemporary Pygmalions – the glamorous scientist surgeon.[10] The result was that those within medicine, and above all those within medical education, who wished to promote the prestige of their profession with the lay public and particularly with those who were guardians of the morals and the dominant norms of the society, did so by creating an image of the doctor as a natural scientist with a humanistic goal or stance. The legitimation of this orientation in medicine was reflected both in governmental support for particular research and teaching approaches, and by mass societal support even if the latter could be said to be due to some hard selling by the mass media. Consequently it began to be accepted without need for further argument that all those who aspired to the role of physician had to acquire, as part of their '*rite de passage*', a basic orientation in the 'hard' sciences.

In short, the magic of the scientific ideology as applied to medicine captured the imagination of the consuming public, influenced its ideas of what to expect from medicine, and hence gave the legitimation of public esteem and acceptance to those inputs to the medical armamentarium which came from the laboratory using all the paraphernalia of modern technology including electronic computers, lazer beams, automated processes and so on.

2. *The Influence of the Power Structure Within the Medical School*

This is not the place to make a detailed analysis of the power structure within the medical schools in Great Britain; but at the risk of being considered guilty of making *ex cathedra* statements I submit that those who have the greatest influence on (a) the selection of medical students, (b) the curriculum and (c) students directly, are precisely those who best reflected the laboratory-based or body systems and organs orientation in medicine.

The evidence for the first statement (a) came from an examination in 1963 of the composition of selection committees which showed them to be disproportionately composed in most London schools of teachers of the preclinical, laboratory-based sciences.[11] Insofar as clinical teachers were concerned with the selection process they tended to be drawn from those who were also involved in teaching about body systems or organ research often at the microbiological level.

The second statement (b) could also be supported by an analysis of the ways in which proposed innovations in the curriculum are treated by those responsible for final decisions on such matters in the medical school. My own observations and my discussions with medical school educators suggest that any change in the curriculum is the outcome of continuous negotiations between a small group of peers who between them control most of the students' time. The resulting balance may shift marginally when innovations are suggested by anyone within the small group or even by someone outside it; but there is a tendency for the small group to resist any major challenge to its collective authority and thus for there to be considerable inertia in the curriculum.[12]

After the report of the Royal Commission on Medical Education and a similar recommendation from the General Medical Council in its decennial review in 1967,[13] most medical schools undertook to review their entire curriculum, a process which went on in many of them over a period of years and resulted in some changes in the length, content and focus of the curriculum and the method of examining. But, by and large, the scale of the changes instituted was not as great as that of the activity generated; and, according to my current information, there is little sign of enthusiasm for any major change in emphasis. The basic orientation of medical education has hardly shifted away from its prior 'hard' scientific microbiological approach at both pre-clinical and clinical levels. Such inertia can be understood if it is appreciated that those who share the decision-making power are not likely to want to reduce their own involvement in the teaching programme. They may contemplate a situation in which one of their colleagues takes a cut in time, power and influence; but the danger of supporting such a move, which would undoubtedly be interpreted as hostile by the colleague concerned, is that they themselves might become the target of the ganging up of others.

It is furthermore clear that, up to the present, those medical educators most likely to favour a social science approach – that is, the psychiatrists, epidemiologists, social medicine experts and general practitioners – are generally low down in the medical school's 'pecking order' of professional esteem. In many schools, psychiatrists have students for only a short clerkship period in the clinical years. Social medicine departments may have time with students in either the pre-clinical or clinical years or in both; but one such department reported that the time allocated to is was the least popular with students (e.g. Friday afternoon at 4:00 p.m. or Monday morning at 9:00 a.m.), moreover, they have not the resources possessed by the clinical departments to undertake effective small group teaching. General practitioners have only recently been given full-time appointments in a few medical schools; elsewhere their contribution is confined to accepting students into their practices for observation for short elective periods.

In short, the position of these medical specialties – psychiatry, social medicine and general practice – has not been sufficiently secure in most medical schools for them to be able to sponsor effectively the exponents of yet another low status academic subject which presents potentially two threats to their colleagues – the first a threat to the time they can spend with their students, and the second, a challenge to the adequacy of their teaching.

The third statement (c), that is, that the educators with the greatest influence on students are those most likely to stress the laboratory-based scientific knowledge, is based on the assumption that the medical student selects a member or members of the medical faculty on which to model himself. This is a general postulate about the adult socialization process as such which has had much supporting evidence in studies of American medical students: there is no reason to suppose that the same process does not apply in the British system.[14] The role models most frequently chosen by students are usually men whose prestige among their own peers is high, and in their turn these peers tend to give greatest esteem to those who employ modern technologies with conspicuous success, and whose expertise lies in an ability to identify and treat the rare diseases in such a way that death is defeated, if only temporarily. Admiration, not unnaturally, leads to a wish to emulate. The value system of the society which sees more merit in snatching a few individuals from the jaws of death than from acting effectively to reduce the level of such known pathogenic behaviour as smoking is reinforced by a parallel value system within the medical school. Those who are seen as role models thus acquire power through their charismatic command of the constituency of students.

I would argue that those characteristics of the hierarchial structure within the medical school which accord recognition and power to those in the basic scientific disciplines and the traditional medical and surgical specialties, have resulted by and large in those with the greatest power having had good reasons for not wishing to implement wholeheartedly the recommendations of the Royal Commission. Conversely, the power within the medical school of those likely to constitute a major thrust towards including the social sciences in the medical curriculum has been comparatively weak and they have not been able to mobilise enough support from outside the school to influence other than marginally the decisions taken about curriculum. The arguments which have been advanced by those medical educators who oppose a reorientation provide merely the rationale for the maintenance of the existing one. Their persuasiveness rests in the fact that the premise from which their arguments start, namely the need to retain (or indeed increase still further) the scientific technical modalities, has not been seriously challenged.

Thus, for example, two consultants writing in 1969 argued that, given the increasing body of knowledge based on natural sciences, the student has his work cut out to cover the essential basis for modern medical practice and cannot afford the time to study disciplines which they described as fashionable but esoteric, that is, disciplines such as "genetics, immunology, social and physical anthropology and behavioural sciences".[15] Another allegation, used one cannot help thinking to appeal to prejudice and fear and not to reason, is that behavioural scientists are predominantly concerned with the pastoral role in medicine, which social scientists are accused of wishing to substitute for technical competence.[16] The distinguished clinicians of the paper putting forward this interpretation of the move to include behavioural sciences in the medical curriculum went on to imply that it was an impertinence to suggest that doctors had anything to learn about humane concerns for patients from sociologists. Other common arguments used by those who defend the *status quo* are that the behavioural sciences, unlike the natural sciences, are 'soft' as opposed to 'hard' sciences, that they deal with temporal rather than fundamental phenomena and that their exponents do not all speak in unison and are given to cannibalistic controversies. Of course, those who argue in these ways, ignore the fact that controversies in the field of the natural sciences are not unknown[17] and that speculation and alternative explanations are often the starting point for useful research.[18] They are on rather firmer ground when they find fault with some of the work which purports to be sociological. Much of it has been methodologically naive and logically inadequate; but to tar all sociological work with a brush which should apply to some of it alone is – to mix metaphors – to throw the baby out with the bath water.

3. The Influence of the Medical Student Culture

Some of the earliest studies of adult socialization suffered from the 'empty vessel' fallacy. They saw the neophytes undergoing the process as essentially passive recipients of the norms of the profession they were joining. Any variations in the way in which individual students absorbed or failed to absorb those norms were attributed to variations in the antecedent characteristics of the students themselves, for example, in their social class origin, previous scholastic records and so on. More recently, following Becker *et al.* in *Boys in White*, sociologists have recognised that there is at least one sub-culture within the medical school system, namely a student sub-culture, and that it has an important influence on medical education.

Studies comparable to that undertaken by Becker have not so far been done in England, but talks which this author has had with medical students in several schools certainly confirm the impression that most medical students feel themselves to be overloaded with work.[19] They cope with overload and the pressure of examinations as well as that of continuing assessment, (if not of a formal of an informal, judgmental kind) by discriminating between what they perceive as important and unimportant for the attainment of their immediate goals, namely passing examinations and finally qualifying. The behavioural sciences, which contribute little or nothing to the material on which students are examined, are likely to be among the first to get short shrift from the students, the more so because some clinical teachers will speak disparagingly of their relevance.

However, while observations similar to those made in the preceding paragraph have been made in many schools in the United States and Britain, there are some indications that in recent years a significant minority of medical students have begun to examine sceptically the exclusive concentration of modern medical education on the biological sciences at the expense of the behavioural sciences, particularly as these apply to understanding health care delivery systems, including such issues as priorities and effectiveness in meeting societal health needs. Reportedly, it is this minority of students which has been exerting pressure on the medical faculty to include social science teaching in its curriculum. The student body, in other words, is not monolithic; even if the dominant culture is one of resistance to social science teaching, it may well be that in the future a substantial proportion of that body will come to represent a challenge to the hegemony of the upholders of current conventional wisdom.

4. The Influence of the Social Scientist

The Royal Commission on Medical Education considered that the behavioural sciences should be taught by sociologists and psychologists with appointments in the university departments of their parent disciplines rather than by those with appointments in the medical faculty.[20] They believed that if the social scientists were employed by the medical school they would inevitably be placed in a department headed by a member of a medical speciality, in which case they would be deprived of the support of their parent discipline and cut off from the possibility of life-long careers, including promotion to the top of the academic ladder, within the discipline's mainstream. They implied that, in such circumstances, only the second rate sociologists would apply for work in the medical school, in contrast to the position where they envisaged sociologists keeping abreast of their discipline by teaching future sociologists but having a specialised interest at the same time in the application of that discipline to medicine.

This author criticised this recommendation of the Royal Commission on Medical Education in a paper on several grounds, among them (1) that medical students would be quick to pick up clues as to the importance accorded the subject by their mentors if it alone were provided from outside the medical school, (2) that a peripheral commitment would always be regarded as of lesser importance than a central commitment and hence evoke less effort, and (3) that success involved providing a symbiosis of sociology with medicine which in its turn depended on the organic growth of sociology through involvement in research on medically relevant questions.[21]

Current information suggests that some medical schools have followed the Commission's recommendation while others have decided to make appointments of social scientists to departments of community medicine or psychiatry. Impressionistically, it seems that neither solution has shown itself to be dramatically superior to the other, but that those schools which have employed social scientists in the medical school rather than relying on the sociology department to provide service teaching have done marginally better.

Accounts of the teaching of social science in American medical schools have drawn attention to the need for teachers in subjects which are not seen by students as central to excel as teachers if they are to exert any influence on their students.[22] This observation is likely to be true of the British scene as well. Indeed, a hypothesis which I predict would be supported by the evidence is that the interest and acceptance of behavioural science teaching by students and by faculty is directly related to the teaching abilities of the educator. Low ability produces low interest and vice versa.

Teaching ability, however, is a complex concept. It is not a characteristic of individuals but of interactive situations between teachers and students. The judgement of ability will always be made in a specific, given context by others, and the teacher may consequently receive different judgements from different students on the same occasion, by the same student on different occasions and by different students on different occasions. There are many factors which would influence such judgements. They include perception of the physical appearance of the teacher (some of the most successful teachers in some medical schools appear to be physically attractive young women); prior conception of the importance of the position occupied by the teacher (students are more disposed to listen attentively and uncritically to professors than they are to readers); mannerisms; humour; and not least perceptions of the relevance of the topic to the achievement of one's immediate goals.

It is my contention that on some of these factors, and particularly on the last, many of those who have been responsible for teaching social sciences to medical students have not scored sufficiently high to be acceptable to more than a small minority of such students.

While the impact that an individual teacher has on his students is not entirely, or indeed mainly in his control, it is more so than is generally appreciated. I believe that the poor rating of sociological teaching would improve if there were to be a change in the attitudes which some sociologists who do the teaching hold to it.

The particular attitude which I have observed and which seems to me to be dysfunctional from the standpoint of teaching medical students is a barely veiled hostility to and contempt for the medical profession. The study of the causes of this hostility and contempt forms part of the sociology of sociology.

First, sociologists have had to fight in Britain for the legitimacy of their subject as an academic discipline. The high prestigious Universities of Oxford and Cambridge have still no established chairs (professorships) in sociology and have only grudgingly allowed its intrusion into their degrees by way of papers in other honours schools. The uphill fight for recognition and status has left 'a chip on the shoulder' of British sociologists. The fight entailed disassociating themselves from the low status, quasi-professional social work occupations, a task not made easier by the presence of a group of academic social scientists, part-sociologists, part-pragmatic economists, unashamedly interested in social policy and administration and in training social workers. Some academic sociologists found it particularly galling that medicine, the faculty which is perhaps most geared to a vocational rather than an academic task, has, if not the highest prestige in the university, a capacity to command the greatest share of limited resources in any academic dog-fight. In short, in academia, sociology is low in the pecking order and medicine high, and this respective order does not seem justified to sociologists by the criterion of contribution to scholarship.

Second, sociology by its very nature is concerned with power structures, with social control and with the distribution of rewards to participants in social systems. The sociological analysis of modern society suggests that doctors have considerable power which is legitimated for them both by the granting of considerable statutory powers and by public acclaim[23] and they are used increasingly to reinforce the social controls through which those with power in the society maintain their hegemony.[24] Sociologists are human and may well feel envious of the esteem in which the medical profession is held. Futhermore, radical sociologists, and many of them are radical, see the medical profession as a conservative force which allows itself to be used, whether consciously or not does not matter, to shore up an ailing society by convincing people that it is they who are ill or mad and not the society which is bad.[25] Since most medical students, unlike sociologists, probably share the public's belief about the essential benevolence of medicine, they may be surprised and shocked by the challenge to the image of the profession they have chosen which is presented to them by the sociologists.

Third, much of the recent expansion in sociology has been due to an acceptance on the part of professional groups of its relevance to their own members. It has been something of a paradox that while sociologists have had to fight an uphill battle to secure resources to undertake research and teach on their own account, they have been courted by doctors, engineers, social workers, architects, teachers, priests and even military men to contribute to the training of their neophytes. Moreover, they have found it easier to secure funds for research if they will agree to participate in collaborative investigations where the problem is set and the terms defined by the particular professional group and not by the sociologists. Some academics, therefore, have been driven unwillingly into service teaching for economic and negative professional reasons. In their teaching they may well show their resentment at the great disparity between the rewards (economic and in esteem) which the medical students will finally achieve and those that they themselves can command.

For all these reasons, therefore, I believe that a number of sociologists now teaching in medical schools are ambivalent about their task. It may be this ambivalence which prevents some sociologists from making the contact necessary for a learning process to take place – namely, a feeling of shared interest between teacher and learner.

Indeed, sociologists have often paid too little at ention to the medical students themselves. Some have prepared syllabuses which were more appropriate to first year sociology students in which there was little which the medical students would recognise as of immediate relevance; others have thought to interest medical students by a popular presentation, but low level from the intellectual point of view, of some dramatic issue such as drug addiction or abortion. I have even detected some perverse satisfaction on the part of sociologists when their courses have been greeted by indifference or hostility. It helps to confirm for them the desired stereotype of the doctor as essentially a self-satisfied, anti-intellectual, anti-humanistic, narrow-minded aspirant to a position in a privileged sector of the social stratum. It has all the trappings of a self-fulfilled prophecy.

THE FUTURE

This analysis of the reasons for the comparative lack of effort to undertake the teaching of the social sciences in the medical curriculum in Britain suggests that a complex of factors has been operating to frustrate the proposals made by the Royal Commission of Medical Education in 1969 and the General Medical Council in 1967. Does the analysis also imply that these proposals are no more likely to be successfully implemented in the future than they have been in the past? And, if this is the case, would it not be more sensible for the advocates of social science teaching to reconsider their policies and cease to 'bang their head against the brick wall' created by entrenched attitudes and statuses within both the medical school and the academic departments of sociology? These questions can only be answered satisfactorily if we can predict with any certainty the roles which the medical profession is likely to perform in the last quarter of the twentieth century. It is to this question, then, that I propose to devote the rest of this paper.

Those who advocate the teaching of behavioural sciences assume that it will have a beneficial effect on the performance of doctors. (Cynically, I suppose, they may also feel that it will give jobs to social scientists who might otherwise not be able to earn a living). The first question, then that needs to be asked is what should the role of doctors be in the next 25 years. We need to answer this question if we are to decide what the objectives of medical education should be and how far it should include the social sciences.

Up to the present, the main emphasis of medical educators has been on training people who will be able to reverse pathological conditions which can cut an individual's life short or give him excessive pain. Training reflects this emphasis. There is an increasing body of knowledge which has to the imparted about the nature of life-threatening or pain-inducing conditions, why they occur, who is most susceptible to them, how they can be prevented by prophylaxis or, more important, reversed by therapeutics. This knowledge comes predominantly from research which has taken place in the laboratory and is backed by clinical trials and epidemiological inquiry. Students of medicine must be able to apply it to human beings. There is too great a body of knowledge for any single doctor to be able to be expert over the whole range. Hence, while there is a modicum which all neophyte physicians must learn, the expanding range of knowledge has to be coped with by a prolongation of the training period in specialties and super-specialties.

However, in the most prosperous countries, the changing pattern of health and disease has meant that medicine is now called upon to deal chiefly with illnesses which prevent individuals from performing selfsupportive activities, from developing their intellectual or physical potential and from achieving an inner sense of well-being. It also has to deal with chronic continuing illness particularly among the middle aged and elderly population. The demand, therefore, has changed and now implies that all sections of the population should have access to services to deal with ills which are not necessarily life-threatening but which cause dependency, limit self-fulfilment and create unhappiness.[26]

While no-one would argue that doctors of medicine should be the only providers of such services – other professions, for example teachers, priests, social workers, nurses, and many other kinds of therapists have knowledge and skills to apply to the solution of such problems – a substantial body of opinion would accept that the medically qualified doctor has a clear role to play in these. The question is whether he should confine his role in these tasks to that of mastering and applying the knowledge which is a spin-off from the traditional task of saving life or relieving physical pain, or whether he should play a part in defining and establishing more precisely the social objectives of medical care, in determining priorities especially where the social objectives may conflict, and in implementing the personal or group-based services which are indicated.

In short, the question is whether the doctor should in the future be primarily an applied scientist or technologist working from his traditional knowledge base – admittedly an extended one – or something else? Should he continue to concentrate on mastery of the physiological, anatomical and biochemical nature of man, the pathogenic agents which can cause a departure from the normal, and the prophylactic or therapeutic procedures and substances which can prevent a departure from or achieve a reversion to normal? Or should he extend his knowledge base and concern himself with psychopathology and social pathology when these are inextricably bound up with physical pathology?

If the doctor's role is conceived in the first way, his need to acquire knowledge of the behavioural sciences will be much more limited than if it is conceived in the second. Other professionals both in and outside the health service will have the main responsibility of acquiring the psychological and sociological knowledge needed and then applying it to people. Doctors will only need to acquire the knowledge and skills in inter-personal relationships which will enable them to see that their own work is effective.

Many doctors will claim that they already acquire such knowledge and skills during their medical apprenticeship, not by formal teaching in the behavioural sciences, but by experimentation and experience and by observing their medical colleagues at work. Social scientists might, however, claim that the absence of theory and of knowledge of the results of empirical studies means that the learning which does occur and is demonstrated in practice is less effective than it could be. Studies in the United States and in Britain have demonstrated that doctors frequently do not understand the problems of communicating with patients of different socio-cultural backgrounds and personality and so fail to make their service as effective as it could be.[27] Other studies have also suggested that failure to understand the structural pressures exerted on themselves and other health professionals is widespread and results in job dissatisfaction and wastage.[28]

It is at least worth seeing whether interpersonal relationships, which must after all accompany the performance of any preventive or therapeutic procedures for an individual and are in themselves likely to have an effect on outcome, would be improved by introducing doctors systematically during training to some of the more relevant concepts in the behavioural sciences. What these concepts are, how they can be learned most effectively, how they can be applied, and how the effects of their application can be tested, will present difficulties. But if there is agreement that the present haphazard way of acquiring skills in doctor-patient or doctor-other professional relationships leads to unsatisfactory results, then, it follows that the way should be open for experiments in providing more systematic learning experiences.

There are many, however, who believe that it is both impossible and undesirable to confine the doctor's role as suggested hitherto to those conditions which are life-threatening or severe pain-inducing.[29] The doctor, it has been argued, has been cast in a role which demands that in the future he take a full part in securing the wider objectives of social well-being. Nor is he himself likely to be content with what must become a more limited role, that of medical technologist and not of full professional.

If this is the case, if the doctor of the future is to take a wider responsibility for the range of human problems which can undermine social functioning and a sense of well-being, then his need to master behavioural sciences is paramount. He must become an applied behavioural scientist and counsellor as well as the possessor of knowledge concerning biological processes, pathogenic agents, and therapeutics.

Clearly, the need and opportunity to function as a behavioural scientist will differ from specialty to specialty. The pathologist and the surgeon will be at one end of a continuum; the psychiatrist and the primary care physician at the other. The needs of doctors responsible for planning and administering health services will differ again from those of the doctor engaged solely in clinical one-to-one practice.

In short, given the perpetuation of a medical education system which seeks to provide a common base of knowledge and skills in all doctors and of a practice situation which encourages diversification and post-graduate specialisation, it is clear that there must be a close examination of the appropriate level and particular aspects of the behavioural sciences needed by various specialties, especially at post-graduate level.[30]

This paper has deliberately not examined the detailed questions of what in the social sciences should be taught and how it should be taught in medical school or in post-graduate training. Rather it has addressed itself to the prior problem of determining what the role of the doctors should be in the future medical care systems of the last quarter of the twentieth century. If the doctor of the future is seen simply as one who is concerned exclusively with the physiochemical properties of man and his organs, then all he may be required to learn at medical student level is enough to enable him to produce interpersonal skills in relationships with patients and other health professionals. If, on the other hand, he is to be concerned with the interface between physiological problems and psychosocial pathology, then he must acquire a considerably greater range of knowledge and understanding of the social sciences and their implications both for the etiology of the illnesses with which he is dealing and for the lives of those who are his patients.

CONCLUSION

Which of these roles is the medical profession most likely to fill in the future – that of technologist, concerned primarily with the physiological, or that of applied behavioural scientist, concerned with the psychosocial as much as with the physiological? I do not know the answer to this question. The odds are evenly balanced. There are pressures in both directions, and the outcome will depend, not only on decisions taken by the medical profession itself – which, in any case, is not a monolitic body speaking with a single voice. While some of the highly prestigious super-specialists will line up for a restriction of concern, newer specialty groups within medicine, such as the psychiatrists and the community physicians as well as revitalised general practitioners, are determined to broaden the medical horizon but to remain within the medical world.

Professional groups outside medicine in the social service sector will also influence the future pattern. Social workers in Britain have already acquired control over considerable resources devoted to the care of the chronically sick and disabled (both physical and mental).[31] They want to have the same power to define the problem and exercise autonomy in deciding on treatment and disposal that the medical profession now enjoys. Their aims may well bring them into conflict with those in medicine who aspire to a behavioural applied scientist and counsellor role.

The public, too, both as electors of governments and as individual consumers will also influence the outcome. They are likely to show much ambivalence. Other things being equal, governments will want to find solutions which are least costly in national resource terms. For this reason, they may want to substitute social workers and nurses for doctors because the latter are a more expensive resource in a system characterised by its labour intensive activity. On the other hand, such a course may make them unpopular with both the medical profession and their own constituency – the electorate composed of consumers of medical services – and they will try to compromise. In the last resort, the doctors are able to wield more power than are social workers, and the support of the former is essential if the National Health Service is to survive and work.

REFERENCES

* This is the original paper given at the Warsaw Conference on the Sociology of Medicine, held under the joint auspices of the Research Committee on the Sociology of Medicine, International Sociological Association, and the Polish Academy of Sciences, Institute of Philosophy and Sociology at Jabłonna, Poland, in August 1973.

The paper with some modifications was published in *International Journal of Health Services* **4** (1974) 549–563.

1 Report of the Royal Commission on Medical Education (1968), Cmnd. 3569 London.
2 *Ibid*, para. 108.
3 *Ibid*, para. 109.
4 University of London, Faculty of Medicine, Syllabus for the degree of M.B., B. S., 1972.
5 These issues are discussed by Rosemary Stevens in her two books: *Medical Practice in Modern England*, Yale Univ. Press, New Haven 1966, and *American Medicine and the Public Interest*, Yale Univ. Press, New Haven 1971.
6 British Medical Association, Planning Unit Working Party Report, *Primary Care*, London 1970.
7 Office of Health Economics, *Information Sheet* **21** (1972).
8 D. Whitteridge and G. W. Harris, *Lancet* (1969) 48–49.
9 World Health Organisation, European Office. Report of a working group on *The Selection of Students for Medical Education* (1973) 14. Copenhagen, mimeo.
10 M. Jefferys, *Social and Economic Administration* **4** (1970) 37–47.

[11] This enquiry was conducted by a small group of D.P.H. Students at the London School of Hygiene in 1963 as part of a wider study concerned with the recruitment of women to medicine. The data on the composition of committees was not used in the publication. M. Jefferys, S. Gauvin and O. Guleson, *Lancet* (1965) 1381–1383.

[12] The incremental nature of change has been considered by George Maddox in relation to changes in policy in the National Health Service: Muddling Through Planning for Health Care in England, *Medical Care* **9** (1971) 439–448; but it is equally appropriate to apply it to changes in professional education.

[13] General Medical Council, *Recommendations as to Basic Medical Education* (1967).

[14] The observation was first made explicit by R. K. Merton, G. G. Reader and P. L. Kendall in *The Student Physician*, Harvard Univ. Press, Cambridge, Mass. 1957. It has been frequently replicated in other studies.

[15] D. Whitteridge and G. W. Harris *op. cit.* (1969).

[16] A. C. Dornhurst and A. Hunter, *Lancet* (1967) 666–668.

[17] J. D. Watson, *The Double Helix*, Weidenfeld and Nicholson, London 1968.

[18] H. Himsworth, *The Development and Organisation of Scientific Knowledge*, Heinemann, London 1970.

[19] Some British medical students who have spent elective periods in American medical schools suggest that American students are harder worked and work harder than do their British counterparts.

[20] Royal Commission on Medical Education, *op. cit.*, para. 249.

[21] M. Jefferys, 'Sociology and Medicine: Separation or Symbiosis?', *Lancet* (1969) 1111–1116.

[22] See R. F. Badgley and S. W. Bloom (in press), *Social Science and Medicine* 1973. Behavioural Sciences and Medical Education: The case of sociology, H. E. Freeman, L. G. Reader, and S. Levine, *The Handbook of Medical Sociology* (1963). Introduction by the Editors to the first edition.

[23] See E. Freidson, *Professional Dominance: The Social Structure of Medical Care*, Atherton, N.Y. 1970.

[24] I. Zola, 'Medicine as an Institution of Social Control', *Sociological Review* **20** (1972) 487–504.

[25] The influence of R. D. Laing and D. Cooper among radical sociologists in Great Britain, especially those interested in the sociology of deviance, the sociology of medicine and labelling theory has been very great.

[26] These statements hardly need documentation. They are well stated in T. McKeown, *Medicine in Modern Society*, Allen and Unwin, London 1965, and more succintly in the B.M.A. Planning Unit Working Party Report on Primary Medical Care 1970, *op. cit.* J. Fry, *Profiles of Disease*, Livingstone, London and Edinburgh 1966, is also useful.

[27] See for example D. Mechanic, *Public Expectations and Health Care*, Wiley-Interscience, N.Y. 1972, p. 203–222 for a review of some of the most important studies.

[28] See for example, R. W. Revans, *Standards for Morale*, Oxford University Press, London 1964.
[29] This is particularly true of those who wish to promote a greater involvement of the medical profession in primary and continuing ambulatory care. See, for example, The Royal College of General Practitioners, *The Future General Practitioner. Learning and Teaching*, B.M.J., London 1972.
[30] The ideas embodied in the last few paragraphs were first developed by the author in a paper in *Acta Socio-Medica Scandinavia* 3 (1971) 157–160 under the title 'What is the Purpose of Learning Behavioural Sciences in Medical Education?'.
[31] Under the Local Authority (Social Services) Act 1970, a professional social work qualification is normally required of those who direct the Social Service Departments of Local Authorities in England and Wales, departments which receive substantial resources for the ambulatory and institutional care of the physically and mentally handicapped or ill, the elderly and children deprived of a normal home life. This has given social workers a power base over the performance of some functions which were once considered to belong to the health care system and controlled by Medical Officers of Health and other medical doctors.

TEACHING MEDICAL SOCIOLOGY TO GRADUATE STUDENTS IN SOCIOLOGY: A THREE-YEAR EXPERIENCE

YVO NUYENS

Department of Sociology, Catholic University of Louvain, Louvain, Belgium

1. INTRODUCTION

The object of this paper is to give a systematic account of a training program in medical sociology, explicitly and exclusively designed for graduate students in sociology. Anyone who in some way or other is familiar with the international sociological scene, as expressed in congresses, symposia, professional journals, readers and other publications, cannot escape the impression that we are dealing here with a highly underdeveloped area. Training in medical sociology is indeed given some attention, but this bears chiefly on methodology, strategy and the development of medical sociology teaching for the benefit of other professional groups, especially medical doctors, nurses, public health officers, social workers, etc. Medical sociologists often have to be content with the statement that a sound and comprehensive academic training in general sociology should sufficiently guarantee the development of competent medical sociologists. Freeman, Levine and Reeder [1] comment on this as follows: "If there is merit in our position that medical sociology is a speciality defined substantively and with theoretical and conceptual roots in general sociology, it follows that medical sociologists must be well trained and competent general sociologists... Sociologists vary in their opinions of the importance of field training to the educational process, but it is doubtful whether any would contest that familiarity with the settings in which they are to work is not useful. A familiarity with the medical field, in one way or another, is essential to the development of the medical sociologist." These authors strongly advocate, quite rightly, in our opinion, the necessity for specific socialization mechanisms for the medical sociologist. It is clear that these socialization mechanisms can be developed either within or alongside or after the graduate training of sociologists. A combination of both formulas probably yields optimum results, but this is, at least in the initial developmental phase of a training program in medical sociology, hard to implement owing to the required investments of manpower and means which, in the present case, may be presumed to be rather extensive. This paper tells of three years' experience with a training program in medical sociology as it was developed within the graduate training of sociology students.

2. SETTING

The training program in medical sociology is set within the larger framework of the K.U.L. (Katolieke Universiteit Leuven) in Belgium. This University is not only an old Catholic university (founded 1452), but with about 17,000 students is also the largest in Belgium. The language of instruction is Dutch, although there is a tendency, particularly on the level of graduate training, to organize some programs entirely in the English language. Since the University is organized according to the traditional 'Faculty' system, we are interested here specifically in the Faculty of Social Sciences. This faculty was only recently developed, as a result of Belgium's rather weak tradition of research in the social sciences. Up to the 'fifties the main emphasis was on a polyvalent, predominantly juridical-philosophical training, in close connection with the Faculty of Law. Mainly because of the development of sociological research early in the 'sixties, attention was shifted to an intradisciplinary and empirical approach. This finally resulted in the establishment of an autonomous Faculty of Social Sciences with three departments, viz. Sociology, Political Science and Mass Communication, each furnishing a separate graduate training program. At present, student recruitment is distributed over the three departments as follows: about 60% for the Department of Sociology and about 20% for each of the other two departments. The academic staff of the Department of Sociology includes eleven full-time professors, four part-time professors, and

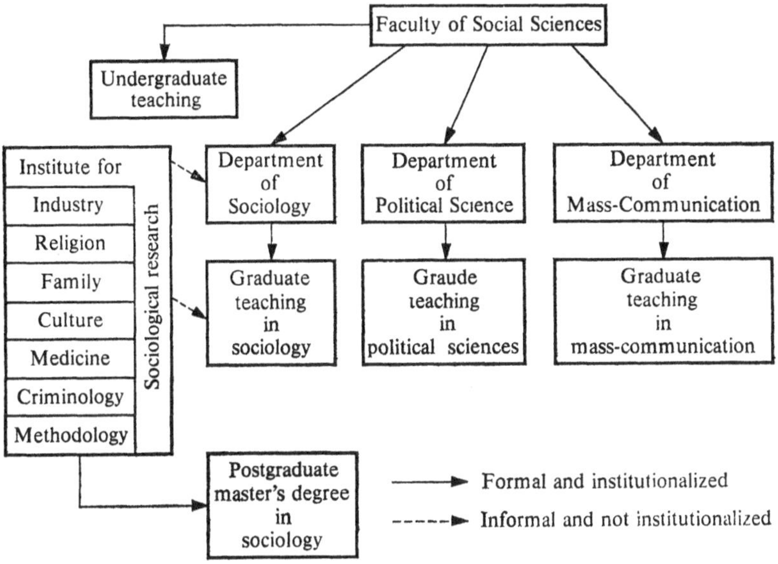

Fig. 1. Organizational structure

thirty teaching and research assistants, the staff-student ratio being about 1/14.

This general setting is represented schematically in Fig. 1. Attention must be drawn to the particular position of the Institute for Sociological Research. Whereas the not very extensive research of the Department of Sociology is financed by university grants, the applied and basic research of the ISR is centred in extra-university funds, i.e. so-called contract research. The latter includes about 80% of all sociological research presently conducted at the university. In matters of both direction and policy the ISR is situated apart from the academic and faculty structures although many actual, informal, and non-institutionalized connections exist between both structures. Internally the ISR is divided into seven separate departments. One of these is the Department of Medical Sociology, which, at the moment, includes one full-time professor, one part-time professor, and four full-time assistants. This staff is actually charged with teaching medical sociology within the framework of the graduate program in sociology.

For further details on the ISR, see Appendix IV.

3. GRADUATE TRAINING IN SOCIOLOGY

Sociology training starts with a two-year undergraduate program which, as we indicated above, is not within the framework of any of the Departments but within that of the Faculty. This undergraduate program aims at a broad academic and multi-disciplinary introduction of the social sciences. Thus a number of general introductory courses such as philosophy, economics, psychology, law, ethics, statistics, social history, etc. are included. Yet even at this level there exists a nucleus of sociology, constituting both formally and in reality the basis of this undergraduate program. We particularly refer to the courses Sociology I+II (delineation of the sociological frame of reference, concepts, theories, models, and a historical survey), Research Methods (general survey of the principal research techniques, research design, and analysis), Society: Facts and Problems (delineation of the social referential framework with special attention to the problem-oriented approach, see Merton). In addition, a practical initiation into sociological research is organized through sociological field exercises. One of the fields occasionally used is health care.

In this article, however, we are chiefly interested in graduate training. The two-year graduate program on the one hand extends the line of undergraduate training: in addition to more directly policy-oriented courses, sociological theory and sociological research techniques remain essential to the training program. On the other hand, a number of application areas are provided in which the students learn to practise the sociological trade. Such areas are, for example, sociology of the family. religion, industry, culture, urban, criminal and MEDICAL sociology, With respect to these application areas, not all of which are equally developed, an important evolution should be indicated. At the beginning, i.e. during the period 1963–1969, the number of application areas was restricted to three, viz. Family, Industry, and Religion. Hence these three areas were developed as complete specialties of sociology, to the effect that through courses, seminars, seminar-courses, etc. students were given a training which was more or less exclusively designed for the sociology of the family, of industry of or religion. Although the training ideally was aimed at producing a general sociologist, in fact this graduate training led to the training of specialists in these fields. Moreover, this training developed chiefly around the dialectical relation between theory and research, while the policy-dimension (social engineering, sociotechnics, clinical sociology) was treated less explicitly and less directly.

Under the influence of a number of factors, this curriculum was modified rather drastically in 1969. The increasing number of students, the limited staff provided for the above-mentioned fields, the development of a number of other fields, and the scarcely articulated and crystallized demand for sociologists on the Belgian labour market indeed raised a number of questions about the organization of sociology training in only three fields of specialization. The following modifications were made:

– The number of fields of sociology was increased from 3 to 9. In addition to the existing fields the curriculum was supplemented with urban, economic, criminal and medical sociology, together with sociology of culture and sociology of population.

– The development of these new fields was limited to the introduction of a basic course in the sociological specialties with the exception of medical sociology. This specialty was developed more extensively according to the pattern of existing specialties., i.e. through lectures, seminars and seminar-courses into a complete field of specialization, in addition to the existing fields of family, industry, and religion.

– In contrast to the former arrangement, students could no longer complete their graduate training in sociology in only one field, but were obliged to combine at least two fields. Students were given freedom of choice insofar as they could choose at least one complete specialization field – viz. family, industry, religion, or medical sociology – and could supplement it with one or more partial fields.

– Finally, in order to give more free scope to the problem-solving approach, the sociology nucleus of the curriculum, as reflected in various sociological specialization fields, was supplemented with a cluster of more directly policy-oriented subjects such as social casework, community organization, social administration, techniques of management, labour relations, health care administration, etc. Students are obliged to include a number of these subjects in their curriculum, but their choice of subjects is free. Since most of these policy-oriented subjects are taken from other training courses, the internal coherence of these subjects is very limited and as such they are scarcely suited to the specific needs of a sociological training.

Summarizing the principal modifications introduced in 1969 it may be stated that the narrow specialist training program was extended towards several fields of sociological application, that a stronger emphasis was put on development of the policy-dimension in training, and that the students were given a higher degree of flexibility and independence in making up their curriculum. After a three-year (experimental) period, the program is now again under discussion and a procedure to modify the curriculum has been started. The design and orientation of these new modifications will later be discussed briefly; first the present situation of graduate training in medical sociology will be commented upon with respect to its content.

For a survey of the present graduate curriculum in sociology see Appendix II.

4. GRADUATE TRAINING IN MEDICAL SOCIOLOGY

As in all graduate training, that of medical sociology is a concrete didactic translation of a number of teaching objectives, which, in turn, are derived from specific job definitions. That is why we first make a few observations on the definition of the role of the (medical) sociologists, then present the teaching objectives, and finally discuss the training curriculum itself.

4.1. Definition of the Role of the (Medical) Sociologist

With Freeman, Levine, and Reeder we may state that "...medical sociology is distinctive only in its subject matter; its boundaries are phenotypic. It makes use of concepts, theories, and methods in sociology for the study of the health and illness of persons... Medical sociology, like all sociology, is concerned with social relationships and social processes, and its theoretical base must of necessity be that of general sociology. The activities of medical sociologists span the various areas of interest to the discipline..." From this it can be inferred that the definition of the medical sociologist's role scarcely deviates from the general definition of the sociologist's role: he is first of all a sociologist, applying his sociological knowledge and skills to one specific subsystem of society. In spite of, on the one hand, the fact that every functional definition is subject to time and place and, on the other hand, the recent, although chiefly academic, international debate about the role of the sociologist (Gouldner, *Frankfurter Schule*), it is generally agreed that three essential dimensions can be distinguished (see, for example, Sokołowska [6]).

These dimensions are:

- research: includes both basic and applied research, even though this division (of scientific research) is debatable;
- teaching: applied to the medical setting teaching is an extremely important function due to the increasing involvement of the behavioral sciences in medical training;
- social engineering: sometimes called clinical sociology, social-technics, or problem-solving sociology; this is a new, rapidly expanding function of the sociologist, defined by Sokołowska as "a theory of socially effective action". To the sociologist, social engineering implies a direct involvement in policy, though in everyday reality this involvement may assume various forms.

This general definition of the sociologist's role can equally be applied to the medical sociologist who, in practice, will usually be confronted with these three dimensions. His specific role consists of actualizing these dimensions in and with respect to the medical setting, which is sometimes characterized as a guild-like structure in which the social fact of professional dominance provides a number of barriers to the involvement of non-medical people (in this setting) [2]. To the medical sociologist the latter is an important feature which should be taken into account while defining the teaching objectives.

4.2. Teaching Objectives in (Medical) Sociology

From role-definition a number of teaching objectives can be deduced. Our attention here is confined to the teaching objectives relative to the functions of research and social engineering, not that of teaching. At Louvain training for teaching functions is the subject of a special training program which the students are free to take separately from and combined with their specific sociological training. This program emphasizes didactic and pedagogic training of future sociology teachers on the college-level. The teaching of medical sociology is covered by this program only occasionally and for purposes of example.

With regard to these teaching objectives two approaches are possible: either a number of more or less abstract and normative reflections on these objectives are given, or an empirically based insight into the actual and concrete objectives as they are attempted and realized by teachers themselves, is aspired to. With respect to the latter approach, we refer to the recently published results of an inquiry held among a hundred sociology teachers on the academic level who were questioned about the objectives of sociology teaching [3]. A scale of 108 items was constructed, to which a factor analysis was applied, resulting in the following dimensions:

1. knowledge and control of research methods,
2. knowledge of sociological theories,
3. sociological analysis of social phenomena,
4. development of opinions on important social problems,
5. ability to handle theoretical concepts,
6. ability to work and think systematically,
7. knowledge of methodological principles,
8. skill in thinking in concrete terms usable in policy-making,
9. ability to comprehend and make use of research reports,
10. insight into the meaning of statistics.

These objectives are closely related to two dimensions which are traditionally distinguished in most teaching objectives, viz. knowledge and skill. It should be noted that these teaching objectives are related chiefly to the research dimension, and only to a much lesser extent to the dimension of social engineering. This can probably be explained by the fact that the latter role has developed only recently and at present is still strongly debated.

These objectives of general sociology teaching can be directly applied to the teaching of medical sociology, to the effect that knowledge and skills are to be actually applied to the medical setting. This implies that medical sociology should define at least two specific teaching objectives, viz.

- thorough knowledge of the morphological substratum of health care in our own society, this includes the empirical delineation of the subsystem of health care in its structural and organizational manifestations, as well as the data, indicators, and sources through which this subsystem is made sociologically observable;

- a primary socialization of the medical subculture; we have already indicated above the guild-like structure of the medical setting, in which the involvement of non-medical people was impeded by numerous barriers. A socialization process built into the training may provide the sociologist with opportunities of partially bridging these barriers.

The latter item in particular draws attention to a dimension which so far has remained highly underdeveloped in the definition of any teaching objectives, namely the development of correct attitudes. So far these were usually left to intuition and good example. Since attitudes determine actual behaviour, we feel that professional attitudes should be made explicit and be included in teaching as an important objective. With respect to medical sociology the following attitudinal characteristics may be considered the object of specific teaching activities:

- balance between the orientation towards research and the orientation towards social engineering;
- readiness to evaluate critically medical scientific results on the one hand and one's own behaviour and achievements on the other;
- readiness constantly to reformulate a given medical definition of a problem into a sociological definition, i.e. readiness to maintain one's sociological identity and authenticity;
- readiness to collaborate with other disciplines;
- readiness to use a long-term perspective with respect to the concrete effects of the professional work produced.

In the curriculum presented below an attempt is made to implement these teaching objectives through a series of specific teaching activities.

4.3. Teaching Medical Sociology

First it must be indicated that training in medical sociology is built into the total graduate program in sociology (see above), the first objective of which is to train sociologists and not various categories of (sub)specialists. This total program is particularly developed around three dimensions, viz. sociological theory, sociological research and social policy. At present the specific program in medical sociology includes the following teaching activities:

4.3.1. Teaching course in medical sociology (60 hours – first year),

4.3.2. Seminar course in medical sociology (60 hours – first year),
4.3.3. Seminar course in medical sociology (60 hours – second year),
4.3.4. Practical training (p.m. – first year),
4.3.5. Memoir (p.m. – second year),
4.3.6. Seminar course in medical sociology and medical psychology (30 hours – second year).

With respect to the above-mentioned functions and teaching objectives these teaching activities show the following features:

	Knowledge	Skills	Attitudes
Research	4.3.1	4.3.2 /4.3.3 /4.3.5	4.3.6
Social engineering	4.3.1	4.3.2 /4.3.3	4.3.4

Fig. 2. Curriculum in medical sociology

It must be noted that we are dealing here exclusively with specifically medical sociological teaching activities. With respect to the dimension of social engineering in particular the students are given the opportunity to supplement their program with a number of more directly policy-oriented subjects: yet as we stated above, these subjects are only slightly related to the various sociological specialties since they are usually taken from other teaching programs. At present this situation is felt to be highly problematic yet, for the time being, there is no adequate solution at hand.

We will now briefly explain the various medical sociological teaching activities.

4.3.1. Teaching Course in Medical Sociology

Object: The first objective of this teaching course is to offer the largest possible introduction to medical sociological theory as it has been shaped in the course of research. Secondly, this course aims at giving elementary morphological information about the health care system as a social fact. Since this course is the students' first systematic contact with medical sociology and health care, the emphasis is on imparting knowledge, while a certain balance between the dimensions of research and social engineering is attempted.

Form: There are 30 weekly two-hour listening and responding lectures. In order to reduce the ex-cathedra character of the lectures and stimulate the students' activity, reading lists are used: small groups discuss one or more articles selected in advance, report on them and submit their report to discussion during the lecture. After the conclusion of each topic, (for example, the hospital, illness behaviour, the doctor-patient relationship, etc.) a synthesis is made in collaboration with the students.

Subject matter: By means of reading lists, the most relevant topics of medical sociology are covered. Criteria of relevance are:

– on the one hand theoretical and scientific; theories on health behaviour (Rosenstock, Mechanic, Suchman), for example, are essential because of their actual significance for medical sociology;
– on the other hand, social-problematic; in connection with the recent medical strike in Belgium, for example, an extensive treatment of the Freidson approach with respect to professional dominance was an indicated topic.

Whereas initially the White model in particular was used [5], at present the concept of 'patient career' as recently developed by McKinlay [4] is frequently employed as an organizing framework. Regardless of the organizational framework or the topic covered, the following three elements are always given full attention:

– introduction of conceptual frameworks, theoretical approaches, and models of analysis;
– insertion of the most important research findings;
– indication of the most essential empirical data, or at least the sources providing these data.

For further details on the subject matter of this course, a survey of the reading list in use at present is given in Appendix III.

Evaluation: Student evaluation of the teaching course is done through an oral exam, consisting of three questions:

– a question on the students' knowledge of the subject matter;
– a critical approach to an article selected by the student himself;
– an application of the matter covered to an actual policy problem.

4.3.2. Seminar Course in Medical Sociology (First Year)

Object: The primary objective of this seminar is to offer students a first confrontation with the practical reality of medical sociological research. The emphasis is clearly on the development of skills and the ability to solve both research and policy problems. A secondary objective is to stimulate and promote the students' readiness for cooperation and team work.

Form: There are 30 weekly two-hour seminars. Individual and team assignments are distributed and the assignments performed are submitted to discussion. An important part of the seminar course takes place in the field where a number of research techniques such as interviewing, participant observation, contacts with priviledged judges, secondary analysis, etc. are actually practised.

Subject matter; The subject matter of this seminar course varies every year. Usually one central theme is selected, which is then elaborated in the form of a piece of teaching research. In the past years such themes were for example:
– sociological profile of the mental hospital patient: empirical investigation of the patient population in three adacemic psychiatric institutions with respect to a number of socio-cultural characteristics;
– analysis of medical consumption: a piece of research based chiefly on a secondary analysis of the factors determining the nature and the extent of medical consumption behaviour;
– preventive health behaviour: exploratory research into the variables explaining participation or non-participation in preventive cancer screening of women in a suburban area.

This last theme in particular yielded good results for both the students and the seminar leader(s). First, the students were offered the opportunity to participate directly in the successive steps involved in sociological research – to design and actively collaborate in solving various problems which constantly arise in the course of a research project. The seminar included a practical exercise in direct problem solving. In view of the very slight participation in preventive cancer examinations in the area studied (about 25% of all women invited), the students were given the opportunity to design a program of action which was to be applied to the next area in which the examination was held. Both factors combined resulted in a relatively high student involvement in the seminar.

Evaluation: In this seminar course no specific test is taken. Individual and collective student performance is constantly evaluated during the entire course. At the end of the course individual written evaluations of the seminar are given by the students themselves.

4.3.3. Seminar Course in Medical Sociology (*Second Year*)

Object: The objectives of this second year seminar course are practically identical to those of the first-year seminar course, except that it is no longer a first confrontation with or introduction to medical sociological research but a further development of the knowledge and skills acquired during the first year. In addition, the instructor's share in this course decreases and the students' share increases, with the intention of bringing the students to a certain degree of self-reliance in medical sociological assignments.

Form; See 4.3.2.

Subject matter: Since this seminar course was started only last year, our experience with it has been extremely limited. It is our intention to change the subject matter of this seminar course every year, so that every second year follows up the theme treated in the first-year seminar course. Thus the first and second-year seminar courses would more or less constitute a unity, allowing more time and attention to be devoted to the various steps of the research. Next year, for example, the investigation into preventive health behaviour, which was started in the first-year seminar course, will be continued.

Last year the seminar course was devoted to the problems of the general practitioner in Belgium. This followed up a finished research project on the same theme conducted by the Institute for Sociological Research. By means of a secondary analysis of the results obtained through this investigation, existing hypotheses were reformulated and new hypotheses were developed and tested through a small-scale experimental investigation. Due to the restricted time-span, an analysis of the results obtained could not be included in the seminar course, which was felt to be a drawback, especially by the students. In order to prevent such situations in the future it will be attempted to link both seminar courses.

Evaluation: See 4.3.2.

4.3.4. Practical Training

Object: This practical training primarily tries to provide students with the opportunity of socializing with the medical subculture and of making direct contact with some policy problems as they appear in everyday (hospital) reality. A secondary goal is the acquisition of further knowledge and skills in the field of health care.

Form: So far this practical training has only consisted of a one-week 'internship' in a teaching hospital attached to the University. The students (usually about 10 in number), whose participation in this practical training is on a voluntary basis, spend an entire working-week in the hospital and follow the work-schedule which applies to most role-groups in the hospital. It is important to note that the students do not primarily participate in hospital activities as sociologists with well-defined observation or research assignments, but rather try to experience hospital reality through directly patient-oriented assignments (to achieve a patient's eye view, as it were).

Subject matter: In consultation with the medical and nursing managers, the students are assigned to various hospital departments and preferably given directly patient-oriented tasks. Departments which have so far qualified are: reception, social services, various nursing departments, mobile library, and out-patient services. As volunteers of a kind, the students perform a number of simple tasks in their departments such as transportation of patients to examinations, distribution of food, elementary hygiene care, conducting conversations with patients and their visitors, distribution of mail, etc. The emphasis – we repeat – is clearly on the experience of hospital reality from the patients' vantage point in order to gain an insight into policy problems within the medical setting and possibly learn to think in a problem-solving manner.

Evaluation: Since participation in this practical training is not compulsory, no specific evaluation of the students' role-performance in the hospital is made. At the end of the internship a large evaluation meeting is organized, in which both the students and the hospital and the department directors (usually head nurses) participate. The students individually evaluate their hospital stay, which often results in hard confrontations with representatives of the departments concerned. Afterwards these confrontations may serve as didactic material in the teaching course.

4.3.5. Memoir

Object: The object of the memoir, with which the graduate training is concluded, is to provide the students with the opportunity of developing independently a sociological definition of a problem. The students are expected to apply the most important dimensions of their graduate training, viz. theory, research and social policy in a personal manner to a part of social reality with or without a socially problematic character.

Form: The memoir is a mimeographed paper of 100 to 150 pages which the student prepares during the second year, under the supervision of a professor of his choice. This supervision is accomplished through regular personal contacts between student and sponsor.

Subject matter: The subject matter or the theme of the memoir is chosen by the student in consultation with the promotor. Whereas formerly the student was completely free to choose his subject, the choice is now somewhat limited since every professor at the beginning of the second year hands out a list of topics for the memoirs he wants to stimulate and promote. However the students still remain free to make a choice outside of these lists. A brief illustrative survey of the memoirs written in recent years in the field of medical sociology is given in Appendix IV.

At this moment memoirs are prepared, for example, on group practice in Belgium, medical training and the choice of a profession, changes in psychiatric institutions, psychiatry's image in the press, antipsychiatry as a social process, death in hospital, professionalization in nursing, illness behaviour, the establishment of a new teaching hospital as a process of decision-making, etc.

Evaluation: On the one hand, continuous evaluation is made through the regular contact between student and sponsor and, on the other hand, a final evaluation is made of the completed memoir which the student is required to present and defend before a closed jury. In the overall evaluation the memoir is given a 1/3 value of the total set of exams.

4.3.6. Seminar Course in Medical Sociology and Medical Psychology

Introductory note: This is a seminar course conducted by the Faculty of Medicine for medical students, of which the author, in his capacity of sociologist is head instructor, together with two psychiatrists. Recently this seminar was also made accessible to graduate students in (medical) sociology. This seminar course is optional for both medical and sociology students.

Object: Being open to both medical and sociology students, this seminar course has a double object: on the one hand, in order to provide a more comprehensive and complete training it attempts to familiarize medical students with the psychological and sociological approach and, on the other hand, for sociology students, it acts as an additional socialization mechanism towards the medical subculture. Hence the emphasis is chiefly on the development of attitudes, more particularly on the development of a readiness among various (future) experts to analyze together a specific problem in its various aspects and possibly to arrive at a joint solution to the problem.

Form: Fifteen weekly two-hour work-meetings are organized in which individual and collective assignments are distributed. This seminar consists predominantly of reading assignments: a number of articles relevant to the theme being treated are selected, presented by the students, and taken as a starting-point for group discussions during the seminar. On exceptional occasions outside experts are invited to the seminar in order to animate the discussion.

Subject matter: The subject matter of this seminar course changes every year. Each time one central theme is selected in advance and then elaborated in the form of an analysis of the literature. In past years the following themes have been treated:
– death and dying,
– the social aspects of illness and health,
– the medical model in medicine and psychiatry.

For next year the medical students especially insisted on choosing the theme: 'Medical Training and the Behavioural Sciences' – a choice not without significance to a medical school where so far behavioural sciences are practically non-existent.

Evaluation: In this seminar course no specific exam is taken. The students' individual and group performance is constantly evaluated during the entire course. It should be observed, however, that as far as the students are concerned, medical students are much more positive in their evaluation of this seminar than are sociology students – an observation susceptible to various interpretations.

5. THREE YEARS LATER: RETROSPECTIVE AND PROSPECTIVE IDEAS

Even though it is very difficult reasonably to evaluate a training program which has been operating for only three years, the following retrospective and prospective ideas can be formulated in conclusion. First it must be stated that at a time of intense social questioning of health care and a tendency towards a more rational and scientifically based development of health care, the organization of a training program in medical sociology is no longer a matter exclusively of academic priorities but also, and primarily, of social priorities. In other words, the present structure, evolution, and problems of health care are sufficient grounds for the introduction of specific training programs in medical sociology. With respect to this training program we offer here the following ideas, possibly assuming the form of theses:

1. A solid general sociological training in which the dimensions of theory, research, and policy are equally represented, is a necessary condition for the training of medical sociologists. This condition, however, is not as necessary for a training in medical sociology.

2. Preparation for medico-sociological professional activities should be actualized in the training program by a number of specific medico-sociological teaching activities.

3. The development of these specific teaching activities has previously been necessarily fostered by research activities in the field of health care. Simultaneously with the start of a teaching program a complete field research program must be developed.

4. The extent of medico-sociological teaching activities is also a matter of academic priorities and will also be determined by the manpower available. In certain cases it will be desirable to develop the teaching of medical sociology in close combination with other sociological specialties in order to establish larger teaching units; those preferred combinations will chiefly depend on personal and not so much on academic factors.

5. As is true for every kind of sociological training, a training program in medical sociology must create, apart from pure research tasks, sufficient room for problem-solving tasks (social engineering). Whereas at the moment training for research roles is scarcely problematic, training for social engineering, for example with respect to medical sociology, remains very much a problem. An attempt at translating this dimension into a set of specific (though borrowed) policy subjects, apart from the actual sociology training, has failed, at least as far as the Louvain experience is concerned.

6. With respect to teaching objectives, attention so far has been given chiefly to knowledge and skills, while attitudes were left aside or, at any rate, were left to the intuition and interpretation of the persons concerned. It seems necessary, especially with respect to medico-sociological training, to devote more attention to this in future, so that a clear definition of teaching objectives with respect to professional attitudes should be achieved, in order to develop appropriate teaching activities.

7. With respect to a training program in medical sociology the absolute necessity for providing a number of socialization mechanisms towards the medical setting must be particularly emphasized. These mechanisms evidently may assume variable forms: common lectures or seminars together with medical students, participant observation in medical settings, full probation in helath care institutions, even a

common basic year for the various disciplines of health care (doctors, nurses, psychologists, social workers, sociologists, etc.). To the sociologist, however, these socialization mechanisms should also guarantee a 'detached concern'.

Whereas previously deductive teaching models were predominantly used, (also in sociology training) the question may be asked whether, in the light of the changed teaching situation at the universities and the changed position of the student therein, it will not be necessary to create more room for more inductive teaching models. When medical sociology manages to actually develop such models, it will make a new creative contribution to general sociology.

BIBLIOGRAPHY

[1] H. Freeman, S. Levine and L. Reeder, *Handbook of Medical Sociology* (second edition), Prentice Hall, New Jersey 1972, p. 518.

[2] E. Freidson, *Professional Dominance*, Atherton Press, New York 1970.

[3] J. Van Kemenade and A. Wyngaards, 'Doelopvattingen van sociologie-docenten', *Sociologische Gids* 1 (1969) 12–22.

[4] J. B. McKinlay, 'The Concept of Patient Carrier as a Heuristic Device for Making Medical Sociology Relevant to Medical Students', *Social Science and Medicine* 5 (1971) 441–460.

[5] Y. Nuyens, *Medical Sociology in Some European Countries*, S.O.I., Leuven 1972, 47.

[6] M. Sokołowska, 'On the Scope of Medical Sociology', *W.H.O., Seminar on the Teaching of the Social Sciences in Medical Education* (1969) roneo, 2–5.

APPENDIX I. SOCIOLOGY CURRICULUM

Undergraduate Program (2 Years)

First Year:

1. Society: Facts and Problems
2. Sociology I
3. Introduction to Sociological Research
4. Statistics with Mathematical Introduction I
5. Historical Introduction to Philosophy
6. Logic

7. Moral Philosophy
8. Private Law
9. History of Social Facts and Institutions
10. Methodology
11. Psychology
12. Seminar Course: Introduction to Scientific Work
13. Practical training in Statistics
14. Language examination: English or French

Second Year:
1. Sociology II
2. Statistics with Mathematical Introduction II
3. Social Philosophy
4. Ethics
5. Economics
6. Social Psychology
7. Current Philosophy
8. Sociological Research I
9. Sociological Research II
10. Demography
11. Social History of Belgium
12. Elements of Public Law
13. Field Work

Graduate Program (2 Years)

1. Sociology III
2. Sociology IV
3. Sociological Research III
4. Sociological Research IV
5. History of Political and Social Theories:
   a) from the Renaissance to the Present Day
   b) Marxism, Origin and Evolution
6. Problems of Christian Political and Social Ethics
7. Social Policy I: General Theory
8. Social Policy II: Special Problems
9. A choice of two sociology courses:
   a) Sociology of Religion
   b) Sociology of Labour and Industry

- c) Sociology of the Family
- d) Sociology of Population
- e) Economic Sociology
- f) Urban Sociology
- g) Criminal Sociology
- h) Medical Sociology (60 hours)
- i) Sociology of Culture

10. Optional Seminary course (first year)
    - a) Sociology of Religion
    - b) Sociology of Labour and Industry
    - c) Sociology of the Family
    - d) Sociology of Population
    - e) Medical Sociology (60 hours)
    - f) Sociology: Special Problems
11. Optional seminar course (second year)
    - a) Sociology of Religion
    - b) Sociology of Labour and Industry
    - c) Sociology of the Family and Population
    - d) Medical Sociology (60 hours)
    - e) Methodology
12. Special Problems of:
    - a) Sociology of Religion
    - b) Sociology of Labour and Industry
    - c) Sociology of the Family
    - d) Sociology of Population
    - e) Social Psychology

APPENDIX II. READING LIST – TEACHING COURSE ON MEDICAL SOCIOLOGY (1972–1973)

I. Medical Sociology: a General Introduction

1. Bibliography: Handbooks, readers, articles, journals, ...
2. E. Freidson, *Substantive Issues in Medical Sociology* (1970).
3. I. Gadourek, *Evaluation Research in the Field of Medical Sociology* (1966).
4. Y. Nuyens, *Medicine and Sociology* (1969).
5. F. Steudler, *Le champ de la sociologie médicale* (1972).

II. Sociology of Health and Illness

6. R. Coe, *Characteristics of Disease* (1970).
7. R. Greyf, *The Role-Model in the Sociological Explanation of the Phenomenon of Illness* (1971).
8. S. Kasl and S. Cobb, *Health Behaviour, Illness Behaviour and Sick Role Behaviour* (1966).
9. D. Mechanic, *Health, Disease and Deviant Behaviour* (1968).
10. Y. Nuyens, *Social Factors in Illness and Health Behaviour* (1972).
11. T. Parsons, *Definitions of Health and Illness in the Light of American Values and Social Structure* (1957).
12. E. Suchman, *Stages of Illness and Medical Care* (1965).

III. Healers and Healing Practices

13. R. Corwin, *The professional Employee: a Study of Conflict in Nursing Roles* (1961).
14. M. Field, *The Doctor-Patient Relationship in the Perspective of Fee-for-Service and Third-Party Medicine* (1961).
15. E. Freidson, *Professional Dominance and the Ordering of Health Services* (1970).
16. Y. Nuyens, *Sociology of the Nursing Profession* (1969).
17. Y. Nuyens and R. Jolie, *The Political Role of the Physician* (1972).
18. R. Wilson and S. Bloom, *Patient-Practitioner Relationships* (1972).

IV. Health Care Institutions

19. R. Coser, *Alienation and the Social Structure* (1963).
20. E. Freidson, *Patterns of Practice in the Hospital* (1970).
21. Y. Nuyens, *Hospitals and Client Evaluations* (1971).
22. Y. Nuyens, *Death and Dying in Hospitals* (1972).
23. C. Perrow, *Hospitals: Technology-Structure and Goals* (1965).
24. M. Seeman and J. Evans, *Stratification and Hospital Care* (1961).
25. A. Wessen, *Hospital Ideology and Communication between Ward Personnel* (1958).

V. Health Care Policy

26. J. Stoeckle and I. Zola, *After Everyone Can Pay for Medical Care: Some Perspectives on Future Treatment and Practice* (1964).
27. A. Strauss, *Medical Organization, Medical Care and Lower Income Groups* (1969).

APPENDIX III. OVERVIEW OF SOME MEMOIRS IN THE FIELD OF MEDICAL SOCIOLOGY (1969–1972)

1. Health professionals

1.1. An analysis of medical ideology. Two case studies.
– Definition of the Problem: How does the traditional professional medical model evolve with respect to changes in health care and society?
– Method: Analysis of the reviews of the most important Belgian medical associations.
– Findings:
1. Some medical groups are more open to evolution than others.
2. With respect to autonomy and 'collegiality' some medical groups have raised the professional model to a universal value by combining it with the medical-ethical code.

1.2. Social Problems of the General Practitioner in Belgium.
– Definition of the Problem: Position and function of the G.P.
– Method: Content analysis of the publications of the principal medical organizations dealing with these problems.
– Findings: The most important element of the re-evaluation of the G.P. appears to be his cooperation with the specialist.

1.3. The framework in which psychiatric nurses try to define the particular purport of their profession.
– Definition of the Problem: The role of psychiatric nurses as defined by various authorities.
– Method: Analysis of documents and interview.
– Findings: Generally the ideologiacl definition of the nursing role only partially corresponds to reality. Yet an evolution is observed.

1.4. Recruitement of nursing staff in general hospitals.

- Definition of the Problem: Which are the various factors underlying the staff composition, both qualitative and quantitative, in hospitals?
- Method: Study of the recruitment of hospital nursing staff; the composition of the staff was examined through the recruitment procedures of general hospitals.
- Findings: In 1968 there was a great shortage, both qualitative and quantitative, of nursing staff. The awareness of the different hospitals and the different evaluation of the attendant potential, the nature of the selection criteria applied, and the degree of selection, are the most important factors underlying this shortage.

1.5. Profile of the nursing student. Exploratory study in three nursing schools.

- Definition of the Problem: This investigation tries to provide a picture of the nursing student in various institutions, and at the same time to answer the question as to why there has been an increase in the number of students in recent years.
- Method: Analysis of the selection tests which the applicants must pass in order to be admitted to nursing courses.
- Findings: The increase in the number of nursing students is explained by the increase in the number of male nurses and the increase of the number of girls continuing their education after secondary school. More than half of these students belong to large families, and only to a small extent to the working class. In only 20% of the cases is the mother professionally employed, more than one third come from urban areas, and at the outset of their studies the majority have strong charitable and idealistic motives.

2. *Health Care and Welfare Institutions*

2.1. Bureaucratic and professional tendencies in the light of the problem of hospital size.

- Definition of the Problem: see title.
- Method: Analysis of the literature and survey research.

- Findings: Conflicts between bureaucracy and professionalism usually occur in large hospitals. Team work is considered a necessary solution.

2.2 Humanization of the hospital.

- Definition of the Problem: Will economic priorities oust humanitarian requirements or are compromises possible?
- Method: Study of literature, and case studies.
- Findings: Some elements of a solution to this problem are proposed.

2.3. Hospital public relations. A means of creating a correct image•

- Definition of the Problem:
  1. Definition of 'public relations'.
  2. Investigation of the extent to which Belgian hospitals practise public relations.
- Method: Study of the literature and exploratory research through written inquiry.
- Findings: Empirical inquiry shows that public relations are for all practical purposes in a state of confusion.

2.4. Social work in hospitals.

- Definition of the Problem: Which factors interfere with the operation of the hospital's social services as a concrete form of medical social work?
- Method: Study of secondary sources.
- Findings: Medical social work is an essential element of comprehensive medicine, but it still encounters many material and non-material impediments.

2.5. The psychiatric hospital as a therapeutic community.

- Definition of the Problem: Can a traditional psychiatric institution be transformed into a therapeutic community?
- Method: Study of the literature and analysis of a few experiments abroad.
- Findings: It is impossible to design a unidimensional model of the therapeutic community. This modification of a traditional institution

is dependent on the degree and the nature of the pathology to be treated.

2.6. A Dutch psychiatric center for delinquent and maladapted youth. A sociological exploration in the light of the 'therapeutic community'.

- Definition of the Problem: Can the ideology of the 'therapeutic community' actually be implemented?
- Method: participant observation.
- Findings:
  1. The center adequately achieves a therapeutic climate, which, however, differs from the definition postulated by M. Jones.
  2. The therapeutic community is a dynamic process.

2.7. Institutes for neglected children. Exploratory study.

- Definition of the Problem: Profile of neglected children and their education in four institutes in Flanders.
- Method:
  1. Analysis of secondary sources.
  2. Interview of privileged witnesses.
- Findings:
  1. These institutes live a socially irrelevant existence.
  2. The definition of negligence and the attachment to institutes are repressive procedures.

2.8. From 'Godshuis' (House of God) to 'Bejaardentehuis' (Old People's Home) in Antwerp.

- Definition of the Problem: How did old people's homes evolve with respect to a changing society and the position of the aged within it? (19th and 20th centuries)
- Method: Ideological criticism of values, ideas and objectives on the basis of secondary sources.
- Finding: The changed position of old people in society has created a qualitative and quantitative shortage of old people's homes, stimulating (profit-seeking) private initiative.

2.9. Modifications in the position and function of Old People's Homes.

- Definition of the Problem: Socio-cultural modifications in the position of the aged affect the institutional solutions of the problem of old age.

– Method: Historical study on the basis of Gurvitch's stratification model; use of secondary sources.
– Findings:
  1. The number of private institutions has greatly increased over the last 20 years.
  2. The old people's home as an ultimate solution is not part of an overall old age policy.

2.10. Telephone samaritan services in our society. Analysis and functioning.

– Definition of the Problem: Ideology of existing telephone samaritan services in Western Europe and accounts of their functioning. Empirical analysis of one service in a Belgian metropolis.
– Method: study of the literature and empirical research.
– Findings:
  1. Services are located exclusively in large cities, where loneliness is thought to be greater.
  2. They do not provide material help but psychological and moral support.
  3. They are operated by volunteers.

2.11. Agencies for problems of living and family problems.

– Definition of the Problem:
  1. Analysis of origin, procedures, and therapy.
  2. Segregation and integration of these agencies.
– Method: Probation and empirical research.
– Findings: There is a tendency towards integration. The segregation rate varies according to the particular character of each agency.

3. Health Problems

3.1. Assistance to the mentally retarded child. An attempt at a sociological approach.

– Definition of the Problem: An attempt is made to set assistance to the mentally retarded child in a sociological perspective in order to reveal the determining factors promoting or interfering with this assistance.

- Method: Theoretical study. Application of sociological knowledge in order to set this problem in the desired perspective.
- Findings: The slight penetration of the problem to the policy-making level and the absence of the necessary channels for this, constitute a first observation. The most important impediments to assistance to the mentally retarded child are the still insufficient development of mental health care in Belgium, the rejection by society at large of the mentally retarded, the difficulties of access to an institution, and the narrow approach practised in the institutions themselves.

3.2. The typology of handicapped children and their reintegration.
- Definition of the Problem: How does our society define the state of 'being handicapped' and how does it organize assistance?
- Method:
  1. Exploratory study of the existing provisions in a certain region.
  2. Analysis of primary and secondary sources.
- Findings:
  1. There is a dual attitude with respect to physically and mentally handicapped persons: mentally handicapped persons suffer discrimination.
  2. The absence of a coordinated policy prevents adequate assistance.

3.3. Traffic accidents in Belgium.
- Definition of the Problem: The starting-point was the social character of the traffic accidents. In particularly the phase preceding the traffic accident is studied. An examination is made of how this social problem is handled by the authorities concerned and of the means employed to prevent such accidents.
- Method: Analysis of traffic statistics and the accident files of the Supreme Council for Road Safety.
- Findings: Accidents must be combatted on both a human and a technical level. While the authorities take action with respect to road construction, educational and preventive measures must equally be expanded.

3.4. Alcoholism and the family.
- Definition of the Problem: The family's influence on the alcoholic.

- Method: Study of former research.
- Findings: Sociological research is almost completely lacking. Research on the problem of alcoholism is more of a psychological nature.

3.5. Analysis of the concepts 'drug user', 'drug scene', and 'drugs' in the Belgian Dutch-speaking press and their confrontation with reality on the basis of a few case studies.
- Definition of the Problem: Does the personality and the environment of the drug user correspond to the image depicted by the press?
- Method: Analysis of newspapers and case study.
- Findings:
  1. The press plays an important role in the stigmatization of the drug user.
  2. The press pictures a negative stereotype.
  3. There is little or no resemblance between the actual drug user and the image depicted by the press.

3.6. Drugs and society. A delineation of drug use by youth.
- Definition of the Problem: Definition of subcultural drug use and its confrontation with reality.
- Method: Study of the literature and empirical exploratory research in a certain region.
- Findings: Description of the influence and the role of the group with respect to its members.

4. *Health Care Policy*

4.1. The care of handicapped persons: an introductory definition of the problem.
- Definition of the Problem: Which rationales determine the legal provisions for the care and integration of disabled persons?
- Method: Analysis of primary and secondary sources.
- Findings:
  1. The problem of the disabled person is gradually becoming a problem of social rehabilitation.
  2. Social rehabilitation is conceived of exclusively as economic and financial, so that new marginal groups are created.

4.2. The drug phenomenon. Social, legal, and political implications.

- Definition of the Problem: Definition of the drug problem from a political point of view.
- Method: Analysis of the content of Belgian laws concerning drugs.
- Findings: The law is very repressive with respect to drugs and drug users and thus increases the contrast between 'normal' and 'deviant'.

4.3. Analysis of the organization of Belgian mutual funds.

- Definition of the Problem: What kind of organization represents the beneficiary of health care? A morphological, ideological, and social analysis.
- Method:
  1. Analysis of the review articles and documents of these organizations.
  2. Interviews with privileged witnesses.
- Findings: External pressure, raising the consciousness of the patient population, is required in order to rouse the mutual funds from their rigidness and reactivate them as the dynamic and democratic representatives of the medical consumer.

4.4. From 'Assistance' to 'Welfare'? Sociological reflections on the reform of the 'C.O.O.' (Committees for Public Assistance).

- Definition of the Problem: How does an assistance agency as a social provision adapt itself to changing problems?
- Method:
  1. Analysis of primary and secondary sources.
  2. Qualitative interviews with privileged witnesses.
- Findings:
  1. Attempts at reform always have the nature of a compromise: the development into a welfare organization is interfered with by external rationales.
  2. The double function – assistance as a participation promoting activity and assistance through the establishment of care supplying institutions – remains.

4.5. Labour relations in the health sector.

- Definition of the Problem: Investigation into the legally ordered relations on the national professional level between organized employers and organized employees in this sector, and analysis of the codification of arrangements for collective agreements on these issues.

- Method:
  1. Analysis of reviews and documents of organizations and official documents.
  2. Interviews with privileged witnesses.
- Findings:
  1. The joint union front tries to obtain higher salaries by means of bilateral discussion and social programming.
  2. In addition, strong professional organizations devote themselves to the revaluation of the profession.

TEACHING MEDICAL SOCIOLOGY TO SOCIOLOGY STUDENTS: A BRITISH VIEW*

MARGARET STACEY

Department of Sociology, University of Warwick, Coventry, England

My approach to this subject is tentative: I graduated in sociology during World War II, but have relatively recently come to the study of medical sociology. Indeed I stumbled upon it about ten years ago by the accident of being a sociologist who became interested in certain aspects of the hospitalization of child patients. It is even more recently that I have had to give serious consideration to the teaching of medical sociology to sociology students.

Sociology is used to embrace many approaches to the social. When I speak of sociology students I am referring to those who study social relations, social institutions, social interactions, culture. Therefore I exclude those whose prime area of study is social administration or social policy or who are training to become social workers. The students I have in mind may later go on to train in these or other areas, but presently they are simply equipping themselves as sociologists, students of society. For them, therefore, medical sociology represents one specialism among many which they may study, others being the sociology of education, of industry, of the family, social stratification for example and sociological theory and methodology.

When I speak of medical sociology I am also distinguishing this subject from social medicine. The latter I take to be a branch of medicine concerned with certain social aspects of health and illness, e.g. the control of infectious diseases, environmental health, epidemiology. A growing minority of British medical schools are now teaching some medical sociology to their students, but these developments are embryonic, the sociology lecturers finding difficulty in achieving an adequate toe-hold in crowded medical syllabuses. Developments such as those taking place at Southampton in the Sociology Department associated with the new medical school are all too rare. But progress is being made slowly. There are in fact few places in Britain where medical sociology proper is taught to social scientists in training. Adjacent disciplines are more commonly taught, such as social policy in health, the organization of health care and health administration. Keele University teaches an option in medical sociology to undergraduates and Leicester an option on the sociology of health. My former department at Swansea University College recently started a course in sociology honours for first degree students. Postgraduate teaching in medical sociology occurs in more centres than these: notably at Aberdeen and Bedford.

A distinction has been made between the sociology of medicine and sociology in medicine (R. Straus, 1957; Freidson, 1970; Wilson, 1970). The latter develops in medical schools as a technical aid to the practice of medicine. In this sense sociology in medicine has some affinity to social medicine, although the former remains sociology while the latter is a branch of medicine. The sociology of medicine develops best outside the medical school and is a more critical discipline. Here the sociologist examines analytically all aspects of health institutions including the social concepts of health and illness themselves. For sociologists such analysis must be part of their attempt to understand social relations and social processes. As citizens sociologists may be inclined to believe that such analyses are an essential part of the review to which any complex society must expect its health institutions and its health professionals to submit.

There is no doubt that it is the sociology *of* medicine which one wishes to teach to sociology students rather than sociology *in* medicine, although they should be aware of the latter and of its content. But the emphasis for sociology students is on the sociology of medicine and this seen as part of the general understanding of society which students must gain. Medical sociology is a valuable discipline for this teaching purpose, for it can include so many aspects of general sociology and be used to test so many aspects of sociological theory as they emerge in the area of health and illness treatment. These can include the relevant belief systems; the organization of health care, both the organization to provide the services and also the organization of professions and occupations concerned; the interpersonal interactions involved in the giving and receiving of care; and the relationships between the society as a whole and all these aspects of health care.

One of the necessary preconditions that must be fulfilled before sociology can be successfully taught to undergraduates is that their preconceptions about society should be made overt to them and that they should acquire a facility to question these assumptions about how society works and what are the 'right' values to hold, assumptions with which they have grown up. In no other way can they learn to look at the social institutions and the social relations of their own society or other societies with anything approaching the necessary detachment. Beliefs and practices relating to health and illness are fundamental aspects of any society. Furthermore, all students not only participate in these beliefs and attitudes but will also have been participants in the health care systems of their own societies. Part of their education as sociologists is to turn them into observers as well as participators (cf. Wright Mills, 1959).

At the outset of a course on the sociology of medicine for sociology undergraduates I would therefore begin with a discussion of the concepts of health and illness and their variability. Here there is cross cultural evidence to suggest that concepts of health and illness vary widely from culture to culture (e.g. Saunders, 1954; Paul, 1955). Objectively definable conditions which put people to bed in one society are tolerated in another such that normal life is continued. There is evidence that pain is differentially felt and certainly that standards of behaviour in relation to pain are variable. I recall the speech made by the ward sister of an antenatal ward in which I once was a patient. The sister addressed all of us who were starting labour saying that if we had heard the screaming from the labour ward (delivery room) the previous night we should know that this was an Italian woman and that it would not be necessary for us to behave like that. The sister did not suggest the woman had suffered exceptional pain of a kind we were unlikely to experience. I don't think she believed that the Italian had suffered worse than average. Here the ward sister was being a guardian of the British culture in relation to childbirth behaviour, a gatekeeper of the values of her society. Until they are introduced to this literature which discusses the variability of health and illness concepts students are inclined to believe that illness as taught in their families and as they have learned to experience it is a physically objective phenomenon common to all mankind.

To describe the variations is easier than to explain them. Explanation can probably only be attempted in relation to the study of many aspects of the societies where the variations are found. Probably therefore only hints can be given in undergraduate courses of what the correlates of these variations might be. As the course progresses and one looks at various aspects of the sociology of health care some partial explanations may emerge. To alert students to this some early study of a book like William Glaser's *Social Settings and Medical Organization: a Cross-National Study of the Hospital* is helpful, for here he relates various major variables to factors associated with the organization of health care (Glaser, 1970).

At this stage too it is important to alert students to the variations with regard to beliefs about health and sickness within their own society. These may arise in association with ethnic differences or in association with social class differences. In such a discussion the general points about ethnicity and stratification which students will have come across in their general sociology can be pointed up in this particular context.

Such variations in the perception of what is illness can also usefully be set against variations in the objectively observable incidence of illness throughout a population when a given measure of illness is used. The Southwark screening study is a useful example of this (Epsom, 1969). In addition people's reactions when symptoms are recognized may vary as Wadsworth *et al.* (1971) have recently shown. No action may be taken, non-medical treatment or medical treatment may be sought. These studies show that by medical standards those who present with an illness are matched by many similar people who do not present. They also show the variation in action taken when people do recognize themselves as ill.

Such a study of illness behaviour naturally leads to a dicussion of the adoption of the sick role on the lines suggested by Parsons (1951) and Mechanic (1968) and recently examined by Robinson (1971). This can show the social processes in which beliefs about illness and feelings about their personal state of health operate within the social constraints people perceive themselves to be in. Here, therefore, one can include some discussion of the value and also the limitations of role theory and notions such as the 'sick role' in analyzing such social processes.

This discussion cannot be taken too far, however, before the students have gained some knowledge of the organization of health care services.

This, it seems to me, may be done in a number of ways. First of all some overall picture is necessary of the provision of services showing for whom and by whom care and treatment are offered and with what goals. Such an analysis would be in terms of the social categories of givers and receivers. Thereafter health care organization and the health care professions can be looked at in some detail. Thus hospitals may be examined as a particular type of large-scale organization and the relevance of the theory associated with the large-scale organizations can be discussed. Many students will be familiar with these theories in their relation to industrial organization. The differences involved, because the work is with people and not objects, must emerge here and various problems associated with the status of the patient perceived by professionals as a person to be processed (Goffman, 1961; Tizard, Raynes and King, 1971).

The relevance of two further important areas becomes clear: one is professions and the process of professionalization and the other is the interactions which take place between professionals and patients in particular organizational settings, the social systems of health care. In considering the professions the study of medical sociology can be particularly valuable for the sociology student. The medical profession is generally accepted as being the most nearly ideal-typical example of a profession. Its use as a model by other health professionals and the constraints they experience in attempting to achieve professional autonomy can be illuminating for the student. There is increasing data becoming available on these professions and occupations (Freidson, 1970, 1972; Folta and Deck, 1966). There is also interesting material on the ways in which the professions modify the structure of the health service and of the health care organizations (Freidson, 1970; Davies, 1972).

Having grasped something of the organization of health care in general and of the hospital in particular and of the health care profession and occupations, the students' attention can then be usefully drawn to the interaction processes and to the transactions which take place in ward, surgery or clinic (Bloom, 1963; Freidson, 1961; Skipper and Leonard, 1965; Cartwright, 1964, 1967). Microsociological studies of for example, in-ward interactions of the consultation process, of interactions in outpatient clinics provide the relevant teaching material. From these face-to-face interactions much of the pattern of the health services is built up, here the order is negotiated (Straus, 1963). For my part, however, I would want the students to be aware that these transactions and the order it is possible to negotiate in ward or clinic are constrained in certain ways by negotiations that have already taken place elsewhere, between professionals (highly organized) and administrators, particularly by negotiations leading to resource allocation. Here the sociology of the health service itself becomes relevant and some attention must be paid to the sociology of the politics of health care. Thus the constraints in a fee-for-service situation compared with a national health service are quite different. Constraints on their choice experienced by physicians and patients operate at different times and places in the transactions in these two systems. In this wy, hopefully, the student can achieve some grasp of the relationship of the micro to the macro sociology.

As a teaching instrument, therefore, in my view medical sociology can be a most valuable sub-discipline, for it can be used to illustrate the strengths and weaknesses of various theoretical and methodological positions in general sociology as they are applied to the health field. It also teaches the student about an important area of belief and organization in society and about professional groups who are apparently being accorded increasing power to manipulate their fellow men. As well as increasing understanding of social relations, a study of medical sociology can also be a most useful preparation for students who will later train in a variety of applied areas, such as health administration and social work. It also has a part to play in increasing citizen awareness of the quality and nature of care being offered.

I would like to acknowledge the help of Mrs. Maureen Chester in the preparation of this paper.

BIBLIOGRAPHY

S. Bloom, *The Doctor and His Patient*, Russell Sage, N.Y. 1963.

A. Cartwright, *Human Relations and Hospital Care*, Routledge and Kegan Paul, London 1964.

A. Cartwright, *Patients and their Doctors: A Study of General Practice*, Routledge and Kegan Paul, London 1967.

C. Davies, 'Professionals in Organizations', *Sociological Review* **20** (1972) 553–567.

J. E. Epsom, *The Mobile Health Clinic – An Interim Report on a Preliminary*

Analysis of the first One Thousand Patients to Attend, London Borough of Southwark, Health Dept., 1969.
J. R. Folta and E. S. Deck, *A Sociological Framework for Patient Care*, Wiley, 1966.
E. Freidson, *Patients' Views of Medical Practice*, Russell Sage, 1961.
E. Freidson, *Professional Dominance: The Social Structure of Medical Care*, Atherton, N.Y. 1970.
E. Freidson, *Profession of Medicine*, Dodds Mead, N.Y. 1972.
W. A. Glaser, *Social Settings and Medical Organization: a Cross National Study of the Hospital*, Atherton, 1970.
E. Goffman, *Asylums*, Anchor 1961.
D. Mechanic, *Medical Sociology*, Free Press, N.Y., Collier Macmillan, London 1968.
C. Wright Mills, *The Sociological Imagination*, N.Y. OUP, 1959.
T. Parsons, *The Social System*, Free Press, New York 1951.
D. Robinson, *The Process of Becoming Ill*, Routledge and Kegan Paul, 1971.
J. Tizard, R. D. King and M. V. Raynes, *Patterns of Residential Care*, Routledge and Kegan Paul, 1971.
J. K. Skipper and R. C. Leonard, *Social Interaction and Patient Care*, Lippincott, 1965.
A. Straus, L. Schatzman, R. Bucher, D. Ehrlich and M. Sabshin, 'The Hospital and its Negotiated Order', in: E. Freidson (ed.), *The Hospital in Modern Society*, Free Press, N.Y. 1963.
R. Straus, 'The Nature and Status of Medical Sociology', *Amer. Soc. Rev.* **22** (1957).
M. E. J. Wadsworth, W. J. H. Butterfield and R. Blaney, *Health and Sickness: the Choice of Treatment*, Tavistock 1971.
R. N. Wilson, *The Sociology of Health: an Introduction*, Random House, N.Y. 1970.

REFERENCE

* Direct reprint requests to: Margaret Stacey, Department of Sociology, University of Warwick, Coventry, England.

GOALS AND FUNCTIONS OF THE DEPARTMENT OF BEHAVIORAL SCIENCE IN THE UNIVERSITY OF KENTUCKY COLLEGE OF MEDICINE

ROBERT STRAUS

Department of Behavioral Science, University of Kentucky, Lexington, Ky. U.S.A.

HISTORY

The Department of Behavioral Science at the University of Kentucky was formally established in 1959 as a basic science department in the College of Medicine – part of a new University Medical Center, planning for which began in 1956.

At that time, behavioral scientists were participating, in a modest way, in the medical education programs of perhaps half of the 85 medical schools in the United States. In nearly every instance, their participation was through departments of psychiatry or of public health and preventive medicine and, in nearly every case, the behavioral scientist's role was preceived as contributing primarily to the educational objectives of psychiatry of or preventive medicine. There were no distinct patterns of content or context which described the role of behavioral scientists in medical education.

It was the conviction of those planning the development of the University of Kentucky Medical Center that a familiarity with the behavioral sciences was extremely important in the practice of medicine and in the understanding of processes associated with the delivery of health care, and that these disciplines were potentially basic to all of the fields of medicine, not merely psychiatry or public health, and to all the health professions. It was also believed that a strong faculty in the behavioral sciences could be recruited only if they were afforded a place in the structure of the University which would recognize the validity of basic research and graduate education along with the applications of behavioral science theory and methods to the education of health personnel and applied research problems in the health and medical field. Furthermore, it was felt that such a group could be most effective within a medical center if it was given a strong organizational base with sufficient status to permit behavioral scientists to participate in the day-to-day decision making process involved in curriculum planning and other key activities and a base for collaboration as equals with faculty in other departments and units of the Medical Center.

The Department of Behavioral Science was formally activated a year and a half before the first medical students arrived at the College of Medicine. During this period, members of the Department who were recruited initiated their own research programs, participated in the committee activity of the College of Medicine, and established relationships with the departments of their basic discipline on the University campus which included the teaching of courses and other participation in graduate education. With the development of the College of Dentistry in 1961, the Department of Behavioral Science also became a basic science department of the College of Dentistry.

As currently conceived, the Department of Behavioral Science has 10 full-time faculty positions representing the disciplines of sociology, cultural anthropology, social psychology, human development, and psychological statistics. Each member of the Department holds a joint appointment in the University department of his basic discipline and there are reciprocal joint appointments from these departments to the Behavioral Science Department. Although the joint appointments do not carry either specific salary or duties, in all instances they have led to significant cross-departmental teaching activity.

TEACHING PROGRAM

The Department of Behavioral Science is involved in five distinct kinds of teaching activity. These include programs in the Colleges of (1) Medicine and (2) Dentistry, (3) some courses offered for students in Nursing and the Allied Health Professions, (4) a program designated 'Concentration in Medical Behavioral Science' offered for predoctoral students and (5) postdoctoral training.

Within the College of Medicine, the Department has its own basic course entitled *Health and Society*. Originally, essentially a lecture course, Health and Society has been modified several times to provide increased opportunities for seminar discussion and laboratory-type student projects. Most changes in the format of the course have reflected the constructive critique of students and colleagues. Since its inception, evaluations of the course have supported the validity of objectives and subject areas but have gradually suggested greater depth and more opportunity for students to observe principles in action. Some such suggestions have reflected the different backgrounds of a new generation of medical students. In 1960, few medical students had taken any courses in the social-behavioral sciences as college undergraduates. In 1975, a majority of the students have had at least one such course and there are several behavioral science majors.

The new Health and Society course, first offered in 1969, and revised annually, is designed to build on student interest and readiness for greater depth and diversity and student motivation for more personal involvement in learning. Following just three plenary meetings of the entire class designed to identify objectives and provide a conceptual frame of references, each student takes two topical seminars, each consisting of nine two-hour meetings in a three week period. Brief resumes prepared by the students are designed to provide for each seminar a written record of the major ideas, the nature of evidence and the significance.

Plenary sessions in 1975 dealt only with a unifying concept of behavior and its application to selected clinical syndromes and with the clustering principle of human pathology.

Seminar topics include:

1. Aging and Health.
2. Human Response to Pain, Stress and Illness.
3. Behavioral Factors in Coronary Heart Disease.
4. Legal and Ethical Problems in Medical Technological Change.
5. Factors Affecting Responses to People in Need of Help.
6. Physicians, Children, Parents and Families.
7. Death and Dying.
8. Medical Care Delivery and Medical Care Organization.
9. Physicians' and Patients' Perceptions of Each Other.
10. The Physician as a Coordinator for Comprehensive Care.
11. Psychosocial Adjustment to Chronic Conditions.
12. Quantification in Medicine.

13. Social Aspects of Mental Illness.
14. Problems of Alcohol and Other Psychoactive Drugs.
15. Population Control and Family Planning.
16. The Hospital Patient: Experiences and Problems.
17. Medical Students and Medical Education.

Coincidental with the Health and Society course, members of the Department of Behavioral Science participate, along with members of most other departments, in a Saturday morning clinical case conference. The case conference is built around problems introduced through patients, with emphasis on the interrelationship among the various basic sciences and the potential application of basic science concepts which the students are studying. Faculty work with students on a tutorial basis helping students prepare for their assigned roles in the case conference.

In the first year, the Department of Behavioral Science also participates in the teaching of communication and interviewing as part of a course on introduction to the Professions. Here, the attempt is to stress the varied forms of human communication, identity barriers and help students come to terms with their own blind spots and deaf spots and develop greater sensitivity in observing, listening, and conveying their own messages to others. Members of the Department work with students in reviewing TV taped practice interview sessions between students and patients and providing constructive analysis and review.

In the third and fourth years of the curriculum, the Department of Behavioral Science has no formal time, but members of the Deparment occasionally participate in an *ad hoc* way as resource persons in the major rounds and management conferences of several of the clinical departments. The Department also offers a series of topical electives in the first and second year.

Within the curriculum of the College of Dentistry, members of the Department of Behavioral Science participate in the teaching of clinical dentistry at numerous points where application of basic concepts can be discussed and illustrated in terms of what the students are doing at the time. This 'chairside' teaching is currently being developed particularly in association with the Departments of Periodontics, Pedodontics and Oral Diagnosis.

The Department has developed three courses which are now being utilized by students in the College of Nursing and in the School of Allied

Health Professions. Two of these are taught at the undergraduate level; one is a course in human growth and development which covers the entire life span; the other is a course entitled 'Behavioral Science Concepts in Health and Disease'. The third course is entitled 'Society and Health' and is taught for upper division undergraduates or graduate students other than those majoring in one of the behavioral sciences. This is being taken by students in vocational rehabilitation counseling, physical therapy, dietetics, public health, by a number of special students in nursing, and some miscellaneous others.

The Department's major graduate program is entitled 'A Concentration in Medical Behavioral Science'. The Concentration is offered to students working toward a doctorate degree in any of the behavioral science disciplines. Such students are expected to meet the basic requirements for a degree in their discipline. In addition, they are given personalized, intensive research training, they take a group of core seminars with members of the Department of Behavioral Science, write a dissertation under the direction of a member of this Department, and spend about two years with office space in the Medical Center experiencing what we call an enculturation to health and medicine. The program has been operating for 12 years and there have been 18 completed degrees.

The postdoctoral training offered by the Department has been adapted to the special needs and interests of the postdoctoral fellow. Thus far, there have been six fellows: a physician from Chile, three physicians from Brazil, a sociologist from Venezuela, and a dentist from the U.S.A. Currently, a proposal is under consideration by the University which would establish a Ph.D. in medical behavioral science for physicians, dentists, and other health professionals.

RESEARCH

The research activities of the Department are varied and numerous. Currently, faculty research interests include: a study of changing values and attitudes of medical students (J. V. Haley); the evaluation of hypovolemia using multivariate procedures and the evaluation of training for advanced radiologic technologists (J. V. Haley); studies of renal dialysis organization and of prenatal and infant health care (E. B. Gallagher); evaluative studies of medical education, including cross cultural study of predictors of clinical performance (J. V. Haley); study of behavioral factors associated with providing complete dentures for previously edentulous patients (J. Cohn and R. Straus); studies of various forms of dependency (R. Straus) and studies of hospital patient care (M. Pearsall and R. Straus); long term studies of Southern Appalachian health problems and health behavior (M. Pearsall); relationship between health and smoking patterns and a study of behavior of a child with spina bifida (P. Moody); lay perception of personality, development of children's self concepts (R. Jones); effects of freedom restriction (R. Jones); the development and testing of methods for training child development, early childhood education, and health personnel in the use of common intervention techniques (J. Archambo); assessment of discrepancies between physician, paraprofessional, and parent perceptions of health problems in preschool children (J. Archambo); physical and behavioral adjustments after heart attack with primary focus on early death and invalidism (T. Garrity); recent life change and its effect on health studies (T. Garrity); physician and lay attitudes toward treatment of the dying patient (T. Garrity); perceptions of illness in a cross cultural setting (J. Wiese and R. Jones); psychological, cultural and organizational factors in tuberculosis detection and treatment (J. Wiese), and cultural aspects of health services planning (J. Wiese). In addition, graduate students during their course programs, each assume a modest research training project and there are ten doctoral dissertation projects currently in progress.

FACILITIES

The Department of Behavioral Science is located quite centrally in the Medical Center complex. This location brings members of this department into daily informal contact with the rest of the faculty. Resources of the department include faculty offices, study areas for graduate students, a small groups laboratory with one-way mirror and closed circuit TV, various desk top calculators, tape recorders, and access to the University's IBM 360-65 computer. Probably the most valuable resource, however, is the Department's central location and access to the Medical Center-at-large as a 'laboratory'. The Department's teaching role – both for students of the health sciences and for our graduate students – is uniquely enhanced by this feature.